Diagnosis and Management of Special Populations

Diagnosis and Management of Special Populations

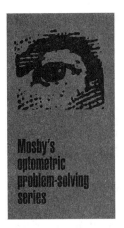

Mosby's optometric problem-solving series

Edited by

Dominick M. Maino
O.D., M.Ed., F.A.A.O.

Professor, Department of Pediatrics and Binocular Vision,
Illinois Eye Institute,
Illinois College of Optometry;
Chief, Optometric Services, IEI at the
Gilchrist–Marchman Rehabilitation Center,
Easter Seal Society of Metropolitan Chicago, Inc.,
Chicago, Illinois;
Adjunct Professor of Pediatric Optometry,
Centro Boston de Optometria,
Madrid, Spain

Series Editor

Richard London
M.A., O.D., F.A.A.O.

Diplomate, Binocular Vision and Perception,
Pediatric and Rehablitative Optometry,
Oakland, California

with 98 illustrations

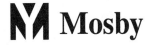 Mosby

St. Louis Baltimore Berlin Boston Carlsbad Chicago London Madrid
Naples New York Philadelphia Sydney Tokyo Toronto

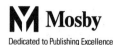

Mosby

Dedicated to Publishing Excellence

Executive Editor: Martha Sasser
Associate Developmental Editor: Kellie F. White
Project Manager: John Rogers
Production Editor: George B. Stericker, Jr.
Series design: Jeanne Wolfgeher
Manufacturing Supervisor: Betty Richmond

Copyright © 1995 by Mosby–Year Book, Inc.

Printed in the United States of America
Composition by Carlisle Communications, Ltd.
Printing/binding by Plus Communications.

Mosby–Year Book, Inc.
11830 Westline Industrial Drive
St. Louis, Missouri 63146

Library of Congress Cataloging-in-Publication Data

Diagnosis and management of special populations / book editor,
    Dominick M. Maino.
        p.   cm.—(Mosby's optometric problem solving series)
    Includes bibliographical references and index.
    ISBN 0-8151-5901-3
    1. Handicapped—Medical care.   2. Optometry.   3. Ophthalmology.
    I. Maino, Dominick M. II. Series.
        [DNLM: 1. Vision Disorders.   2. Disabled.   3. Health Services
    Needs and Demand.   4. Optometry.   WW 140 D5365 1994]
    RE952.5.H35D53 1994
    617.7'0087—dc20
    DNLM/DLC
    for Library of Congress   94-38762
                                                                       CIP

94 95 96 97 98/ 9 8 7 6 5 4 3 2 1

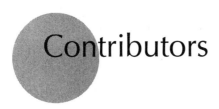

Contributors

Sandy Block, O.D., M.Ed., F.A.A.O.

Associate Professor,
Chief, Department of Pediatrics and
  Binocular Vision,
Illinois Eye Institute,
Illinois College of Optometry,
Chicago, Illinois

Gerhard W. Cibis, M.D.

Chief of Ophthalmology,
Children's Mercy Hospital;
Department of Ophthalmology,
University of Missouri,
Kansas City, Missouri

Steven Cool, Ph.D., F.C.O.V.D.

Professor,
College of Optometry,
School of Occupational Therapy,
School of Professional Psychology,
Pacific University,
Forest Grove, Oregon

Robert H. Duckman, O.D.

Professor,
College of Optometry,
Department of Clinical Sciences,
State University of New York,
New York, New York

Ellen Richter Ettinger, O.D., M.S., F.A.A.O.

Associate Professor,
College of Optometry,
Department of Clinical Sciences,
State University of New York,
New York, New York

Kelly Frantz, O.D., F.A.A.O., F.C.O.V.D.

Associate Professor,
Department of Pediatrics and Binocular
  Vision,
Illinois Eye Institute,
Illinois College of Optometry,
Chicago, Illinois

Stanley W. Hatch, O.D.

Assistant Professor,
New England College of Optometry,
Boston, Massachusetts

Frederick Hecht, M.D.

Hecht Associates, Inc.
Jacksonville, Florida

Dominick M. Maino, O.D., M.Ed., F.A.A.O.

Professor, Department of Pediatrics and
    Binocular Vision,
Illinois Eye Institute,
Illinois College of Optometry;
Chief, Optometric Services, IEI at the
    Gilchrist–Marchman Rehabilitation
    Center,
Easter Seal Society of Metropolitan
    Chicago, Inc.,
Chicago, Illinois;
Adjunct Professor of Pediatric Optometry,
Centro Boston de Optometria,
Madrid, Spain

Joseph H. Maino, O.D., F.A.A.O.

Low Vision Consultant,
Kansas State School for the Blind;
Clinical Associate Professor,
Department of Ophthalmology,
University of Kansas Medical Center,
Kansas City, Kansas;
Chief, Regional Low Vision Rehabilitation
    Center,
Kansas City VA Medical Center,
Kansas City, Missouri

Janice Emigh Scharre, O.D., M.A., F.A.A.O., F.C.O.V.D.

Coordinator, Rehabilitative Services,
Professor, Department of Pediatrics and
    Binocular Vision,
Illinois Eye Institute,
Illinois College of Optometry,
Chicago, Illinois

Darrell Schlange, O.D.

Associate Professor,
Department of Pediatrics and Binocular
    Vision,
Illinois Eye Institute,
Illinois College of Optometry,
Chicago, Illinois

Don Seibert, O.D.

Huntington VA Hospital and Medical
    Center,
Huntington, West Virginia

Michael D. Wesson, O.D., M.S., F.A.A.O.

Associate Professor of Optometry,
University of Alabama at Birmingham,
School of Optometry/Medical Center;
Past Director, Division of Optometry,
Chauncy Sparks Center for
    Developmental and Learning
    Disorders,
Civitan International Research Center,
Birmingham, Alabama

Michael Zost, O.D., F.C.O.V.D.

Assistant Professor,
Illinois Eye Institute,
Illinois College of Optometry,
Chicago, Illinois

*This text is dedicated
with love to those I love,
Sylvia, Dominick III,
Christina, and Dominick Sr.*

Preface

What's so special about special populations? Are they special because many of these individuals walk, talk, and think differently from the rest of us? Perhaps. Are they special because they may act or behave in an unusual or curious fashion? Perhaps. Are they special because there are so few of them? Definitely not! It's been estimated that more than three million individuals have one or more handicapping conditions that affect their ability to work, worship, and recreate. If any one thing makes this group special, it is a lack of access to health and vision care.[1]

Are we addressing the vision care needs of special populations? One mechanism of assessing this is to ask several questions of our schools and colleges of optometry. How well do the schools and colleges of optometry prepare our students to work with special populations? How many have residencies designed to work with this group? How many have didactic and clinical courses devoted specifically to working with individuals deemed special? How many schools and colleges have established clinics to serve this population and have faculty with the necessary expertise? Although no optometric research has addressed these issues, my impression is that few of our academic institutions have considered establishing such programs or clinics.

One institution that has developed programs in this area is the Illinois College of Optometry (ICO). Over the last 3 years ICO (in conjunction with the Easter Seal Society of Metropolitan Chicago)* has provided eye and vision care for thousands of individuals with

* This project was supported by grants from the United Way of Chicago, the Amoco Foundation, and the Washington Square Health Foundation.

developmental disabilities. This group has ranged in age from a few months to 92 years. The children and adults examined have been diagnosed as having Down syndrome, cerebral palsy, mental retardation with nonspecific etiology, head injury, psychiatric disorders, behavior disorders, and various anomalies induced by substance abuse. Preliminary findings[2] strongly suggest that this population has a much higher incidence of moderate to high refractive errors, strabismus, amblyopia, and ocular health abnormalities than the general population.[3] For many of the handicapped children and adults who received care this was their first experience of a full-scope optometric evaluation. With legal blindness 200 times more frequent in individuals with handicaps than in the nonhandicapped,[4] this should not be their only experience. It is my hope that this text will aid private practitioners, faculty, and students in providing the high quality eye and vision care that special populations require.

At this time I'm not convinced that special populations are all that special. They need optometric vision care just as much as any other group you may serve. I am convinced that as an optometrist you can become special by meeting the health and vision care needs of persons with disabilities.

References

1. Kastner T, Luckhardt J: Medical services for the developmentally disabled. *New Jersey J Med* 87:819-22, 1990.
2. Maino D: An eye care delivery service model for children and adults with developmental disabilities: a program of the Easter Seal Society of Metropolitan Chicago and the Illinois College of Optometry. Access to Health Care Symposium presented at the American Association on Mental Retardation 116th Annual Meeting. New Orleans, La 5/29/92.
3. Maino D, Maino J, Maino S: Mental retardation syndromes with associated ocular defects. *J Am Optom Assoc* 61:316-23, 1990.
4. Geering J, Maino D: The patient with mental handicaps: a primary care perspective. *South J Optom* 10:23-7, 1992.

Acknowledgments

I wish to thank the Easter Seal Society of Metropolitan Chicago, the National Fragile X Foundation, The Fragile X Research/Clinical Group (Elizabeth Berry-Kravis, MD, Ph.D., Bill Pizzi, Ph.D.; Rita Brusca, Ed.D., June Barnhart, Ph.D.; Terry Treitman, Sandy Block, OD, M.Ed., and Peter D'Aloia, D.D.S); and the Sotos Syndrome Support Association for their continued support and encouragement. I also thank Rick London, series editor, for his support of this project. I also wish to acknowledge Deanine Mann, M.A., CCC-SLP; Sue Hill, OTR; Kathleen Zayner, OTR; Sylvia Maino, RN; and Kris Razma, OTR; for teaching me what **SPECIAL** really means. Last (but not least), I need to acknowledge the outstanding support for my many **special** projects given by David Greenberg, OD, MPH (Dean/Vice President of Academic Affairs, Illinois College of Optometry), and Janice Scharre, OD, MA (Chief of Rehabilitative Services, Illinois College of Optometry). All of the individuals and organizations named above are indeed **SPECIAL!**

Dominick M. Maino

Contents

Diagnosis and Management of Special Populations

Normal and Abnormal Visual Development: Clinical Implications of Neurobiological Research

Steven J. Cool

Key Terms

Neurobiological research	Brain plasticity	Critical period
	Rehabilitation	Sensitive periods
Visual development	Language of	Selective inhibition
Brain development	"clinical metaphor"	Disuse atrophy

In general, the research findings of what one might characterize as basic sciences (biochemistry, physiology, neurobiology) and the treatment outcomes of front-line clinicians rarely find a common forum of expression and integration. There is, however, a great deal that the basic scientist and the clinician can learn from each other if the opportunity presents itself and both are open to nonjudgmental discourse. It is in the spirit of such discourse that this chapter is offered, in the hope of building a modest bridge from the esoterica of basic science to the usefulness of clinical application.

In the broadest sense, vision is the global ability of the brain to extract, process, and act on information presented to the retina. From appropriately focused patterns of light reflected from objects in the environment, the adult brain is able to make meaningful and useful interpretations and predictions about the nature of the world. Relevant questions we need to ask include: How does the brain develop this ability to process visual information? What do we know of the neurobiological processes underlying brain development? What do we know of the neurobiological processes associated with the development of abnormal visual processing? Does nature dominate, or is nurture given a major role to play? What role does brain plasticity play in normal visual development, and in the rehabilitation of visual dysfunction? Is brain plasticity age-related? How can the development and/or redevelopment of visual information processing be facilitated? These are the primary questions that will be addressed in this chapter. It is hoped that clinicians can apply the basic science laboratory lessons of the past decade to their specific patient populations.

At this point I beg the reader's indulgence of a minor digression to make clear the particular biases I bring with me to this writing. Joseph Campbell devoted his life to the study of myth, and in his final two books[1,2] (transcripts of interviews with Bill Moyers and with Michael Toms, both published posthumously), he redefined the meaning of "myth." What he said was that myths are not made-up fiction or fantasy (make-believe) stories but rather are truths told in the language of metaphor because the language of a scientific database is unavailable to the myth maker. When one discovers some truth about the world, Campbell says, but has no scientific data-based language with which to communicate that truth, the language of metaphor is used in "truth saying," and it is this metaphoric truth saying that makes up myths.

With apologies to Professor Campbell, I would offer the following as an example of what he means by "metaphoric truth telling." Suppose you know someone (John) who is a fleet and agile runner of the high hurdles, and you want to describe his athletic ability to someone else. You could use a scientific data-based language and give a full description of his skeletal mechanics, his musculoskeletal biomechanics, his neuromuscular physiology, and you would be providing an accurate and truthful description. If, however, you live in a time or place in which you do not have access to this scientific data-based language, you could merely say, "John is an antelope." At a scientific, data-based level, he is not an antelope; but in the language of metaphor this statement conveys a great deal of truth about John, despite its being factually false. When the underlying facts are unknown or inaccessible, the language of metaphor becomes a powerful means of passing truth from one generation to the next.

And I would suggest that, in the realm of human neurobiology, most of the major discoveries of how the nervous system receives, processes, and uses information have been made not by basic scientists but by clinicians in their daily interactions with patients and clients. Lacking a clear scientific data-based language with which to communicate their discoveries, these workers communicated in "clinical metaphor" or "clinical mythology," which is a language full of truths about the human nervous system but is without strong scientific verification. I fervently hope that what follows will provide ample scientific ammunition to enable clinicians to defend their clinical truths against the oft heard challenge "But where's the scientific proof?"

Historical Context of Today's Neurobiology

Historically, the nature of the brain's processing of sensory and motor information was understood to be primarily a genetic preprogramming. The cerebral hemispheres were seen as subdivided into anatomically localized major functional continents, with their activities programmed by genetic inheritance into the growth and development of the central nervous system. Until some 30 years ago, virtually no one in the scientific community of biologists (and few in the community of experimental psychologists) believed that any brain functions (except the so-called "higher executive functions"—learning, memory, thought, cognition) were subject to major influence by the environmental situations in which the individual was raised. Specifically, the retinogeniculostriate pathways were thought to be invariantly "wired" into the embryological codes of the individual and not to be amenable to experimental modification.

More recently, however, we have come to understand that the strictly nativist position on brain development is probably wholly true only for the cold-blooded vertebrates. Mammalian brains gain their superiority over the brains of other vertebrates by having an increased level of flexibility, which is a function primarily of brain plasticity—the ability to program the brain's circuitry in accordance with environmental needs and dictates. Primates have developed this programmability to a high degree. *Homo sapiens* (literally "wise, knowing, sensible man") is the dominant creature on our planet because he possesses the most programmable brain of all. Research during the past 30 to 35 years has shown the way to an entirely new discipline, developmental neurobiology, which gives us transformational insights into the depth and breadth of brain programming.

During the past 50 to 75 years, theoretical physics has led to the discovery that there are few scientific absolutes. Thus, for example, the absolute laws of Newtonian physics have been found to be merely high-probability statements about physical world relationships under usual and normal conditions of observation. A case in point is the "optics law," which states that light striking a plane mirror will be reflected at the same angle as the angle of incidence (angle of incidence = angle of reflection law). Despite the fact that this appears to be an unvarying and absolute truth, Richard Feynman[3] (among others) has shown it to be otherwise. He has demonstrated that, whereas the angle of incidence = angle of reflection pathway is indeed the very high-probability outcome, under the right, precisely controlled conditions, light can be reflected from a mirror so the angle of reflection is *different from* the angle of incidence. He stresses the importance of understanding that "low-probability outcome" does not mean "impossible," and he urges that all workers—scientists and nonscientists alike—search for improbable possibilities in their worlds.

CLINICAL PEARL

Search for improbable possibilities.

I would like to suggest a direct parallel between this law (of optics) and the law of localization of function in neurobiology. The nativist, invariant, localization-of-function argument is the statement of a high-probability outcome under normal and usual conditions of development. However, rarely do patients or clients with special needs present themselves in the clinic under normal and usual conditions. They are there precisely because something is abnormal or unusual; and yet, most often, they are evaluated and treated according to the rules for normal and usual conditions of function. Long before research scientists began to understand this paradox, clinicians realized that a new set of rules was necessary for dealing with the abnormal and unusual conditions of patient/client symptoms. The plasticity or flexibility of the nervous system was long ago recognized by practicing clinicians as an important feature of treatment; and over the past 30 years, research in developmental neurobiology has focused a great deal of energy on studying the improbable possibility of plasticity/flexibility in the brain.

Foundations of Developmental Neurobiology

In 1949 D.O. Hebb[4] published a revolutionary book on CNS function. A central concept of this work that was the synaptic connections between nerve cells in the mammalian brain (especially the cerebral cortex), are formed on the basis of "functional stimulus interactions with the environment." In other words, the brain is literally programmed by experience, especially experiences that occur early in life. A colleague of Dr. Hebb, Hans Selye,[5] formalized his landmark ideas on stress in a book entitled *The Stress of Life.* Selye maintained that stress plays a major role in determining the efficiency and effectiveness with which people are able to interact in the world. Positive stress (what Selye called "eustress") makes behavioral interactions with the environment easier and more efficient. Negative stress ("distress") makes those interactions more difficult and less efficient. Putting Hebb's and Selye's ideas together leads to the notion that the brain is programmed by functionally relevant environmental interactions and that levels of stress play a significant role in determining what and how this programming will occur. The literature of the past 3 decades supports these ideas.

Starting with the work of David Hubel and Torsten Wiesel, in the early 1960s, there has been a steady stream of research into the developmental neurobiology of vision. Much of this has been devoted to studying the behavior and formation of connections among individual brain cells, and from it has come a great deal of information about the global function of vision. Initially Hubel and Wiesel[6] explored the various stimulus features that were most likely to elicit activity in cells of the visual cortex of normal adult mammals. What they found was that each cell seemed to have its own constellation of stimulus preferences. Some were activated most by a dim light stimulus. Others showed maximum activation to a moderate light level. Still others responded maximally to a very bright light. Some cells responded best to a vertical bar of light moving in a horizontal direction across the retina, others to a horizontal bar moving vertically. Some cells responded best to combinations of these orientations and directions of movement. Some responded to a rapidly moving stimulus, others to a slowly moving light, etc. Thus, by the late 1960s, it appeared that visual neurophysiologists might be buried under a morass of data points.

However, a number of visual cortex cellular response characteristics stood out in Hubel and Wiesel's mind. Foremost among these was the fact that, although each cell had a unique constellation of stimulus response characteristics, there were some commonalities: (1) each cell responded best (or only) to a straight edge or bar of light moving across the retina; (2) some 75% to 80% of the cells responded to binocular stimulation; (3) each cell had an exact set of requirements for eliciting a response. Hubel and Wiesel asked the following questions about these features: Did the cells possess stimulus-response characteristics as a result of innate genetically predetermined growth and development mechanisms? Or, were there some experiential components in the way they responded? The answers to these questions came as a distinct surprise to many, and the consequences are still being puzzled over and researched today.

Experiential Basis for Brain Programming

To begin to explore the subject, Hubel and Wiesel[7-9] elected to study binocularity. They asked whether the 75% to 80% of visual cortex cells normally activated binocularly were that way at birth or whether experience played a role in programming them. They raised cats and monkeys in which vision was restricted in one eye from birth by means of an opaque contact lens or suturing of the lids. When the animals were 3 to 6 months old, data from individual cells of the visual cortices were recorded. No longer did 75% to 80% of the cells respond to binocular stimulation; rather only a few in the eye that had been deprived of light responded. The vast majority of cells reacted only to stimulation in the eye that had not been subject to the early months of deprivation. Virtually none showed any tendency to be binocularly sensitive.

What these authors, and many others after them (Hirsch and Spinelli[10,11] and von Noorden et al.[12,13]), corroborated was that, far from being preset and preprogrammed by genetic mechanisms, the information-processing characteristics of the visual cortices seemed to be an outcome of the kinds of experiences encountered in early life. Indeed, in November 1981, when the Nobel Prize for Physiology/Medicine was awarded to Hubel and Wiesel, the awarding committee of the Karolinska Institute made the following statement (as quoted by a United Press International article [November 7, 1981]):

> [Hubel and Weisel] ... found that the capability of the visual system to interpret images is developed after birth and that a prerequisite is for the eyes to be exposed to varied visual stimuli. It is only a slight exaggeration to say that what we see today, in other words, how we perceive the visual world around us, depends on the visual experiences we had during the first stages of our lives. If those [early experiences] are dull and distorted—for example, through errors in the lens system of the eye—it may lead to permanent impairment of the brain's ability to analyze visual impressions.

CLINICIAL PEARL

The capability of the visual system to interpret images is developed after birth.

All this information is pretty well understood by most vision/eye-care specialists today. The clinical ramifications are, of course, extremely far reaching. As Herrin[14] has underscored, the importance of early detection and treatment of visual dysfunction cannot be overemphasized. This is especially true for patient populations who have to deal with multiple dysfunctional systems. Unfortunately, our understanding of the unfolding developmental neurobiology vision story seems to end abruptly in the middle 1970s. Yet the basic research of the past 15 years has enormous implications for clinical practice.

By 1975 the brain-programming story, as told by Hubel and Wiesel and others, was that the first 3 to 6 months of a cat's or monkey's life

constitutes a "critical period" for the development of normal programming of the visual cortex. During this time the animal's brain is
building the capacity to respond to salient visual features of the
environment. If these environmental stimuli are, in some way, compromised (as by unilateral eye occlusion, strabismus, ammetropia,
etc.), then the information processing of the animal will also be
compromised. Hubel and Wiesel developed, and most other investigators accepted, the idea that this compromising of cortical programming was a function of what they called "disuse atrophy." If certain
information-processing capacities were prevented from developing
during this critical period, the corresponding processing connections
from the visual pathways to the visual cortex would atrophy through
lack of use. So, the researchers reasoned, it was essential to correct
visual system abnormalities/dysfunctions before the critical period
had passed (Fig. 1-1).

Thus much of the research in the early to middle 1970s—such as
that by von Noorden et al.[7,8]—concentrated on this critical period. The
findings, which were widely published and understood in the vision-
care community, suggested that the total length of the critical period
was 3 to 6 months for cats and monkeys, 18 to 24 months for higher
nonhuman primates (chimpanzees and gorillas), and 3 to 6 years for
humans. During this period it was reasoned that infants and children
should receive ample visual inputs so the normal neural connections
in the brain could be made. If some visual system anomaly evidenced
itself during this time, it was believed to be absolutely critical that it
be corrected quickly. If it were left uncorrected, it would likely
produce disuse atrophy of potential neural connections in the visual
system, thereby rendering the individual permanently unable to
process visual information normally.

By 1975 there was a strong emphasis on the necessity for early intervention and treatment of any visual system anomaly. This had to occur
before the ending of the critical period so there could be some hope of
developing normal vision. The evidence and line of reasoning pointed to
the "fact" that at the end of the critical period, whatever experiences had
been programmed into the visual cortex were permanently cemented in
place and could not be changed or modified. The used connections were
thought to be permanently represented in synapses of the visual cortex,
and the disused connections were thought to atrophy. And it was, of
course, an article of faith among the research community that any attempt at vision rehabilitation beyond the age of 6 to 8 years was a waste
of time, energy, and money. This certainly underscored the importance
of early detection and treatment of visual dysfunction; but any good
rehabilitation clinician could also have told you that remediation of
neural dysfunction (that is, reversal) is possible, though more difficult,
in older patients. Nevertheless, the basic science position in 1975 was
that the end of the critical period signaled the absolute end of brain

VISUAL DEVELOPMENT INVENTORY

	Newborn	1 Month	2 Months	3 Months	6 Months	9 Months	12 Months	18 Months	24 Months	3 Years
OCULOMOTOR										
Fixation	To face	→								→
Saccades H	(+)	(−)	(+)(+)	(+)					One shift to target	→
V	(−)	(−)	(−)	?						→
Pursuits / Visually directed reaching	(−)	(−)	(−)	(+)	(+)					→
Face regard	(+)									→
OKN: T-N and N-T response	Asymmetric (+)	Asymmetric	Asymmetric	Asymmetric	Symmetric	→				→
ACUITY										
Preferential Looking OU	20/400 to 20/1200	20/300 to 20/1200	20/150 to 20/600	→	20/50 to 20/200			20/40 to 20/100	20/30 to 20/80	20/20
Electrophysiological			20/120		20/25					
BINOCULARITY										
Alignment								Adultlike levels of angle lambda		
Near pt of convergence	up to 10 in	→			To nose					
Fixation of moving target		(+)		Response + →						→
10 Δ response	(−)(−)	(−)(−)		→	70% of time / Well developed		→			
Stereopsis	None				Well developed					
ACCOMMODATION										
Accuracy	Accurate for 30 cm (12 in)			Well developed	Accurate for 75 to 150 cm	→				
Lag				+0.75						
PUPIL RESPONSES										
Chromatic discrimination			Well developed unable to do	Basic trichromatic (+)	Well developed					
Blink response to visual threat	(+) Sluggish				Near normal					Normal
Contrast sensitivity function				Adultlike low frequency attenuation	→					Adultlike btwn 3–5 yr

FIGURE 1-1 A visual development inventory. (Courtesy Dr. Janice Scharre, Illinois College of Optometry, Chicago.)

programming in the primary, sensory, and motor cortices. However, in 1976, two studies[15,16] appeared that literally turned the critical period/disuse atrophy story on its ear.

Sensitive Periods Replace Critical Periods; Selective Inhibition Replaces Disuse Atrophy

Duffy et al.[15] performed a simple experiment, following the Hubel and Wiesel monocular deprivation model, in which they definitively showed that disuse atrophy does not occur as a result of early visual system anomalies. They repeated the Hubel-Wiesel type of study, making the visual cortex completely responsive only to inputs from the nondeprived eye but nonresponsive to inputs from the deprived eye. Then, while recording the electrical activity of individual visual cortex cells, they administered intravenous bicuculline. When this drug enters the CNS, it blocks the receptor molecules for one specific neurotransmitter, gamma-aminobutyric acid (GABA), the principal inhibitor in the CNS. Wherever GABA is active, it reduces nerve cell excitability; in other words, it turns nerve cells off. On the other hand, because bicuculline blocks the action of GABA, it also has the tendency to release nerve cells from their inhibited state; that is, it turns nerve cells back on that have been turned off by GABA. It was found that when bicuculline was administered the cells were able to resume their activity. What Duffy et al.[15] demonstrated was that dysfunctional early visual experiences do not necessarily result in anatomical loss of visual pathway connections; rather, the brain actively inhibits connections that are not used early in life while maintaining the anatomical connectedness.

What occurs during the critical period (perhaps better termed *sensitive* period) seems to be similar to what occurs embryologically during cellular differentiation. Initially each embryonic cell is undifferentiated; that is, it has the full genetic complement and is capable of becoming any type of tissue in any organ. However, as the embryo develops, each cell undergoes differentiation. This is the process wherein it takes on certain structural and functional capacities; in other words, it goes from being undifferentiated to being fully (and only) a liver cell, a big toe cell, or an earlobe cell. In the process none of the genes is lost; rather, for example, the differentiated liver cell status occurs by active repression of all genes that are not liver cell genes and by active derepression (turning on) of all genes that are liver cell genes. Under normal circumstances, once this active differentiation has occurred, the cell forever remains a liver cell. However, as recent genetic research into cloning and recombinant DNA has shown, under extraordinary circumstances these turned-off genes can be turned back on again and an entire new organism cloned.

The recent data on nervous system development indicate that a similar mechanism is responsible for the sensitive period effects of brain programming. As Duffy et al.[15] and Kratz et al.[16] have demonstrated, during the sensitive period of development the visual cortex actively turns off the possibility of responding to aspects of the environment to which it is not exposed (as by deprivation of stimuli to one eye) and actively turns on the responsiveness to stimuli to which it is exposed. Under normal conditions of development these possibilities of processing (programmed by early experience) remain constant throughout life. However, it might then be asked: "If it is possible to 're–turn on' a cell's genes through the process of cloning, should it not also be possible to re–turn on a visual cortex cell's information-processing possibilities?" And, indeed, the literature of the past decade seems to respond with a resounding yes.

The implications for clinical practice are many. Clearly if the sensitive period (first 6 to 8 years of life) is the time when the foundation building blocks of visual perception are being laid (or programmed into the brain), it would behoove the clinician to do his or her utmost to ensure that normal visual sensorimotor capabilities are attained by the pediatric patient. Beyond the early detection and treatment of dysfunction, however, research thus far has elucidated little more than the salient psychosocioemotional and behavioral variables involved in awakening and maintaining brain plasticity throughout a person's life.

Attention and Brain Plasticity During and After the Sensitive Period

As the research just mentioned has shown, brain cells of the visual cortex are very plastic or programmable during the sensitive period of development. Our experiences early in life set the stage for the way our cortex responds to environmental stimulation. At some point, however, the brain decides that it needs to stop programming the visual cortex and start using the stored information for more complex information-processing tasks. This is what has been termed the *end* of the sensitive period in development. Research during the past 10 to 15 years has concentrated on exactly what the mechanisms of cortical plasticity are and what means there are for allowing this plasticity to recur after the end of the sensitive period.

Late in the 1970s and early in the 1980s, a number of studies[17-19] converged on one line of reasoning—that cortical plasticity is linked to mechanisms of arousal, attention, motivation, and emotion. A particular region of the brain stem reticular activating system, called the *locus coeruleus*, was believed to be involved in these mechanisms, and the research of Pettigrew,[17] Kasamatsu,[18] and others found that the locus coeruleus is indeed closely tied to mechanisms of cortical plasticity both during and after the sensitive period. What these workers discovered was that if the selective attention mechanisms of the locus coeruleus are disturbed or turned off; it is possible to completely eliminate plasticity during the normal sensitive period (in other words, if the action of the locus coeruleus is suppressed, so also will be cortical programmability). In addition (and perhaps more important), they found that, if an individual is allowed to develop through the sensitive period (either normally or with special programming conditions) and then the locus coeruleus is stimulated (chemically or electrically) into a higher-than-normal level of activity, this cortical plasticity can be re–turned on, even months or years after the sensitive period has ended.

CLINICAL PEARL

Cortical plasticity is linked to mechanisms of arousal, attention, motivation, and emotion.

Thus the role of the locus coeruleus in cortical plasticity was demonstrated. Singer's work[19] has shown that arousal, attention, motivation, and emotion are all relevant (psychological) variables correlating with actions of the locus. Accordingly, the past 10 years have seen much attention directed toward the neuroanatomical, neurophysiological, and biochemical functionings of the locus coeruleus. Work by Kasamatsu,[20] Aoki and Siekevitz,[21] and others (summarized by Gordon et al.[22]) has shown the following to be true:

1. Cells of the locus coeruleus are virtually the only cells in the CNS which use norepinephrine as their neurotransmitter.
2. These few cells send out billions of bifurcating axons to make noradrenergic connections with cells in the remainder of the CNS.
3. An important biochemical action of these connections (synapses) is to set up intracellular conditions in the post-synaptic cells for the formation of new synapses.

In short, it was shown that the neurotransmitter norepinephrine is essential to the processes of cortical plasticity and of learning and memory.

The importance of this finding cannot be overemphasized, because as a result of it the solid link between brain plasticity and stress (which Hebb[4] and Selye[5] had hypothesized 35 to 40 years earlier) was explicitly demonstrated. Although norepinephrine has been known to be a CNS neurotransmitter for only 15 to 20 years, it has been recognized for some 50 to 75 years as one of the adrenalinelike hormones secreted by the adrenal glands in response to stressful stimuli. Now we see that norepinephrine is also intimately tied to cortical plasticity, learning, and memory.

If we stop for a moment to consider some of our own experiences, it will become clear that we have been affected by this linkage on a number of occasions. Nearly all of us of a certain age can recall the events on the day that John Kennedy was assassinated or, if not that old, then perhaps on the day that the space shuttle Challenger exploded. The remarkable thing is not that we remember the assassination or the actual explosion but that we also remember very inconsequential details of events around the same time. For example, I can remember clearly the restaurant where I was having dinner the night I received an emergency phone call telling me that my father had died suddenly of a heart attack. Although I had not been in that restaurant before, and have not been there since, I remember many incidental details of its interior—the draperies and chandeliers, the phone booth where I took the call, even some phone numbers scrawled on the wall above the phone.

Why do we remember such details associated with these important attentional and emotional events? Precisely because they *are* powerful attentional/emotional events and are accompanied by a systemic flood of adrenal response stress biochemicals, including a large amount of norepinephrine. This is not synaptic norepinephrine from the reticular activating system; but, nevertheless, in the amounts secreted from the adrenal glands it reaches sufficient concentrations in the circulation to pass into the CNS and trigger the cortical plasticity functions that lead to our remembering things for some short length of time after the initial shock of the event has hit. The biochemistry of cortical plasticity and the biochemistry of stress both involve norepinephrine. So, as Selye[5] suggested, stress can play a major role in how efficiently and effectively we learn and remember.

The developmental neurobiology research of the past decade and a half has demonstrated that the CNS biochemistry (and the endocrine/ immune system biochemistry) associated with arousal, attention, motivation, emotion, and stress is intimately tied up with the capacity of the CNS to be plastic, to be able to learn and remember, and to be capable of reprogramming when the initial programming is dysfunctional. Since this work is so closely tied to biochemical analyses and neurotransmitter functions, one might rightly ask whether it means that we can merely take a pill or a shot of the right chemicals and suddenly be "plastic" again. The answer would be "yes," but with some very serious restrictive qualifications.

Remember that traumatic life events essentially do give us a systemic shot of the right biochemicals, and the result is that we are replasticized; but we are so plastic that we learn and remember everything in a very unselective manner. And herein lies the problem:

systemic biochemical infusions are very nonspecific in their actions whereas the synaptic actions of cells in the locus ceruleus are extremely specific and locally defined. Thus, although it is the biochemistry of norepinephrine that is responsible for the plasticity (that is, programmability) of cortical nerve cells, it is the synaptic selectivity of the CNS that makes it possible to learn and remember only certain details (to selectively program or reprogram) only a specific target set of cells. These synaptic interaction mechanisms of selective plasticity act like a lawn sprinkler whereas a systemic dose of the same biochemicals acts more like a fire hose. Both give the cortical biochemical activity needed for plasticity, but the former does so very precisely and selectively while the latter does so on a broad, general, and nonselective basis. The crucial question for clinical intervention strategies seems to be how can this discrete plasticity biochemistry be activated within the context of efficacious therapeutic treatment.

CLINICAL PEARL

Arousal, Attention, Motivation, Emotion
The key to efficient and effective clinical interventions is finding a way to engage these mechanisms in each patient and to capitalize on that engagement as one rehabilitates the dysfunctional CNS.

Clinical Implications from Developmental Neurobiology

The answer to the above question is, of course, clear to any practicing clinician who has ever engaged in some form of rehabilitative treatment. It is always said that the alert, aroused, motivated patient who is paying attention to and is emotionally engaged in the treatment strategies is the patient who will make the greatest gains most rapidly. So, can the brain be reprogrammed in an individual beyond the sensitive period of age? The answer is clearly a resounding yes, both for the clinical metaphorical truths and for the data-based truths. And, in addition, the mechanisms involved in setting up conditions for the reprogramming are the same as are involved in the initial development of the programs—arousal, attention, motivation, and emotion. The key to efficient and effective clinical intervention is finding a way to engage these mechanisms in each patient and to capitalize on that engagement as we rehabilitate the dysfunctional CNS.

How does an optometric clinician engage these plasticity mechanisms? The answer is, I think, twofold. Clearly, the core strengths of optometric practice are critical to awakening cortical plasticity. You use lenses, prisms, low vision devices (optical and nonoptical), diagnostic pharmaceutical agents, therapeutic pharmaceutical agents, vision therapy, and the entire optometric armamentarium to provide single, clear, comfortable, binocular, pathology-free vision for the patient. This, alone will produce arousal and attention in the patient, and quite often the improvement will be enormously motivating and emotionally positive for the patient. So, the provision of sound, full-scope, optometric services can have a profound effect on the mechanisms of cortical plasticity and brain programming.

CLINICAL PEARL

Having single, clear, comfortable, binocular, pathology-free vision is enormously motivating and emotionally positive for the patient.

Second (and perhaps more important), the clinician must always remember to practice the art as well as the science of vision care. And what is the art of clinical care? It is the taking of time to sit down and say "Hello" to your patient, to remove the stainless steel and technology from between you and the patient, and to get to know something about just who this particular person is. Thus you, the clinician, can come to know what is attentionally sustaining for this particular person—what is motivationally relevant, emotionally important, and functionally appropriate—and this knowledge can be used to engage the patient in whatever treatment regimen is decided on. In exactly the same way as the old country doctor used to know that Ellie May, down the road, had to have a pill in order to believe she was going to get well, so the modern clinician can practice the art of health care. By fully co-opting the patient into the treatment strategies, the internal biochemistry of plasticity (of health and well-being) can be optimally engaged so the science of health care has its maximal effect.

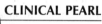

CLINICAL PEARL

If the clinician fully co-opts the patient into the treatment strategies, the internal biochemistry of plasticity and of health and well-being can be optimally engaged so the science of health care can have its maximum effect.

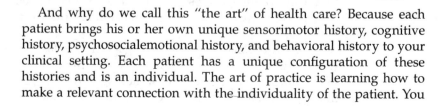

And why do we call this "the art" of health care? Because each patient brings his or her own unique sensorimotor history, cognitive history, psychosocialemotional history, and behavioral history to your clinical setting. Each patient has a unique configuration of these histories and is an individual. The art of practice is learning how to make a relevant connection with the individuality of the patient. You truly become the full-scope, full-service clinician when you practice both the art and the science of health care, engaging what Albert Schweitzer called "the healer within,"[23] setting up the internal biochemistry of health and well-being, and allowing for maximum efficiency and effectiveness of treatment.

REFERENCES

1. Campbell J, Moyers B: *The power of myth,* New York, 1988, Doubleday.
2. Campbell J, Toms M: *An open life,* New York, 1989, Harper & Row.
3. Feynman RP: *QED: The strange theory of light and matter,* Princeton NJ, 1985, Princeton University Press.
4. Hebb DO: *The organization of behavior,* New York, 1949, John Wiley.
5. Selye H: *The stress of life,* New York, 1956, McGraw-Hill.
6. Hubel DH, Wiesel TN: Receptive fields, binocular interaction, and functional architecture in the cat's visual cortex, *J Physiol* 160:106-154, 1962.
7. Wiesel TN, Hubel DH: Single-cell responses in striate cortex of kittens deprived of vision in one eye, *J Neurophysiol* 26:1003-1017, 1963.
8. Wiesel TN, Hubel DH: Comparison of unilateral and bilateral eye closure on cortical unit responses in kittens, *J Neurophysiol* 28:1029-1040, 1965.
9. Hubel DH, Wiesel TN: Brain mechanisms of vision, *Sci Am* 241:150-162, 1979.
10. Hirsch HVB, Spinelli DN: Visual experience modifies distribution of horizontally and vertically oriented receptive fields in cats, *Science* 168:869-871, 1970.
11. Hirsch HVB, Spinelli DN: Modification of the distribution of receptive field orientation cats by selective visual exposure during development, *Exp Brain Res* 12:509-527, 1971.
12 Baker FH, Grigg P, von Noorden GK: Effects of visual deprivation and strabismus on the response of neurons in the visual cortex of the monkey, including studies on the striate and prestriate cortex in the normal animal, *Brain Res* 66:185-208, 1974.
13. Crawford MLJ, Blake R, Cool SJ, von Noorden GK: Physiological consequences of unilateral and bilateral eye closure in macaque monkeys: some further observations, *Brain Res* 84:150-154, 1975.
14. Herrin S: Don't let kids end up like me, *Optom Manage* 27:11, 1992.
15. Duffy FH, Snodgrass SR, Burchfiel JL, Conway JL: Bicuculline reversal of deprivation amblyopia in the cat, *Nature* 260:256-257, 1976.
16. Kratz KE, Spear PD, Smith DC: Post–critical-period reversal of effects of monocular deprivation on striate cortex cells in the cat, *J Neurophysiol* 39:501-511, 1976.
17. Pettigrew JD: The locus coeruleus and cortical plasticity, *Trends Neurosci* 1:73-74, 1978.
18. Kasamatsu T: Enhancement of neuronal plasticity by activating the norepinephrine system in the brain: a remedy for amblyopia, *Hum Neurobiol* 1:49-54, 1982.
19. Singer W: The role of attention in developmental plasticity, *Hum Neurobiol* 1:41-43, 1982.
20. Kasamatsu T: Norepinephrine hypothesis for visual cortical plasticity: thesis, antithesis, and recent development, *Curr Top Dev Biol* 21:367-389, 1987.
21. Aoki C, Siekevitz P: Plasticity in brain development, *Sci Am* 259:56-64, 1988.
22. Gordon B, Allen EE, Trombley PQ: The role of norepinephrine in plasticity of visual cortex, *Prog Neurobiol* 30:171-191, 1988.
23. Schweitzer A. Quoted in Cousins N: *Anatomy of an illness,* New York, 1979, Bantam Books, p 69.

2

Oculovisual Findings in Children with Down Syndrome, Cerebral Palsy, and Mental Retardation without Specific Etiology

Michael D. Wesson
Dominick M. Maino

Key Terms

Down syndrome	Developmental	Education for All
Cerebral palsy	Disabilities	Handicapped
Mental retardation	Assistance	Children Act
Developmental disabilities	Bill of Rights Act	Fragile X syndrome

Developmental disabilities (DD) are severe, chronic, mental or physical impairments that occur at conception or soon after birth. They are likely to continue indefinitely and have a pervasive effect on an individual's functional abilities and need for special education, health, and rehabilitation services.[1] According to Public Law (PL) 95-602 (The Developmental Disabilities Assistance and Bill of Rights Act), there are more than 2 million persons with DD in the United States. Depending on the definition of DD used, this figure is probably a gross underestimation. According to other sources,[1] DD affect more than 5 million

17

children. Individuals with disabilities that occur during the developmental period are more vulnerable and less able to reach an independent level of functioning than handicapped individuals who have had a normal developmental period. Early identification and intervention will reduce the impact of developmental delay, improve cognitive outcome, and often promote academic success.[2-4]

CLINICAL PEARL

Developmental disabilities affect more than 5 million children.

Two important public laws have been enacted based on the study of early identification and intervention. In October 1986 Congress passed PL 99-457, which was an amendment to PL 94-142 (The Education for All Handicapped Children Act). These two broad pieces of legislation required that all infants and children with DD be identified and provided with appropriate services. PL 99-457 stipulated that there be identification and early intervention services from birth to 5 years of age whereas PL 94-142 stipulated that special services be offered through ages 6 to 18 years.

CLINICAL PEARL

PL 99-457 and the Education for All Handicapped Children Act require that every infant and child with developmental disabilities be identified and given appropriate services.

The goal of these laws was to bring family-centered, community-based, coordinated health care, along with development, educational, and social services, to American children[5]—which meant providing health-care delivery within the community, not within institutions. From an optometric perspective, it meant that children with DD would be seeking care more often in private offices than in clinics. This is important, because children with DD appear to have significantly more eye problems, including moderate to high refractive errors, binocular vision dysfunctions, and numerous ocular diseases[6] (Table 2-1). For optometrists this means a greater responsibility for diagnosing and treating eye conditions in children categorized as having developmental delays or being at risk for such delays.

This chapter will review the conditions commonly associated with developmental delays and their general and ocular characteristics and will provide primary-care optometrists a framework for their assessment. Much of this information has not been published. Most of the patients

TABLE 2-1

Relative Occurrence of Ocular Problems in Children (1950 to 1992)

	Refractive error (%)	Strabismus (%)	Other (%)	Total
Normal	15 to 30[7-9]	2 to 4[10,11]	—	—
Cerebral palsy	21 to 76[10]	15 to 60[10]	1 to 25[10,11]	50 to 78[10,11]
Mental retardation	52[12,13]	16 to 40[12,13]	21[13]	50 to 80[14]
Down syndrome	42 to 73[15,16]	23 to 44[7]	33*	—
Fragile X syndrome	59[17]	30 to 50[17-19]	13†	—
Deafness	29[9]	13[9]	9[9]	45 to 55[9,20]

Adapted from Gnadt & Wesson.[6]
*Blepharitis.
†Maino,[19] Maino et al.,[17] and King et al.[18] have not reported the presence of any major ocular health abnormalities. The 13% here represents the presence of nystagmus found in Maino's[19] study.

examined received care at the Chauncey Sparks Center for Developmental and Learning Disorders, a division of the Civitan International Research Center, University of Alabama at Birmingham, and the Illinois College of Optometry Eye Care Service at the Easter Seal Society of Metropolitan Chicago, Inc., Gilchrist-Marchman Rehabilitation Center. The information obtained included a differential description of procedural and refractive, binocular and ocular disease characteristics found with three distinctive diagnostic entities, including Down syndrome (a chromosomal disorder), cerebral palsy (a motor disorder secondary to brain trauma), and mental retardation (MR) with a nonspecific etiology (in other words, not secondary to any other diagnosable condition). A summary of the basic epidemiological data of the first three entities in our study appears in Table 2-2.

Down Syndrome

Langdon Down[21] first described the clinical entity that bears his name in 1866. At the time, because of the uniformly common upward slanting of the temporal palpebral fissures and the presence of epicanthal folds, this chromosome 21 anomaly was referred to as "mongolism." Today the term *mongolism* is considered archaic. A review by Catalano[22] has summarized the chromosomal dysfunction as having three etiologies. Up to 95% of the cases demonstrate nondisjunction of one chromosome during meiosis. Nondisjunction also may occur in later stages of cell division, giving rise to mosaicism in about 1% of persons with trisomy 21 syndrome. This mosaicism decreases the effect of the condition as it relates to intellectual impairment. Finally, there may be a translocation of one chromosome

TABLE 2-2

Basic Epidemiological Data for the Initial Visits of Patients with One of the Three Types of Developmental Disability

	Number	Average age (mo)	Race White (%)	Black (%)	Other (%)	Sex Male (%)	Female (%)
Down syndrome	134	56	93(73)	33(26)	1(1)*	74(56)	59(44)†
Cerebral palsy	91	48	59(69)	25(29)	1(1)	51(56)	40(44)
Mental retardation	14	64	10(71)	4(29)	—	91(64)	5(36)
TOTALS	239		162‡	62	2	134	104

*Unknown.
†1 Unknown.
‡Totals do not equal 239 because of missing data.

to another chromosome pair. The carrier is normal physically and mentally but passes the unusual chromosome structure to his or her offspring (2% to 3% of individuals with the syndrome).

Down syndrome is one of the most common chromosomal abnormalities encountered, occurring in about 1 of every 600 live births (see box on page 21). For women 44 years or older the incidence increases by a factor of 12 (1 in 50). Some 50% of the fetuses abort spontaneously in early pregnancy. The planned termination of a pregnancy may occur more often now that improved diagnostic techniques (such as ultrasound imaging and α-fetoprotein monitoring by amniocentesis) are allowing the family a choice as to whether or not to continue the pregnancy.

Interestingly, the prevalence of Down syndrome is *increasing,* most likely due to the application of better medical technology during the first 10 years of life, which has led to improved survival rates for infants with the syndrome. Congenital heart defects, pneumonia, and acute leukemia are the leading causes of death in individuals with Down syndrome. Heart defects are found in 30% to 50% of affected persons. Many of those children have an abnormal thymus gland, which results in greater susceptibility to infection. Acute leukemia strikes at a rate 15 times that in the general pediatric population. Premature aging, a high incidence of Alzheimer's disease, arteriosclerosis, and fenestrated heart valves typically are seen in adults with the syndrome.

Universally, individuals with Down syndrome and nondisjunction of chromosome 21 will be mentally retarded. The average intelligence quotient by standardized testing is about 50. Mental retardation is generally defined as an IQ less than 70. A score of 50 is in the mild range. Children with Down syndrome due to mosaicism will have a higher level of intelligence. Neurological evaluation often reveals the presence of hypotonicity and poor motor coordination, which can

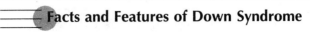

Facts and Features of Down Syndrome

Facts
  Occurring in 1:600 live births
  1:50 with women older than 44
  Detected with ultrasound and amniocentesis
  Associated with congenital heart defects
  Acute leukemia 15 times more common than in the general population
  Mental retardation is universal*
  Good socialization skills

Common identifying features
  Short stature
  Brachycephalic skull
  Flat occiput
  Low-set ears
  Flat nasal bridge
  Protruding tongue
  Dental anomalies
  Short stubby hands and feet
  Very dry skin
  Abdominal protuberance

Common ocular features
  Oblique palpebral fissures
  Strabismus
  Moderate/high refractive error
  Keratoconus
  Broad epicanthal folds
  Brushfield spots
  Iris hypoplasia
  Spoked vessel pattern emanating from optic disc
  New observation: Retinal pigment epithelial disturbances at disc margin

  *Mosaicism is an exception.

further complicate intelligence testing. In fact, the socialization skills of individuals with Down syndrome may far exceed their measured problem-solving ability, giving rise to the impression that the individuals have a higher level of cognitive ability than is actually present.

Clinical Assessment

General physical characteristics

Patients with Down syndrome have physical features that distinguish them (Fig. 2-1). Peculiar characteristics of the head and body accompany the syndrome at different stages of life. There is the short stature with brachycephaly (Fig. 2-1, *D*), often accompanied by a flat occiput,

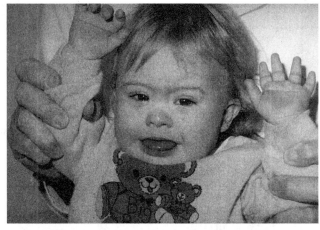

A

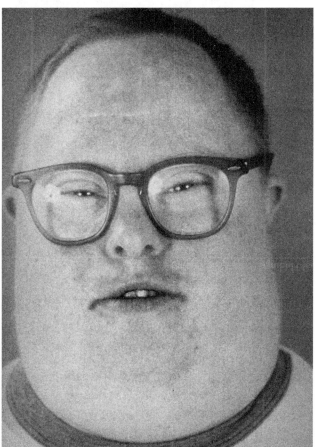

B

FIGURE 2-1 Characteristics of the head and body that accompany Down syndrome at different stages of life include (**A, B**) brachycephaly, flat occiput, low-set ears, flat nasal bridge, and protruding tongue.

Continued.

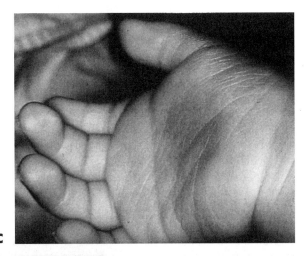

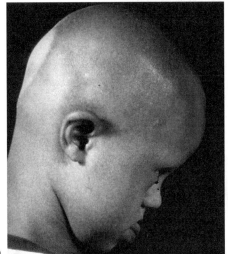
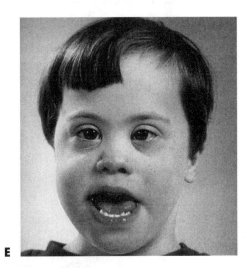

FIGURE 2-1, Cont'd. C, Individuals with Down syndrome show clinodactyly and a prominent simian crease across the palm. **D** and **E,** Brachycephaly, flat occiput, low-set ears, and a flat nasal bridge are also frequently noted.

low-set ears, flat nasal bridge, and protruding tongue (Fig. 2-1, *A* and *E).* The tongue is usually too large for the oral cavity, causing the individual to habitually hold the mouth open. Dental anomalies include a high-arched narrow palate and underdeveloped maxilla with delayed dentition. The hands and feet are short and stubby, with multiple dermatoglyphic irregularities. The major abnormalities include clinodactyly (inward turning of the fifth digit) and a prominent simian (full-width) crease across the palms (Fig. 2-1, *C),* which occur in about half of all affected individuals. The skin is dry, scaly, and inelastic. The hair is almost always straight and soft.

Abdominal protuberance is often seen and most likely is the result of hypotonic muscles. Duodenal obstruction is a frequent abnormality.

Ocular abnormalities

Gross and detailed examinations of the eye and adnexa reveal many differences between individuals with Down syndrome and those in the general population. As mentioned, the hallmark of Down syndrome is the laterally displaced and oblique palpebral fissures (narrow pupillary distance) accompanied by prominent epicanthal folds (Fig. 2-2). Brushfield spots are also common, appearing in about 85% of patients and consisting of pale gray irregular discolorations in the midperipheral irides.[24] They are made up of connective tissue condensations of the anterior stromal layer and should not be confused with Wolfflin nodules, which are found in 10% to 24% of non-affected individuals. Wolfflin nodules are smaller, about 0.5 mm in diameter, less well defined, and more peripherally placed in the irides than Brushfield spots. In addition, Wolfflin nodules are usually found in the last or next-to-last roll of the iris, never in a furrow or crypt.[25] Brushfield spots are more numerous, more distinct, and closer to the pupillary margin.[24]

Another feature is iris hypoplasia.[26] As many as 95% of persons with Down syndrome exhibit hypoplasia of the iris whereas only 2% to 9% have this in the general population.[25,26] Microscopic cross-

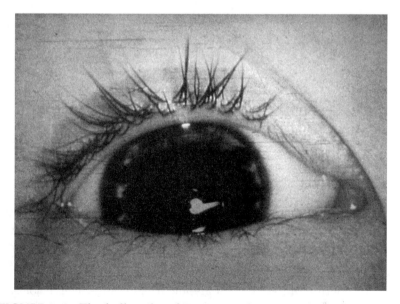

FIGURE 2-2 The hallmarks of Down syndrome are laterally displaced, oblique, palpebral fissures with epicanthal folds and Brushfield spots.

sectional evaluation reveals a thinning of the peripheral iris stroma with large empty spaces and a thickening of the anterior border layer.[24]

The major aberrant fundus feature appears to be extra vessels leaving or crossing the margin of the disc, forming a spoked pattern.[27] This contributes to a hyperemic appearance of the disc[28] and has been documented in about 20% of our patients (although the literature[27] indicates a higher prevalence). The etiology appears to be early bifurcation of the vessels before they cross the disc margin. We have observed that in about 30% of children with Down syndrome there is a disturbance of the retinal pigment epithelium (RPE) at the disc margin. In addition, about 8% exhibit RPE dropout. To our knowledge, this has not been reported previously as a significant feature of the condition, although there is some hint of this in the literature.[23] No other consistent retinal signs appear with the syndrome. It has been suggested,[29] however, that optic disc elevation without a specific cause may occur in at least some patients.

Visual acuity determination

Working with any population that exhibits developmental delay places a significant responsibility on the examiner. A most critical feature of any vision examination is the determination of acuity. The assessment of visual acuity is mandatory for obtaining assistance under PL 99-457. Although specially trained personnel (such as nurses, psychologists, educators, and occupational therapists) screen these patients, the optometrist is often called on to determine visual acuity in difficult-to-test children. A report stating merely "unable to determine visual acuity" or "he/she has usable vision" makes proper placement much more difficult. Optometrists should have a working knowledge of which acuity tests are most appropriate for these special populations.

Based on our experience at the Sparks Center and the Gilchrist–Marchman Center, a comparison is presented of the different methods for acuity determination at far point in patients with Down syndrome, cerebral palsy, or mild mental retardation without specific etiology (Table 2-3). *Far point* usually means 6 meters (20 feet), but this may not be the best distance for many children with disabilities. In fact, the distance used varies as a function of the capacity of the child to attend (Table 2-4). Of the patients with Down syndrome or cerebral palsy, 50% had to be evaluated at a distance of 3 meters or less; and of the patients with mental retardation without specific etiology, 28% needed a closer distance.

Among the patients with Down syndrome, 76% required using the Teller Visual Acuity cards* or the Optokinetic Nystagmus (OKN)

---

*VisTech Consultants, Dayton, Ohio.

TABLE 2-3

Methods of Testing Far Point* Visual Acuity

	Cerebral palsy (%)	Down syndrome (%)	Mental retardation (%)
Teller Visual Acuity cards	63 (40)	29(41)	12(20)
Broken Wheel test	11 (7)	5 (7)	12(20)
Optokinetic nystagmus test	47 (30)	25(35)	3 (5)
Symbols for Children	1(<1)	0	0
Snellen (Tumbling E or Alphabet)	12 (8)	2 (3)	25(42)
Candy bead test	2 (1)	3 (4)	1 (2)
Allen cards	0	2 (3)	3 (5)
Other (raisin test, etc.)	21 (13)	5 (7)	4 (7)
Total	157	71	60
	(100)	(100)	(100)

*Testing distance a function of each child's ability.
Percentages of use are reported with available data on the methods.
Teller Visual Acuity Cards (VisTech, Dayton, Ohio); Broken Wheel Test (Bernell Corp, South Bend, Ind.); Symbols for Children (Lighthouse for the Blind, New York, N.Y.); Allen Cards (Bernell Corp, South Bend, Ind.); Candy Bead Test (Michael D. Wesson, OD, MS, University of Alabama at Birmingham School of Optometry, Birmingham).

TABLE 2-4

Distances at Which Far Point* Visual Acuities Were Successfully Measured

	Number with Cerebral palsy (%)	Number with Down syndrome (%)	Number with mental retardation without specific etiology (%)
less than 100 cm	39 (36)	15 (27)	12 (20)
100 to 199 cm	14 (13)	9 (16)	3 (05)
200 to 299 cm	5 (05)	4 (07)	2 (03)
300 cm	13 (12)	12 (21)	15 (25)
600 cm	37 (34)	16 (29)	28 (47)
Total	108 (100)	56 (100)	60 (47)

*600 cm or less, depending on the ability of the child.

drum[†] for determination of their visual acuity; whereas only 3% responded to the Snellen chart (Table 2-5). The average acuities were 20/68 OD, 20/40 OS, and 20/50 OU—significantly less than for patients with mental retardation without specific etiology (20/28 OD, 20/29 OS, 20/29 OU). This difference most likely reflects the greater degree of overall dysfunction in patients with Down syndrome.

Refractive characteristics

Refractive errors, especially high myopia,[15,26] are associated with Down syndrome. One report[23] notes the presence of substantial

---

†Bernell Corporation, South Bend, Ind.

TABLE 2-5
Average of Best Corrected Visual Acuity at Far Point for Patients with Down Syndrome (I), Cerebral Palsy (II), and Mental Retardation without Specific Etiology (III)

TYPE	I				II				III			
	N*	VA OU$_b$†	Low range	High range	N*	VA OD‡	Low Range	High Range	N*	VA OS¶	Low range	High range
Down syndrome	63/121	20/50	20/1000	20/20	40/121	20/68	NLP‖	20/20	42/121	20/44	NLP‖	20/20
Cerebral palsy	91/213	20/71	NLP‖	20/20	71/213	20/49	NLP‖	20/20	65/213	20/51	NLP‖	20/20
Mental retardation	41/71	20/29	20/154	20/20	58/71	20/28	20/200	20/20	58/71	20/29	20/286	20/20

*Number of observations, regardless of visit, per total number of visits.
†Visual acuity, both eyes open.
‡Visual acuity, right eye only.
¶Visual acuity, left eye only.
‖No light perception.

astigmatism in 18% to 25% of patients. Hyperopia of >1.00 D does not seem as prevalent, with estimates of its occurrence ranging from 8% to 23%. Our experiences, however, do not support these observations. (See Table 2-6 and Fig. 2-3.)

Of 24 children below the age of 25 months, 88% were an average 2.03 D hyperopic and 12% an average 1.00 D myopic (see Fig. 2-6 for cross-sectional data). The amount of hyperopia tended to stay rela-

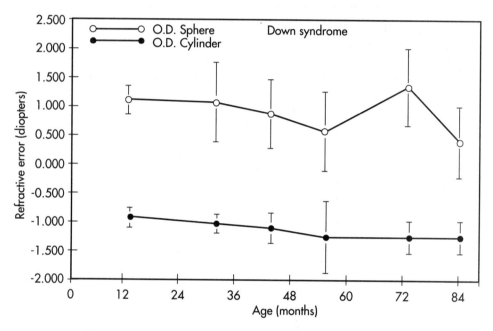

FIGURE 2-3 Refractive errors in Down syndrome. Note that spherical data is separate from astigmatic values.

TABLE 2-6

Cross-sectional Data for Spherical Refractive Error and Astigmatism in the Right Eye of Patients with Down Syndrome*

Age range (mo)	N†	Average OD sphere	SEM‡	N†	Average OD cylinder	SEM‡
0 to 24	37	+1.13	0.24	18	−0.90	0.15
25 to 36	16	+1.09	0.65	8	−1.03	0.15
37 to 48	22	+0.90	0.57	11	−1.09	0.25
49 to 60	13	+0.60	0.67	5	−1.25	0.63
61 to 84	15	+1.35	0.64	5	−1.25	0.27
Over 84	17	+0.40	0.62	12	−1.25	0.27

*Left eye data were similar and therefore not reported.
†Number of Down patients examined at the first visit for each age range.
‡Standard error of the mean.

tively constant throughout the years, displaying some increase in older patients. The degree of myopia, however, appeared to rise significantly although the *number of patients* with myopia was much lower. This may explain why the literature is so confusing on the subject of refractive error for Down syndrome. In other words, there are many more hyperopes than myopes among Down patients, but those who are myopic tend to be more severely affected.

CLINICAL PEARL

There are many more hyperopes than myopes in the Down population, but those who are myopic tend to be more severely affected.

Astigmatic refractive error was found in 49% of the children and adults examined. The amount was relatively constant, averaging 1.09 D across the age groups and ranging from 0.25 to 3.75 D (Fig. 2-3). We would normally expect to find a higher number of healthy children having with-the-rule (WTR) astigmatisms in the early years. The older Down children and adolescents appear to have less WTR and slightly more against-the-rule (ATR) astigmatism (Fig. 2-4). The number of patients with an oblique (OBL) astigmatism also increases in the older age

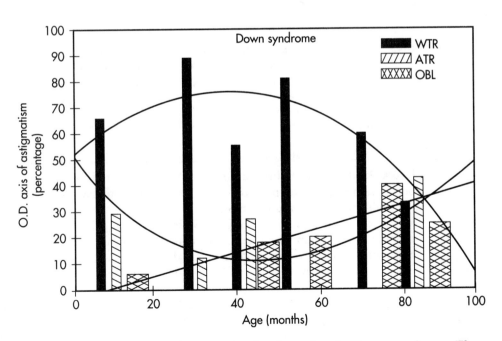

FIGURE 2-4 Right eye axis of astigmatism in Down syndrome. The solid lines are trends in axis position. (*WTR* = with the rule; *ATR* = against the rules; *OBL* = oblique.)

groups. For the oldest population there appears to be a more or less even distribution among the three types of astigmatism.

Binocular vision characteristics

Strabismus is a major binocular dysfunction in patients with Down syndrome. Whereas the prevalence in the general population is only 2% to 4%, in persons with Down syndrome it is 23% to 44%.[7] Combining all visits of Down patients in our sample, we found that 38% had strabismus at near. An extremely large number of the strabismic Down patients (88%) had esotropia, with 83% (better that 2 to 1) displaying a constant deviation. Thus the profile of the Down child with strabismus is of an individual with a constant unilateral esotropia of less than 20 prism diopters (PD or Δ) at near point. At far point the incidence of strabismus (all esotropes) is 12%, which suggests that the etiology of this ocular deviation is a high accommodative-convergence to accommodation ratio (AC/A) rather than a basic esotropia.[32]

CLINICAL PEARL

An extremely large number (88%) of Down patients with strabismus have esotropia, with better than 2:1 displaying a constant unilateral deviation.

The only other binocular feature that should be mentioned is the presence of nystagmus. In one report[32] nystagmus was noted in 16% of the Down population. Earlier reports[26] suggested that the figure might be closer to 10%. Catalano's recent review of the literature[22] pointed to the fact that nystagmus is present 5% to 30% of the time. In a total of 123 visits by our Down patients, 13% presented with nystagmus.

Ocular disease characteristics

Ocular health abnormalities are frequently encountered in the Down population (see box on page 31). Blepharitis/blepharoconjunctivitis is the most often reported condition (about 33%), probably due to impaired lacrimal drainage coupled with eye rubbing.[26,30,31] The eye rubbing may explain why blepharoconjunctivitis is so common in this population. Standard treatment includes daily eyelid scrubs combined with encouragement of the child to cease rubbing his or her eyes.

CLINICAL PEARL

Blepharitis is the most frequently reported condition in patients with Down syndrome, occurring in about 33%.

Keratoconus is another often reported corneal abnormality.[32,33] It is estimated[26] to affect less than 0.1% of the general population but to be present in 1% to 8% of the Down population. We have diagnosed it in

---

Common Ocular Diseases in Down Syndrome

Blepharitis/blepharoconjunctivitis (33%)
Keratoconus (1% to 8%)
Cataracts (flake opacities) (2%)

---

two patients (6%). In both cases the corneal reflex from retinoscopy was the first hint of the condition. In one patient the keratoconus had been previously misdiagnosed as cataract. This person's visual acuity deteriorated during the 6 months from the time of our initial diagnosis. He eventually had a successful keratoplasty.

Cataracts are frequently associated with Down syndrome. Their incidence, however, appears to be age related[23] (as part of the premature-aging complex associated with the syndrome). When we have observed cataracts in younger patients, they have been more dustlike in appearance and are described in the literature[22,26] as flake opacities. In general, cataracts are found in children with Down syndrome over the age of 9 years.

Cerebral Palsy

Cerebral palsy is the name given a group of conditions characterized by a general nonprogressive locomotor dysfunction of varying severity due to a defect or lesion in the immature brain (that is, a central neurological disorder).[34] It is not a disease and it is only rarely inherited.[35,36] Cortical involvement leads to delayed physical development with movement abnormalities, disturbed balance, and (in about half the patients) mental retardation[37] (Table 2-7). Individuals with the disorder who walk have an awkward gait and impaired motor control for such activities as eating, drinking, personal grooming, and writing.

Abnormal muscle tone is the hallmark of infants, children, and adults with cerebral palsy. Occasionally, during the neonatal period, muscles will be hypotonic.[38] This is the basis for the term "floppy baby syndrome." Hypertonicity then follows, generally becoming evident 6 to 9 months later as antagonist muscles co-contract. In all cases a consistently reliable marker is an increase in the deep tendon reflexes.[38] Delayed developmental milestones are always evident, but seldom is there *regression* of motor function.

TABLE 2-7

General Signs of Cerebral Palsy

	Percentage of Patients
Locomotor difficulty	100
Speech disorders	90
Visual disorders	70+
Mental retardation	50
Seizures	35
Scoliosis	15
Swallowing and drooling	10

Disorders of vision and hearing are commonly found in persons with cerebral palsy. Wiklund and Uvebrant[39] have stated that lesions of the white matter surrounding the posterior horns of the lateral ventricles, or subcortical lesions in the occipital lobes, "may affect the visual pathways and cause restriction of the visual field and cortical blindness."

It is estimated[40,41] that more than 90% of individuals with cerebral palsy have the condition as a direct result of factors related to the course of pregnancy. A premature infant (less than 37 weeks of gestation) is five times more likely to develop cerebral palsy than a full-term infant. Some 35% of infants born with cerebral palsy have a low birth weight (under 1500 g or 3.3 pounds), which increases the risk by a factor of 20.[42]

CLINICAL PEARL

Low birth weight increases the risk of cerebral palsy by a factor of 20.

Intraventricular hemorrhage is a frequent occurrence in low–birth weight infants and leads to depression of motor function as well as to sensory deficits. Although the location of the lesion is not always anatomically well defined, the increased intracranial pressure sets the stage for the particular classification of cerebral palsy. The lesion is considered to be nonprogressive and generally occurs early in the pregnancy rather than at the time of delivery or within the neonatal period (first 28 days after birth). Prematurity, however, is not the only major factor. Another is perinatal asphyxia in full-term infants, which accounts for 25% to 30% of the new cases of cerebral palsy.[35] In fact, the risk of developing cerebral palsy increases 250 times when clinical asphyxia occurs (as measured by an Apgar score of 3 or less at the end of 20 minutes).[43] Congenital and perinatal infections (cytomegalovirus, rubella, toxoplasmosis, neonatal meningitis) and poisoning (lead, etc.) are the major etiological factors in patients developing cerebral palsy.[44] Other factors include intrauterine ischemic events, congenital brain anomalies, perinatal metabolic conditions, and (in 2% to 5%) genetics.[45]

Incidence

The prevalence of cerebral palsy is about 2 in every 1000 live births, with little variation in developed countries. In the United States it is about 1 per 1000, with approximately 4000 new cases annually.[35,40,45] The number of cases has decreased because of better prenatal care and intervention procedures. About 10% of the cases, however, are acquired and due to head trauma from accidents in the home or automobile. Other etiological factors include infection, poisoning, malnutrition, and neglect. Individuals who are born with or acquire cerebral palsy often survive to live normal lifespans. Approximately 40% live to reach the age of 40, many living up to 70 years of age. The latest estimate is that some half million people in the United States have cerebral palsy.

Clinical Assessment

General physical characteristics

There are three major classifications of cerebral palsy. Each is characterized by a set of signs and brain lesion locations. Although the classifications can be defined, in reality their identification is often difficult because of the presence of a mixed condition. Table 2-8 shows the classifications with lesion locations and basic signs for each class. The size of the lesion and the severity of impairment have not been statistically correlated.[39]

To make matters even more confusing, the location of the lesion by computed tomography does not always express the predicted behavioral dysfunction since other parts of the cortex may be involved.[39]

The most frequently occurring classification is *spastic*. Hypertonicity is its hallmark. Spastic quadriplegia occurs when both arms and both legs are involved. If only the lower half of the body is affected, the condition is spastic diplegia (the most common type of CP in preterm infants).[46] Spastic hemiplegia involves one side of the body and is the most common form occurring in children born at term.[39] Microcephaly is a frequent finding in cerebral palsy[38] with these individuals being at increased risk for the development of mental retardation. Spastic cerebral palsy may be mild, moderate, or severe. Mild cases are often difficult to diagnose and require the expertise of a competent pediatric neurologist, developmental pediatrician, or pediatric orthopedic surgeon.

The second most frequently occurring classification is *athetoid*. Slow writhing movements are its hallmark. Individuals with athetoid (or choreoathetoid) cerebral palsy manifest unsteady balance and gait,

TABLE 2-8

Summary of The Major Classifications of Cerebral Palsy

Classification	Lesion Locus	General Signs
Spastic	Pyramidal cells and tracts	Muscle stiffness
		Muscle spasticity
		Depressed inhibition
		Muscle co-contraction
		Muscle hypertonicity
		Muscle irritability
Athetoid	Basal ganglia	Interference of voluntary by involuntary motion
		Extraneous motion causing misdirection
		Extraneous motion becoming habituated
		Major signs
		Grimacing
		Lurching
		Drooling
		Superior gaze paresis
Ataxic	Cerebellum	Equilibrium disturbance
		Depressed motion awareness
		Direction sense disturbance

with involuntary and irregular head, neck, and facial movements. Rh incompatibility is the most important etiological factor in athetoid cerebral palsy. Before the mechanism was completely understood, neonates with Rh incompatibility would usually develop kernicterus (a serious condition marked by high levels of bilirubin in the blood with bile pigment deposits in the nuclei of the brain and spinal cord). In most cases the mother's blood was Rh negative and the fetus's blood Rh positive. This incompatibility was not a problem during the first pregnancy. Once diagnosed, it could be minimized by treating the mother within 3 days of the end of her pregnancy. Without such treatment, however, subsequent pregnancies would result in fetuses with hyperbilirubinemia,[47] which led to pigmentary degeneration of the basal ganglia, dentate nuclei, and other structures of the brainstem, with subsequent mental retardation. Routine treatment early in pregnancy has produced a marked decline in the number of infants born with athetoid cerebral palsy.

The third most frequently encountered classification is *ataxic* with muscle hypotonicity as its hallmark. Its major sign is fine motor dysfunction with general unsteadiness. Ataxic cerebral palsy has been noted accompanying cerebellar lesions[48] and cerebral atrophy.[49] Gustavson et al.[36] have found that at least one form of ataxic cerebral palsy may be due to consanguinity.

Visual characteristics

Visual acuity testing of children and adults with cerebral palsy can be particularly challenging since about half the population is mentally handicapped and has motor impairment. As late as 1977 Lo Cascio[50] reported that visual acuities could be obtained in only about 34% of individuals under the age of 13 years. His sole means of measuring acuity at that time was the Illiterate E. An excellent follow-up study[51] utilized picture identity cards as the method for acuity evaluation. Preferential looking behavior, a relatively new form of assessment, has greatly increased the level of response. Often it is the only method that provides consistent information concerning a particular patient's visual acuity. The comparison of assessment methods in our study (Table 2-3) confirmed this observation. Of those we tested, 40% required the Teller Visual Acuity Cards whereas only 30% required the Optokinetic Nystagmus drum. This compares favorably with the results obtained when individuals with Down syndrome were tested. Only 8% of the patients with cerebral palsy were able to give satisfactory responses to Snellen-type charts. With alternate forms of assessment, binocular visual acuity could be evaluated in 45% of individuals below the age of 13, which is a 25% increase in acuity responses over those of Lo Cascio's study.

Testing distances for the acuities varied significantly, from 15 to 600 cm (median, 212 cm). The median for Down syndrome was 270 cm, considerably farther than for cerebral palsy. These testing distances and acuity values reflect the degree of involvement and the difficulty of obtaining reliable responses (direct comparisons can be made from Tables 2-4 and 2-5). In patients with cerebral palsy the best average visual acuity for either eye was 20/50, with binocular acuity significantly lower (20/71). The most likely reason for these differences is that the monocular acuities were attempted when the binocular could not be obtained or when behavior would not permit occluding one eye. A comparison of the median binocular visual acuities between cerebral palsy and Down syndrome patients reveals that the acuities for CP are 20/100 and for DS 20/50, suggesting that for CP acuities are generally decreased compared with those for DS. This might be due to the much higher incidence of ocular disease and neurological compromise within the cerebral palsy population.

Refractive characteristics

There have been several studies detailing the refractive characteristics found within the cerebral palsy population. Scheiman[52] indicated that more than 60% of his subjects had significant hyperopia, myopia, or astigmatism. He ascertained that hyperopia of greater than +1.50 D was 3 times as common in the cerebral palsy group as in non-affected schoolchildren. Black[53] discovered that 50% of his patients with cerebral palsy had refractive errors exceeding 1.00 D. Breakey et al.[54]

concluded that 64% of their patients with spastic cerebral palsy and 35% of those with athetoid CP had refractive errors greater than 1 D. Using these authors' criteria, Duckman[55] found that about 40% of his patients with CP had significant refractive errors. One of the most detailed analyses of refractive data conducted to date has been that by Lo Cascio.[50,51] Data from 128 patients were analyzed and showed that 61% had refractive errors exceeding 0.75 D. When the data for 224 eyes with refractive errors of 1.00 D or greater were reanalyzed, they showed 30% of patients with significant hyperopia, 9% with myopia, and 20% with astigmatism. Data from our initial visits of 91 patients with cerebral palsy revealed that 63% had significant hyperopia while 22% showed myopia. This suggests that hyperopia is much more likely to be present than myopia (in this instance by a factor of 3:1).

Does refractive error vary with age in patients with cerebral palsy? An indication can be found by looking at Figure 2-5. Spherical refactive error shows a small increase in hyperopia (up to about 5 years of age) and then declines for the oldest age category. Astigmatism is virtually unchanged over the same age range. Figure 2-5, B, demonstrates that approxmiately 50% of patients have WTR astigmatism. An increase in OBL astigmatism is evident for the older ages. When refractive error is divided into the two classes (hyperopia and myopia) with more than 1.00 D or more (Fig. 2-6), the incidence of hyperopia peaks at about 40 months of age. Myopia shows a much larger fluctuation. A possible interpretation of this, from a clinical perspective, is that it is the same as has been uncovered for the Down syndrome.

In other words, there are many more hyperopes than myopes; and yet the average amount of significant myopia is greater and fluctuates more widely in persons with cerebral palsy. This can be easily seen by looking at Figure 2-6, in which the data for CP and DS are superimposed.

Binocular characteristics

Binocular abnormalities are commonplace among individuals with cerebral palsy (Fig. 2-7). Duckman[55] reviewed the literature and summarized the data with respect to strabismus. A re-analysis of his review is presented in Table 2-9, along with our data. Generally the prevalence of strabismus in the cerebral palsy population exceeds (by at least 10 times) that in the general population. In addition, there appears to be slightly more esotropia than exotropia. Note that an average 43% of persons with CP were strabismic (27% esotropes, 16% exotropes). In our study a higher percentage were also noted as being esotropic (27%) (Table 2-9). This is almost twice the number of exotropes (11%) and is the same as the average cited from other studies. The wide variation in individual studies is most likely due to the conditions for measurement (such as testing at far point or near point, with or without

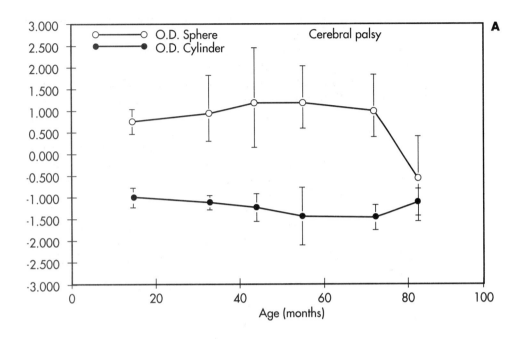

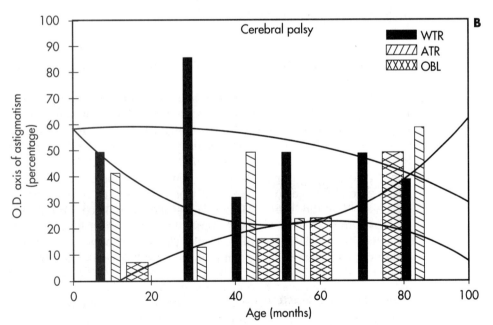

FIGURE 2-5 **A,** spherical and, **B,** astigmatic refractive error in individuals with cerebral palsy. Note that for the 75th month samples no ATR astigmatism was found. At the oldest age, no OBL was observed. Solid lines represent data trends. (*WTR* = with the rule; *ATR* = against the rule; *OBL* = oblique.)

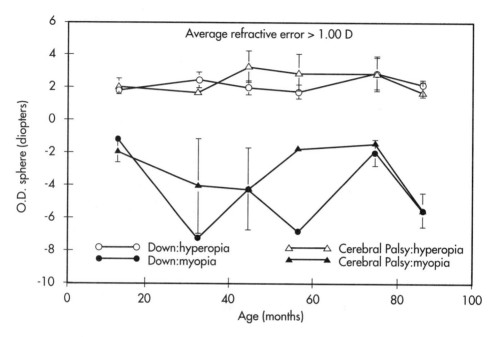

FIGURE 2-6. A comparison of spherical refractive error >1 diopter in Down syndrome and cerebral palsy.

spectacle correction). All testing in this study was conducted at near without correction.

In a small percentage of cases dyskinetic strabismus can be seen. This is manifested when there is a slow tonic deviation similar to a vergence movement. The result is a change from a manifest esotropia to an exotropia. Such a strabismus may be the first clinical sign of cerebral palsy and is usually associated with the athetoid classification.[64] About 4% of our strabismic patients show this condition.

Gaze limitations also are frequently associated with cerebral palsy. Lo Cascio[50] found that 12% of his patients had such limitations. Breakey[58] found 18% of his CP population to manifest gaze paresis. Schieman[52] and Black[53] identified only 4% of their patients with this condition. Our data on gaze limitations (14%) are similar to those of Lo Cascio and Breakey.

Ocular disease characteristics

Of the conditions discussed in this chapter, cerebral palsy displays the greatest proportion of ocular disease characteristics (Table 2-10). Approximately 12% of patients with cerebral palsy have nystagmus and another 8% show optic nerve atrophy (ONA). Grade 3 ONA is the most prevalent within our clinic population, occurring in almost 50% of patients. Some 4% of our patients were identified as not having any usable vision because of ONA, cataracts, or microphthalmos. Optic

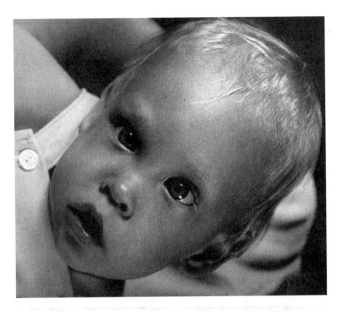

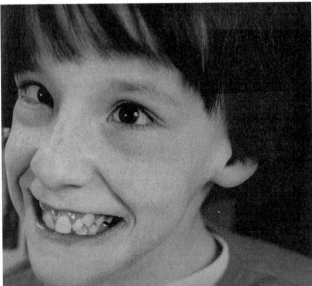

FIGURE 2-7 Binocular abnormalities (such as strabismus) are frequently found in individuals with cerebral palsy.

nerve colobomas and chorioretinal lesions from cytomegalovirus and toxoplasmosis were noted as well. Few studies have recorded visual field defects associated with cerebral palsy. (We have been using a technique that allows for the qualitative assessment of visual field limitations [Fig. 2-8].*)

---

*Balafire, Kyp-Go Inc, St Charles, Ill.

TABLE 2-9

Comparison of Studies for the Presence of Esotropia, Exotropia, and Overall Strabismus in Persons with Cerebral Palsy

	N*	Overall (%)	Esotropia (%)	Exotropia (%)
Jones and Dayton[56]	28	60	24	36
Guibor[57]	147	60	51	0
Breakey[58]	100	48	40	8
Schrire[59]	73	15	11	4
Schachat et al.[60]	98	43	22	21
Lossef[61]	88	34	17	17
Wiesinger[62]	75	51	32	19
Altman et al.[63]	64	44	30	14
Wesson and Maino (this study)†	91	31	20	11
AVERAGE	85	43	27	16

*Total number of subjects in each study.
†Data based on the first visit of 91 patients.

TABLE 2-10

Ocular Anomalies and Disease Associated with Cerebral Palsy

	Studies					
	Lo Cascio[51] (%)	Scheiman[54] (%)	Breakey et al.[54] Breakey[58] (%)	Black[53] (%)	Wesson and Maino* (%)	Average (%)
Nystagmus	8.6	18	4		17.0	11.9
Optic atrophy	6.2	4.0	9	10	12.4	8.3
Visual field defect	3.9	1.0	12			5.6
Blindness (cortical)	3.1				4.1	3.6
Cataract	2.3			3	1.4	2.2
Fundus anomaly	0.8			12	5.5	6.1
Microphthalmos	0.8			4	12.9	5.9
Corneal opacity	3				1.4	2.2

*This study.

Positioning in Cerebral Palsy

A factor frequently overlooked during the assessment of visual systems in individuals with cerebral palsy is the correct positioning of the patient during the examination. Appropriate positioning will minimize stress on the general and ocular muscle tone, as shown in Figure 2-9, A-C.

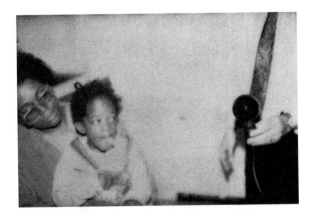

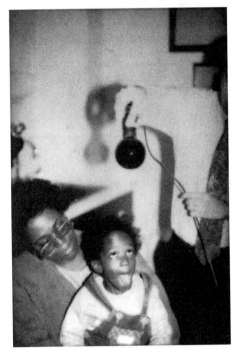
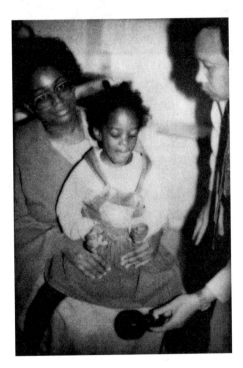

FIGURE 2-8 To qualitatively assess visual fields, the examiner brings in a flickering light from behind the patient and notes their first reaction to the presentation of the stimulus.

Mental Retardation without Specific Etiology

Mental retardation is not "worn on the sleeve" (that is, most patients do not *look* retarded). When we think of mental retardation, we often picture an individual with a condition such as those that have already been described. In this chapter mental retardation is defined as a

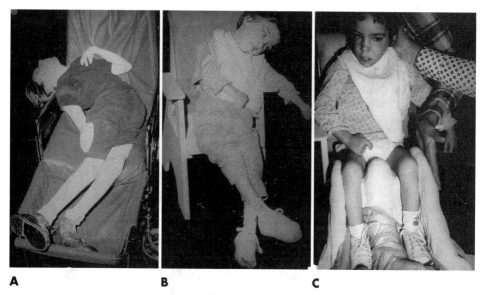

A   **B**   **C**

FIGURE 2-9 **A,** and **B,** show inappropriate positioning of the patient. **C,** demonstrates good patient positioning with the use of supportive seating.

TABLE 2-11

Levels of Mental Retardation and Number of Facilities in the United States Providing Care for Elderly Patients with Mental Retardation

	AAMD* IQ range (%)	Foster care (%)	State institution (%)
Borderline/mild	50 to 70	43	11
Moderate	35 to 55	26	22
Severe	20 to 40	22	29
Profound	Below 20 or 25	9	38

Adapted from Lakin KC, Anderson DJ, Hill BK, et al: *Ment Retard* 29:65-74, 1991.
* American Association for Mental Deficiency.

decreased capacity for problem solving and general academic success. As mentioned earlier, an individual is diagnosed as having mental retardation if the intelligence quotient is below 70 and if poor adaptive skills are demonstrated during the developmental period (birth to 18 years of age) (Table 2-11). Most of these individuals fall into the borderline/mild (educable mentally handicapped) or moderate (trainable mentally handicapped) category. Since there is a clear upward trend in survivability of persons with mental retardation,[65] health care professionals working in nursing homes or other residential facilities are increasingly likely to have contact with this population.

TABLE 2-12

Nomographic Determination of Visual Acuity Utilizing the Teller Acuity Cards at Expanded Distances*

Cycles/ centimeter	Distance tested in feet (centimeters in parentheses)							
	1.25 (38)	2.0 (61)	3.0 (91)	4.0 (122)	5.0 (152)	7.0 (213)	9.0 (274)	10.0 (305)
38	20/24	15	10	7	6	4	3	3
26	35	22	15	11	9	6	5	4
19	48	30	20	15	12	8	7	6
13	70	43	29	22	17	12	10	9
9.8	92	58	39	29	23	16	13	12
6.5	139	87	58	43	35	25	19	17
4.8	188	117	79	59	47	34	26	23
3.2	283	176	118	88	71	50	39	35
2.4	377	235	157	117	94	67	52	47
1.6	565	352	236	176	141	101	78	70
1.3	696	434	291	217	174	124	97	87
0.86	1052	655	439	328	263	188	146	131
0.64	1413	881	590	440	353	252	196	176
0.43	2103	1310	879	655	526	375	292	262
0.32	2826	1761	1180	881	707	504	392	352

*The values within this table represent the denominator of the Snellen fraction.

Visual Characteristics

Visual acuity determination

The measurement of visual acuity in persons who exhibit developmental delay can be exceedingly difficult. Patience, imagination, and alternative forms of testing are needed. (See Table 2-3.) We have been able to assess acuity about 42% of the time using Snellen-type acuity tasks (the Tumbling E or Alphabet). Compared to the figures for cerebral palsy (8%) and Down syndrome (3%), this represents a significant improvement in the management of patients with nonspecific mental retardation. Individuals with mental retardation were able to use the Broken Wheel Visual Acuity Test approximately 3 times more often than those with cerebral palsy or Down syndrome. The Teller Visual Acuity cards, however, have been used successfully only about half as often, which suggests that reliable results can be obtained with standard visual acuity–measurement techniques. Recently Wesson and Peaslee[66] have been able to expand the clinical utility of Teller cards by using a nomogram (Table 2-12). For patients with mild to moderate mental retardation and/or significant motor impairment, pointing techniques and looking behaviors allow quantifiable acuity determination (Fig. 2-10).

It should be noted that extraordinary means of assessing visual acuity are not always necessary with this population. The candy bead

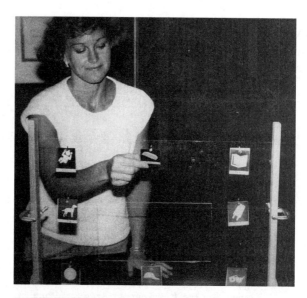

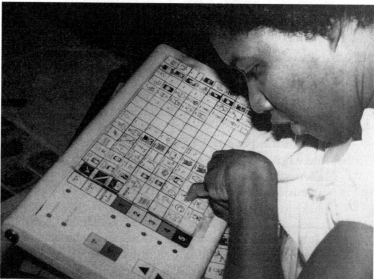

FIGURE 2-10 For patients with mild or moderate mental retardation, pointing techniques allow quantifiable acuity determination.

test, Allen cards, and Optokinetic Nystagmus drum, together, represent only 12% of the tests performed. The preceeding techniques should be available, however, when they are needed. (A conversion chart for the candy bead test and other small symmetrical testing objects is given in Table 2-13.) When using this technique, the examiner places a small candy bead (nonpareil) in one hand and has

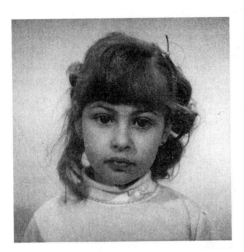
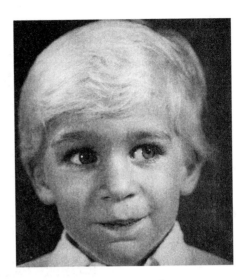

FIGURE 2-11 Both of these children have severe mental retardation, but appear physically unaffected. Conversely, you may work with patients who exhibit substantial physical disabilities, but are unaffected cognitively.

the child pick it out and eat it (with parental permission, of course). Once the child realizes it is candy, the distance can be increased and quantified as he or she responds. The chart (Table 2-13) is based on a 1-minute-of-arc separation rather than on the overall size of the object subtending 5 minutes of arc. This appears to give a more reliable result and is not likely to overestimate acuity. It should be understood that bead color, contrast, and luminance all play an important role in this visual acuity assessment procedure. This may work well as a first approximation of visual acuity.

CLINICAL PEARL

Reliable results can often be obtained for individuals with mental retardation without a specific etiology by using standard visual acuity assessment techniques.

Refractive characteristics

Based on data for both Down syndrome and cerebral palsy, one would expect the same level of significant refractive error to apply to patients with mental retardation. This is *not* supported by our analyses. Table 2-14 compares the three types of developmental disabilities at the initial visit with respect to spherical and astigmatic refractive error

TABLE 2-13
Candy Bead Testing Distance and Visual Acuity

Object size (mm)	Distance in centimeters (inches in parentheses)						
	25(10)	30(12)	35(14)	40(16)	60(24)	120(48)	180(72)
0.5	137	114	98	85	57	29	19
0.7	192	160	137	120	80	40	27
0.9	247	206	176	154	103	51	34
1.1	302	252	216	189	126	63	42
1.3	357	297	255	223	148	74	49
1.5	412	343	294	257	171	85	57
1.7	467	389	333	292	195	98	65
1.9	522	435	373	326	218	109	72
2.1	577	481	412	360	240	120	80
2.3	632	527	451	395	263	131	88
2.5	687	572	491	429	286	143	92
2.7	742	618	530	464	309	155	103
2.9	797	664	569	498	332	166	110
3.1	852	710	608	532	355	177	118
3.3	907	756	648	567	378	189	126
3.5	962	802	687	601	401	200	137
3.7	1017	847	726	635	423	211	141
3.9	1072	893	766	670	447	223	150
4.1	1127	939	805	704	469	234	156
4.3	1182	985	844	739	492	246	164
4.5	1237	1031	883	773	515	257	172
4.7	1292	1077	923	807	539	269	180
4.9	1347	1122	962	842	561	280	187
5.1	1402	1168	1001	876	584	292	194

To put into Snellen equivalent, place the numbers in the table as the denominator of the Snellen fraction. For example, a 1.3 mm test object located at 25 cm (10 inches) has a Snellen fraction of 20/357. (Information based on 1 minute of arc resolution.)

(Fig. 2-12). Inspection of this table reveals that the average spherical refractive error at the first visit for 13 individuals with mental retardation only was 0.15 D, some 6 times less than that for individuals with cerebral palsy or Down syndrome. The error range was also limited (−0.50 to +1.00 D). This 1.50 D spread is 10 to 13 times smaller than for the other two conditions. The average astigmatic error was about half that found in Down syndrome or cerebral palsy, with a variance 4 times less. It is interesting to note, however, that the axis of astigmatism was about the same as found in cerebral palsy and Down syndrome. Generally speaking, when persons with mild or moderate mental retardation without specific etiology are being examined, one should not expect to find significant refractive error different from that normally encountered in routine practice.

TABLE 2-14.

Comparison of Three Types of Developmental Disability at the Initial Visit with Respect to Right Eye Spherical and Astigmatic Refractive Error and the Axis of Astigmatism*

	N+	Age‡	Sphere range				N	Astigmatic range				Axis of astigmatism		
			OD sph§	SEM‖	Low	High		OD cyl¶	SEM‖	Low	High	WTR	ATR	OBL
Down syndrome	120	39	+0.95	0.21	−8.50	+6.50	59	−1.09	0.10	−0.25	−3.75	35(60)	14(24)	9(16)
Cerebral palsy	81	37	+0.90	0.31	−8.50	+11.00	38	−1.15	0.13	−0.25	−3.75	21(55)	12(32)	5(13)
Mental retardation	13	45	+0.15	0.17	−0.50	+1.00	5	−0.45	0.05	−0.25	−0.50	3(60)	2(40)	0

*Left eye results not reported because they were similar to the right eye results.
†Number of cases in which data are available.
‡Median age (in months).
§Right eye spherical refractive error
‖Standard error of the mean.
¶Right eye astigmatic refractive error.
WTR = with the rule; ATR = against the rule; OBL = oblique.

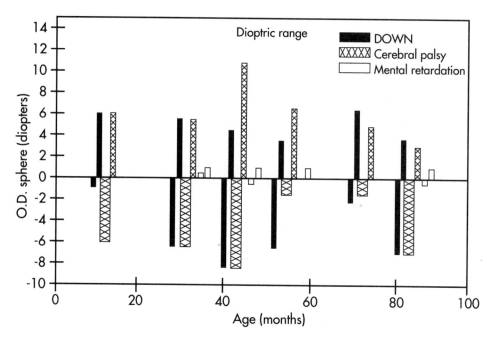

FIGURE 2-12 Spherical and astigmatic refractive error in Down syndrome, cerebral palsy, and mental retardation.

CLINICAL PEARL

When examining patients who are mildly or moderately retarded without specific etiology, you should not expect to find significant refractive error rates different from what you would normally note in routine practice.

Binocular characteristics

Based on our refractive data results, one might expect that the prevalence of binocular dysfunction would be no greater in the mental retardation population than in non-affected clinical population. We have found, however, that this is not true. Of the 13 mentally retarded children in our study, 23% displayed strabismus at 6 meters whereas 38% demonstrated it at near. Most of these patients were exotropic.

One could speculate that birth defects were responsible for this high incidence. It is not clear from such a small sample, however, why strabismus was so prevalent. The only other binocular anomaly noted was extraocular muscle restriction, in 15% of the patients tested. Although other oculomotor/binocular anomalies might have been present, an accurate assessment was often limited by our patients' decreased cognitive abilities (average IQ 38, range 11 to 54).

TABLE 2-15

Characteristics of Fragile X Syndrome

Facts	Common Ocular Features	Common Identifying Features
Occurs in 1:1200 to 1:2000 live births	Moderate to high refractive error*	Learning disabilities
Linked to X chromosome	Strabismus*	Mental retardation
FMR-1 gene cloned	Nystagmus	Large ears
Detected by cytogenetics and direct DNA analysis	Ptosis	Large testes
Multiple family members affected (e.g., siblings, uncles, aunts.)	Few ocular health abnormalities	Hyperactivity Attention deficit Shyness Speech/language dysfunction Hand flapping/biting Gaze avoidance

---

*Should be considered as *associated conditions* of fragile X syndrome. A child with mental retardation of unknown etiology who demonstrates a strabismus should be referred for fragile X genetic screening.

Ocular disease characteristics

Of the 13 mentally retarded patients in our sample, one had bilateral anterior uveitis and exhibited vessel sheathing, two were found to have a choroidal nevus, and one a tigroid fundus. No other anomalies were detected. It is important that all individuals with disabilities undergo a complete eye health evaluation, including dilation. A cycloplegic/mydriatic spray has been used[67,68] that appears to be both fast and effective. Maximum dilation and cycloplegia occur in 25 to 30 minutes. The spray can be applied with the eyes open or closed and seems to cause no sensitivity/adverse reactions.

Fragile X Syndrome

Any discussion of developmental disabilities would be incomplete without mention of the fragile X syndrome. Fragile X is the most frequently encountered form of inherited mental retardation. Approximately 3000 infants are affected yearly (1/1200 boys, 1/2000 girls), without predilection for race or ethnicity. It is an X-inherited genetic disorder, and the first human disease shown to be caused by a nucleotide repeat sequence (cytosine, guanine, guanine). It affects cognitive, physical, and sensory/behavioral development.[69,70] Few papers have discussed the ocular anomalies associated with it. Maino et al.[17] and Storm et al.[71] have noted moderate to high amounts of refractive error, strabismus, and nystagmus. Recent presentations[18,19,72] support these findings. King et al.[18] and Maino and King[72] noted that, of the 50 subjects they examined, nearly half exhibited a strabismus (50% esotropic, 50% exotropic), 7 had an amblyopia, 3 showed a congenital jerk nystagmus, and 2 demonstrated a ptosis. It was also noted that accommodative and convergence insufficiency might be common. Although no major ocular health abnormalities have been documented for this population, King et al.,[18] Maino and King,[72] and Amin and Maino[73] have each reported seeing a single patient with chorioretinal atrophy. It has also been suggested[18] that any individual with mental retardation of unknown etiology who presents with a strabismus should be referred for a fragile X screening (Table 2-15).

Summary

In summary, the following should be noted:

For children with Down syndrome
1. There are many more hyperopes than myopes, but those who are myopic typically show moderate to high magnitudes.
2. The profile of a child with Down and strabismus is that of a constant >20 prism diopter unilateral esotropia at near.

For children with cerebral palsy
1. Visual acuities are decreased compared to those in children with Down syndrome.
2. Hyperopia of a significant degree is much more likely to be found (by a factor of 3 to 1) than myopia.
3. There are many more hyperopes than myopes, but the average amount of significant myopia is greater and fluctuates more widely over time.

For children who have mental retardation without a specific etiology
1. Do not expect to find a significant refractive error different from what is normally found in routine practice.
2. Expect to find a higher incidence of strabismus.
3. Routine examination techniques can often be used.

For children with the fragile X syndrome
1. Expect to find moderate to high amounts of refractive error (hyperopia), strabismus (esotropia), and other learning-related vision disorders.
2. Routine examination techniques must be supplemented with diagnostic procedures suitable for individuals with moderate to severe cognitive disfunction.
3. Specific ocular diseases (i.e., cataract) do not appear to be any more common in fragile X than in the general population.

In closing, patients with developmental delay exhibit numerous oculovisual abnormalities[70] that require using all appropriate diagnostic and therapeutic techniques.[19] Each diagnostic classification exhibits its own characteristic oculovisual profile with which the optometrist should be familiar.[73,74] Special populations are heterogeneous in nature, with their own strengths and weaknesses and must be approached as individuals with unique vision care needs.

REFERENCES

1. Prentice RR, Spencer PE: *Project Bridge. Decision-making for early services: A team approach,* Elk Grove Village, Ill, 1985, American Academy of Pediatrics.
2. Ramey CT, Yeates KO, Short EJ: The plasticity of intellectual development: insights from preventive intervention, *Child Dev* 55:1913-1925, 1984.
3. Martin SL, Ramey CT, Ramey S: The prevention of intellectual impairment in children of impoverished families: findings of a randomized trial of educational daycare, *Am J Public Health* 80:844-847:1990.
4. Ramey CT, Campbell FA: Poverty, early childhood education, and academic competence: the Abecedarian experiment. In Huston A (ed): *Children in poverty,* New York, 1992, Cambridge University Press, 190-221.
5. Berman C, Szanton E: *The intent and spirit of PL 99-457: a source book.* Washington, D.C., 1989, National Center for Clinical Infant Programs.
6. Gnadt G, Wesson MD: A survey of the vision assessment of the developmentally delayed and multihandicapped in university affiliated programs (UAPs), *J Am Optom Assoc* 63:619-625, 1992.
7. Committee on Practice and Ambulatory Medicine: Vision screening and eye examination in children, *Pediatrics* 77:918-919, 1986.
8. Sullivan L: How effective is preschool vision, hearing, and developmental screening? *Pediatr Nurs* 14:181-204, 1988.
9. Regenbogen L, Godel V: Ocular deficiencies in deaf children, *J Pediatr Ophthalmol Strabismus* 22:231-233, 1985.
10. Maino JH: Ocular defects associated with cerebral palsy: a review, *Rev Optom* 116(10):69-72, 1979.
11. Black PD: Ocular defects in children with cerebral palsy, *Br Med J* 281(6238):487-488, 1980.
12. Woodruff ME, Cleary TE, Bader D: The prevalence of refractive and ocular anomalies among 1242 institutionalized mentally retarded persons, *Am J Optom Physiol Opt* 57:70-84, 1980.
13. Bankes JL: Eye defects of mentally handicapped children, *Br Med J* 2(918):533-535, 1974.
14. Tuppurainen K: Ocular findings among mentally retarded children in Finland, *Acta Ophthalmol* 61:634-644, 1983.
15. Gardiner PA: Visual defects in cases of Down's syndrome and in other mentally handicapped children, *Br J Ophthalmol* 51:469-473, 1967.
16. Fanning GS: Vision in children with Down's syndrome, *Austral J Optom* 54:74-82, 1971.
17. Maino DM, Wesson M, Schlange D, et al: Optometric findings in the fragile X syndrome, *Optom Vis Sci* 68:634-640, 1991.
18. King R, Hagerman R, Sargent R, Houghton M: Ocular findings in the fragile X syndrome. Presented at the Third International Fragile X Conference, Snowmass, Colo, June 1992.
19. Maino D: Ocular findings in fragile X syndrome. Presented at the Third International Fragile X Conference, Snowmass, Colo, June 1992.

20. Woodruff ME: Differential effects of various causes of deafness on the eyes, refractive errors, and vision of children, *Am J Optom Physiol Opt* 63:668-675, 1986.
21. Down JLH: Observation of ethnic classification of idiots, *London Hosp Rep* 3:259-262, 1866.
22. Catalano RA: Down syndrome, *Surv Ophthalmol* 34:385-398, 1990.
23. Gaynon MW, Schimek RA: Down's syndrome: a ten-year group study, *Ann Ophthalmol* 1493-1497, 1977.
24. Donaldson DD: The significance of spotting of the iris in mongolism: Brushfield's spots, *Arch Ophthalmol* 65:26-31, 1961.
25. Schmidt I: The Wolfflin spots on the iris, *Am J Optom Arch Am Acad Optom* 48:573-585, 1971.
26. Lyle WM, Woodruff ME, Zuccaro VS: A review of the literature on Down's syndrome and an optometrical survey of 44 patients with the syndrome, *Am J Optom Arch Am Acad Optom* 49:715-727, 1972.
27. Williams EJ, McCormick AQ, Tischler B: Retinal vessels in Down's syndrome, *Arch Ophthalmol* 89:269-271, 1973.
28. Ahmad A, Pruett RC: The fundus in mongolism, *Arch Ophthalmol* 94:772-776, 1976.
29. Catalano RA, Simon W: Optic disk elevation in Down's syndrome, *Am J Ophthalmol* 110:28-32, 1990.
30. Warshowsky J: A vision screening of a Down's syndrome population, *J Am Optom Assoc* 52:605-607, 1981.
31. Ginsberg J, Bofinger M, Roush JR: Pathologic features of the eye in Down's syndrome with the relationship to other chromosomal abnormalities, *Am J Ophthalmol* 6:874-880, 1977.
32. Falls HF: Ocular changes in mongolism. In Apgar V (ed): Down's syndrome (mongolism), *Ann NY Acad Sci* 171:627-636, 1970.
33. Cullen JF, Butler HG: Mongolism (Down's syndrome) and keratoconus, *Br J Ophthalmol* 47:321-330, 1963.
34. Bax CO: Terminology and classification of cerebral palsy, *Dev Med Child Neurol* 6:295-297, 1964.
35. Vining EPG, Accardo PJ, Rubenstein JE, et al: Cerebral palsy: a pediatric developmentalist's overview, *Am J Dis Child* 130:643-649, 1976.
36. Gustavson KH, Hagberg B, Samver C: Identical syndromes of cerebral palsy in the same family, *Acta Paediatr Scand* 58:330-340, 1969.
37. Cohen ME, Duffner PK: Diagnostic indicators in hemiparetic cerebral palsy, *Ann Neurol* 9:353-357, 1981.
38. Barabas G, Taft LT: The early signs and differential diagnosis of cerebral palsy, *Pediatr Ann* 15:203-214, 1986.
39. Wiklund LM, Uvebrant P: Hemiplegic cerebral palsy: Correlation between CT morphology and clinical findings, *Dev Med Child Neurol* 33:512-523, 1991.
40. Sternfeld L: Cerebral palsy. In Grove CM, Gustaitis J, Hantula R, Kenny C (eds): *The new book of knowledge: medicine and health,* Danbury, Conn, 1991 Grolier, 196-199.
41. Holst K, Andersen E, Philip J, Henningsen I: Antenatal and perinatal conditions correlated to handicap among 4-year-old children, *Am J Perinatol* 6:258-267, 1989.
42. Ellenberg J, Nelson KB: Birthweight and gestational age in children with cerebral palsy or seizure disorders, *Am J Dis Child* 57:116-134, 1984.
43. Nelson KB, Ellenberg J: Apgar scores as predictors of chronic neurologic disability, *Pediatrics* 68:36-44, 1981.
44. Peristein MA, Attola R: Neurologic sequelae of plumbism in children, *Clin Pediatr* 5:292-297, 1966.

45. Paneth N: Etiologic factors in cerebral palsy, *Pediatr Ann* 15:191-201, 1986.

46. Hagberg B, Hagberg G, Olow I, von Wendt L: The changing panorama of cerebral palsy in Sweden. V. The birth year period 1979-82, *Acta Paediatr Scand* 78:283-290, 1989.

47. Scheidt PC, Bryla DA, Nelson KB, et al: Phototherapy for neonatal hyperbilirubinemia: six-year follow-up of the national institute of child health and human development clinical trial, *Pediatrics* 85:455-463, 1990.

48. Yoshikawa H, Sakuragawa N, Nitta H: Congenital cerebellar ataxia: a comparative study of clinical data and morphometrical findings of CT and MRI, *No To Hattatsu* 22:9-15, 1990.

49. Miller G, Cala LA: Ataxic cerebral palsy-clinico-radiologic correlations, *Neuropediatrics* 20:84-89, 1989.

50. Lo Cascio GP: A study in cerebral palsy, *Am J Optom Physiol Opt* 54:332-337, 1977.

51. Lo Cascio GP: Longitudinal study of vision in cerebral palsy, *Am J Optom Physiol Opt* 61:689-692, 1984.

52. Scheiman MM: Optometric findings in children with cerebral palsy, *Am J Optom Physiol Opt* 61:321-333, 1984.

53. Black P: Visual disorders associated with cerebral palsy, *Br J Ophthalmol* 66:46-52, 1982.

54. Breakey AS, Wilson J, Wilson BC: The relationship between visual disorders and visual perceptual deficits in cerebral palsy, *Dev Med Child Neurol* 10:251-252, 1968.

55. Duckman R: The incidence of visual anomalies in a population of cerebral palsied children, *J Am Optom Assoc* 50:1013-1016, 1979.

56. Jones MH, Dayton GO: Assessment of visual disorders in cerebral palsy, *Arch Ital Pediatr* 25:251-264, 1968.

57. Guibor GP: Some eye defects seen in cerebral palsy, with some statistics. *Am J Phys Med Invest* 32:342-347, 1953.

58. Breakey AS: Ocular findings in cerebral palsy, *Arch Ophthalmol* 53:852-856, 1955.

59. Schrire L: An opthalmological survey of a series of cerebral palsy cases, *S Afr Med J* 30:405-407, 1956.

60. Schachat WS Wallace HM, Palmer M, Slater B: Ophthalmolgic findings in children with cerebral palsy, *Pediatrics* 19:623-628, 1957.

61. Lossef S: Ocular findings in cerebral palsy, *Am J Ophthalmol* 54:1114-1118, 1962.

62. Weisinger H: Ocular findings in mentally retarded children, *J Pediatr Ophthalmol* 1:37-41, 1964.

63. Altman HE, Hiat RL, Deweese MW: Ocular findings in cerebral palsy, *South Med J* 59:1015-1018, 1966.

64. Buckley E, Seaber JH: Dyskinetic strabismus as a sign of cerebral palsy, *Am J Ophthalmol* 91:652-657, 1981.

65. Lakin KC, Anderson DJ, Hill BK, et al: Programs and services received by older persons with mental retardation, *Ment Retard* 29:65-74, 1991.

66. Wesson MD, Peaslee AG: Expanding the limits of the Teller acuity cards, *J Am Optom Assoc* 61:400-403, 1990.

67. Wesson MD, Bartlett JD, Swiatocha J, Woolley T: Mydriatic efficacy of a cycloplegic spray in the pediatric population, *Invest Ophthalmol Vis Sci* 33 (suppl):1095, 1992.

68. Bartlett JD, Jaanus SD (eds): *Ocular pharmacology*, ed 2, Boston, 1989, Butterworths.

69. Martinez S, Maino D: A comprehensive review of the Fragile X syndrome: oculo-visual, developmental, and physical characteristics, *J Behav Optom* 4:59-64, 1993.

70. Maino DM, Maino JH, Maino SA: Mental retardation syndromes with associated ocular defects, *J Am Optom Assoc* 61:707-716, 1990.
71. Storm R, PeBenito R, Ferretti C: Ophthalmologic findings in the fragile X syndrome, *Arch Ophthalmol* 105:1099-1102, 1991.
72. Maino, D, King R: Oculo-visual dysfunction in the fragile X syndrome. In Hagerman R, McKenzie P (eds): *International Fragile X conference Proceedings,* Dillon, Colo, 1992, Spectra Publishing, pp. 71-78.
73. Amin V, Maino D: The fragile X female: visual, visual perceptual, and ocular health anomalies. (Submitted, *J Am Optom Assoc.* Schedule for publication, Fall 1994.)
74. Geering J, Maino DM: The patient with mental handicaps: a primary care perspective, *South J Optom* 10:23-27, 1992.

Acknowledgment

We would like to thank Gwen Gnadt, OD; and the staff, families, and clients of the Easter Seal Society of Metropolitan Chicago Gilchrist–Marchman Rehabilitation Center and the Chauncey Sparks Center for Development and Learning Disorders, University of Alabama, Birmingham, for their assistance in the preparation of this manuscript.

This chapter was supported in part by grants from the United Way of Chicago, the Amoco Foundation, and the Washington Square Health Foundation.

3

Low Vision Evaluation of the Child with Multiple Disabilities

Joseph H. Maino

Key Terms

Low vision rehabilitation	Visually impaired multihandicapped	Mental retardation

Because of improvements in neonatal health care, many at-risk infants with congenital life-threatening disorders are now being saved. Additionally, with the development of trauma centers staffed by emergency medical response teams, drowning and head trauma victims also are surviving in greater numbers. As the lives of these patients are sustained, many experience irreversible brain damage that leads to multiple physical, mental, and visual handicaps.

The need for low vision rehabilitation for the visually impaired multihandicapped child is great. Although few studies specifically address how these patients could benefit from low vision rehabilitation, several[1,2] hint at the usefulness of low vision prosthetic aids for the partially sighted child with multiple disabilities.

Unfortunately, rehabilitation of more obvious physical or mental problems may be addressed while the eye and vision problems are all but ignored. Caring for the multihandicapped child is an interesting challenge for the low vision specialist. Perhaps the greatest hurdle the clinician must overcome is reluctance to prescribe more than a pair of spectacles. Each patient must have the necessary tools to function at his or her highest level. Obviously, correction of the patient's refractive error and medical eye problems is important; but it is a mistake to underestimate the child's ability to benefit from low vision rehabilitation.

Individual Differences

Every person with multiple handicaps is unique. The term *multihandi-capped* does not automatically imply mental retardation. Many patients with cerebral palsy or head trauma have normal or near normal intelligence. Even if mental retardation is present, it does not necessarily preclude the prescribing of low vision aids. All individuals with mental retardation are educable to some degree. Many of these individuals can be taught to use simple low vision devices.

Numerous studies[3-7] have described the many ocular abnormalities associated with physical and mental disabilities. These abnormalities include (but are not limited to) strabismus, ptosis, cataract, glaucoma, optic nerve atrophy, keratoconus, and chronic blepharitis. Vision problems include high refractive errors, unusual amounts of astigmatism and accommodative dysfunction. By understanding the associated ocular and vision anomalies, the clinician can more easily anticipate the patient's needs.

Many multihandicapped individuals have normal or near normal vision. For these patients it is only a matter of obtaining an accurate refraction. However, in many cases standard refracting techniques are not adequate to correctly determine the best spectacle prescription. In addition, patients with certain kinds of disabilities are more likely to have a particular type of refractive error. By knowing the nature of the patient's disability and by using special refracting techniques, the clinician can properly determine the most appropriate spectacle prescription.

Many handicapping conditions are a result of injury to the motor areas of the brain. A child is diagnosed as having cerebral palsy when the injury occurs before, during, or shortly after birth.[6] Adults acquire motor deficits primarily because of trauma or stroke. The specific type of motor problem must be taken into consideration when the low vision rehabilitation treatment plan is being formulated.

Access and support are two additional considerations in dealing with multihandicapped patients. The optometrist who provides care should have an office that is accessible to persons in wheelchairs and electric carts. Doorways and hallways must be wide enough to allow the patient to move about effortlessly. A special examination area without an examination chair and stand will allow the clinician to deal with wheelchair-using patients. Portable equipment (such as a hand-held tonometer and slitlamp) can also aid in the examination.

Be sure that the office staff is prepared to offer support. The secretary and clerk must understand and try to anticipate the special needs of the children and their parents. For some, you should schedule morning appointments, whereas other patients may do better with an appointment scheduled in the afternoon. The office must be flexible. If a child has a behavior problem, for example, it may be better to set an appointment for the first or last one of the day so as not to disturb other patients.

Special Considerations

The congenital visually impaired child has many special qualities. These children have no history of normal vision and thus have no means of building up a reserve of visual memories. Basic concepts such as "rectangle" or "red" may be totally foreign to them. This lack of visual experience is compounded if the child also has a motor or cognitive impairment.

Many partially sighted children possess adequate amounts of accommodation; but this may not be true for children with multiple disabilities.[8-10] The lack of age-normal focusing ability can directly affect the type of near low vision aids you prescribe.

CLINICAL PEARL

The low vision child with multiple disabilities may simply reject an aid because it is something novel and therefore frightening.

Care of the visually handicapped child who has motor impairment presents several unique challenges for the low vision specialist. There may be spasms or tremors that make it impossible for the patient to use hand-held devices, and thus the practitioner may be forced to use stand-supported or head-borne aids. Partially sighted children generally have a no-nonsense approach to the use of low vision aids. If the devices work, they use them; if not, they don't. The cognitively low impaired vision child, however, may simply reject an aid because it is something novel and therefore frightening. In certain instances the opposite will be true. The child may appear to be using an aid but in reality is only curious about a new and interesting object that has been placed in his hand.

Low vision training is an important part of rehabilitation. It becomes even more important when dealing with a multihandicapped visually impaired child. You should enlist the support of the child's parents, teachers, physical therapists, rehabilitation specialists, and vision teachers to help in educating the patient on how to successfully use the aids.

CLINICAL PEARL

Low-vision training is a very important part of low-vision rehabilitation.

Before the Evaluation

The evaluation of a multihandicapped child with low vision should begin long before the child enters the examination room. Information concerning his or her medical, genetic, developmental, social, educational, and rehabilitative history should be reviewed before the examination. This information will be useful in formulating the appropriate plan of action.

CLINICAL PEARL

Information concerning the child's medical, genetic, developmental, social, educational, and rehabilitative history should be reviewed before the examination.

CLINICAL PEARL

It is important to establish a rapport with the child, care-givers and teachers.

It is important to establish a rapport with the child and care-givers, teachers, etc. to find out what they expect from the examination and what type of information they need. Many parents merely want to know how much vision their child has left. Teachers usually need information on the child's ability to see printed material and information written on the blackboard.

It is a good idea to have a pre-evaluation conference with all those involved in caring for the child. During the conference, you can discuss the tests you will perform and the accuracy of those tests. You may also want to provide the parents and teachers with pre-evaluation homework for the child. You might give them, for example, a set of visual acuity cards so the child can practice naming the test pictures, letters, or numbers.

CLINICAL PEARL

Reasonable goals should be set for the evaluation.

Finally, you should set reasonable goals for the evaluation. If a child has several physical and/or mental handicaps, it might be appropriate to simply attempt to establish his or her level of functional vision and determine whether spectacles are indicated. If the child has normal or near normal intelligence, however, and functions at a high visual level, then a full low vision evaluation is required.

The Evaluation

The eye health evaluation is an integral part of the low vision examination. Obviously, any active disease process that might require treatment needs to be ruled out. It is also important for the practitioner to actually evaluate the abnormal eye to be better able to understand the impact that the eye disease has on visual function.

The timing of the eye evaluation, however, can be problematical. From the practitioner's point of view, it is usually better to perform the evaluation before attempting to assess the need for treatment. When this is done, the decision as to whether an active problem should be treated can be made before low vision rehabilitation commences. Retinoscopy with cycloplegia can also be attempted at this time, although from a management standpoint it is usually more convenient to dilate the eye after the low vision evaluation has been completed.

Visual fields should also be assessed. Confrontation fields can be completed using toys or other objects of interest to the child. Older children may be able to respond to the Amsler grid or tangent screen. This information is important for determining the extent of a central scotoma and whether mobility training will be needed.

Low Vision Distance Refraction

The cornerstone of the low vision evaluation is the distance refraction. It is the foundation on which the entire rehabilitation plan is built. The appropriate equipment must be used, including a pediatric trial frame, hand-held Jackson cross cylinders (JCC), Halberg clips, trial lenses, lens bars, and pediatric low vision near and distance visual acuity charts[11,12] (Figs. 3-1 to 3-3).

CLINICAL PEARL

The cornerstone of a low vision evaluation is the distance low vision refraction.

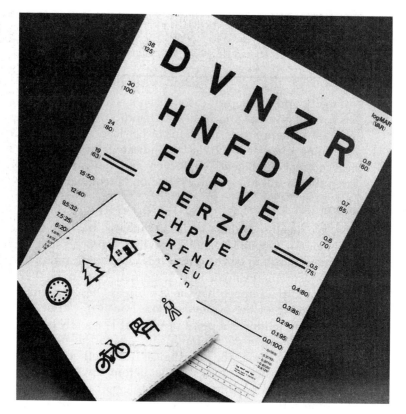

FIGURE 3-1 Distance low vision charts.

Start the low vision refraction by considering the child's optical history. If that includes surgery for congenital cataracts, then you know that the patient will require an aphakic prescription. Children with Down syndrome are more likely to have keratoconus and hyperopia. Cerebral palsy patients are known to exhibit higher amounts of astigmatism and hyperopia. Children with Marfan syndrome or other disorders that result in dislocation or subluxation of the lens may benefit from both an aphakic and a phakic prescription.[3,6-8,13]

Another place to look for clues concerning a child's refraction is the old spectacle prescription. Remember, however, that it can be extremely difficult to perform an accurate refraction on some of these patients; hence, the old spectacles may not be correct.

Keratometry is also a very important refraction tool, especially when the patient has a history of ocular surgery, trauma, corneal scarring, or keratoconus. If cooperation is a problem, you can still obtain significant information by using a Placido disk.

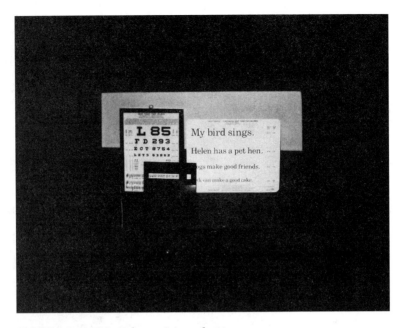

FIGURE 3-2 Near low vision charts.

Once all the above has been gathered and analyzed, it is time to perform retinoscopy. The child should be comfortable. If the examination chair causes anxiety, the child may sit in a parent's lap. In many cases it is a good idea to have a mechanical toy or flashing light at the end of the room to help hold the child's attention. As the retinoscopy light sweeps across the pupil, use hand-held lenses to neutralize the reflex. A lens bar may also be used in place of the trial lenses.

Depending on the child's behavior and/or the ocular disease present, it may be necessary to perform "radical retinoscopy," that is, employ different working distances and positions to neutralize the reflex. It is not unusual to have to kneel on the floor with the patient to determine the best retinoscopic prescription. Cycloplegic retinoscopy may be easier to perform and more reliable in these cases.

CLINICAL PEARL

If the child is hyperactive or has a dense media opacity, it may be necessary to perform "radical retinoscopy," which simply means employing different working distances and positions to neutralize the reflex.

When the child is severely disabled, retinoscopy may be the best "refraction" you can obtain. The final prescription should be based on

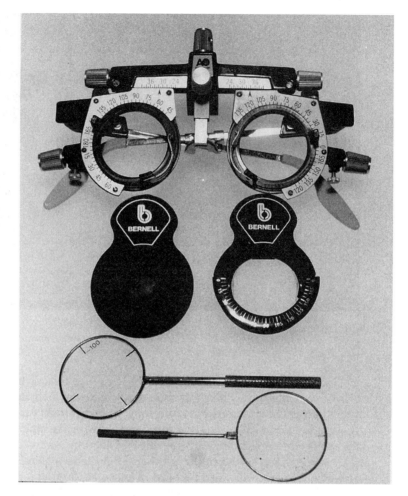

FIGURE 3-3 Trial frame, Halberg clips, and Jackson Cross Cyclinder (+/−1.00 D minimum).

keratometry findings, the patient's subjective reaction to the retinoscopy, the previous information on the eye's refractive state, and your own retinoscopy confidence level. Keep in mind that for many of these patients a margin of error of 2.00 D may be acceptable.

If the patient can cooperate, you are now ready to perform the subjective low vision refraction. The first step is to throw away your phoropter! Trial frame refraction is quicker and more accurate than phoropter refraction in evaluating multihandicapped patients. The acuity chart should be placed close enough so that the larger pictures or numbers can be easily seen. For most adult low vision refractions the test distance will be 3 meters (10 feet). However, it may be better to use a chart distance of 1 meter when testing children. This will make it easier to control their attention and direct their pointing to the numbers or pictures you want identified. (Remember to subtract one diopter from the refraction to compensate for the one meter test distance).

The next step is to place the pediatric frame comfortably on the child's face (a head band may be needed to keep it from slipping). The room light is then dimmed while the acuity chart is illuminated, and either the retinoscopy prescription or the patient's own current prescription is placed in the trial frame. The spherical lens should be positioned in the rear lens well (especially if it is more than 3 D), and the cylinder correction in the front well. Trial lens refractions will be easier to perform if the lenses are placed in the wells so their handles can be readily grasped. Lenses for use in the right trial lens frame well should be taken from the left column of the trial lens set, and lenses for use in the left lens well should be taken from the right column of the trial lens set.

The patient is then asked to read the chart, starting with the larger numbers or figures. This entrance visual acuity is the starting point for the low vision refraction. Next, the spherical lenses are introduced. The lens power should be appropriate for the child's level of vision. The lenses chosen must be of sufficient magnitude that the child can appreciate the difference between them. If the child's visual acuity is 20/400 or worse, start with a 2.00 D difference between the lenses. If the acuity is between 20/100 and 20/50, use 0.50 D changes. The point of this bracketing technique is to make it easy for the patient to tell the difference between lenses. If the child cannot tell the difference between 2.00 D, do not be afraid to try stronger lenses until a response is obtained.

Start with plus lenses. Introduce the first lens and ask the child if the figures are easier to see. If the answer is yes, increase the plus lens until there is no improvement. If the answer is no, ask the child to try to read the chart anyway. Be careful not to over-minus. If the plus lens makes the acuity worse, use minus lenses.

Once the spherical correction is determined, it is time to refine the cylinder axis and power. As with spheres, the Jackson Cross Cylinder power should be appropriate for the patient's acuity level. If the acuity is less than 20/100, use a 1.00 D JCC; otherwise, use a 0.50 D.

To refine the cylinder axis, place the JCC so its handle coincides with the axis of the cylinder in the trial frame. Flip the JCC and ask the patient which is clearer. For minus cylinders, rotate the trial cylinder until its axis is turned toward the red dot. Continue to refine the axis until a reversal is obtained.

After the axis is determined, it is necessary to find the cylinder power. Rotate the hand-held JCC so its minus cylinder axis corresponds to the minus trial cylinder lens axis. Flip the JCC to determine whether more or less cylinder power is required. If the patient requires additional minus cylinder, be sure to increase the plus spherical power to maintain the spherical equivalent. If less minus cylinder is needed, reduce the amount of plus sphere. For example, if the patient requires 2 D more minus cylinder, you must increase the plus sphere by +1.00 D to maintain the proper spherical equivalent. The last step is to refine the spherical power. You would then add plus or minus lenses to the sphere to obtain the best acuity.

Near Low Vision Refraction

For presbyopic low vision patients the determination of a near prescription is straightforward. You simply place a +2.50 D lens over the distance prescription and instruct the patient to read down the Lighthouse Near Acuity test card held at 40 cm. Once that M rating is obtained, it is easy to select the appropriate add that should allow the patient to read 1 M print (about 20/50). For example, if 2 M single-letter text can be read with the +2.50 D add at 40 cm, it should be possible to read 1 M single-letter text with a +5.00 add. Keep in mind that this method was designed specifically for presbyopic patients with low vision. A different approach may be called for in patients with adequate accommodation.

Many preschool phakic children whose only disability is visual impairment maintain normal or near normal accommodation. They usually do not require a reading addition until fourth or fifth grade, when their accommodation lessens and the amount of near work increases.[14] Visually impaired multihandicapped children, however, present an interesting dilemma, because they may not retain their full accommodative ability.[8-10]

When determining the near refraction for multihandicapped visually impaired patients, start by measuring the amplitude of accommodation by performing near retinoscopy or use the push-up technique. If it is significantly below normal for the patient's age, a bifocal prescription may be indicated. A bifocal should also be considered if the patient complains of eyestrain or ocular fatigue after reading for a few minutes.

To determine the power of the required add, have the patient bring a sample of his or her near work to the examination appointment. Ask that the material be held at their normal reading distance and measure the distance between the patient's eye and the text. This will tell you the amount of accommodation the patient uses to see the print. The power of the add should be set so the patient uses about half to two thirds of his or her own accommodation.[15] For example, if the reading material is held at 10 cm, then 10 D of accommodation is being used; if the measured amplitude of accommodation is 12 D, you should prescribe a reading add of +4.00 D. The patient will still hold the material at 10 cm but will be using only half his own accommodation with the bifocal add making up the difference.

If the amplitude of accommodation cannot be obtained, simply measure the distance between the text and the patient's eye. Then place the full add for that working distance over the distance prescription. If the patient complains of blur, the plus should be reduced until the text clears and reading is comfortable.[15]

The design of the bifocal lens is also important. If the bifocal is set too low, the child will simply look over the top of it. Make sure that it is fit so the top is at the lower edge of the pupil.

Low Vision Aids

Prescribing low vision aids for the visually impaired multihandicapped child is a challenge. Multiple disabilities, however, should not automatically stop you from evaluating these patients for low vision devices. First, there must be the clear need for such a device. Second, the patient should be able to hold and manipulate the device. Third, the patient must have the ability to learn how to use the device and benefit from it.

CLINICAL PEARL

First, there must be a clear need for a low vision aid. Second, the patient should be able to hold and manipulate the aid. And third, the patient must have the cognitive ability to learn to use and benefit from the aid.

The simplest low vision aid is the hand magnifier. The power of this device should be about the same as the amount of accommodation required to perform a near task. For example, if the patient must hold printed material at 20 cm to be able to read it, he or she uses 5 D of accommodation to focus the material; therefore the strongest hand magnifier you would want to prescribe would be 5.00 D. Most children require less than the calculated amount of accommodation because they can combine the hand magnifier power with their residual accommodation.

When demonstrating the hand magnifier to a child, have him place it on the reading material and slowly lift it off the page until the material becomes large and clear without distortion. You can also show the patient how the field of view increases in size as the eye comes closer to the lens of the magnifier. Children like to use hand magnifiers to look at maps and pictures, read the small print commonly found in dictionaries and telephone books, and inspect science class specimens.

Stand magnifiers should be considered if the patient has tremors or muscle spasms. These children do well with bar magnifiers and devices such as the +9.00 Jupiter StandLupe (Fig. 3-4). Keep in mind,

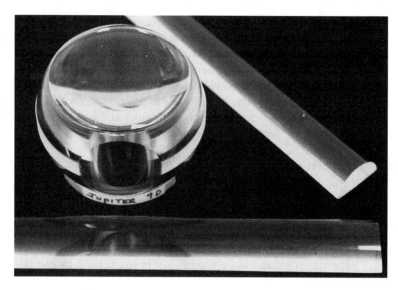

FIGURE 3-4 Jupiter StandLupe and bar magnifiers.

however, that the stand magnifier is manufactured so its lens is closer to the page than its focal length. Although this reduces peripheral distortion, the light rays emerging from the lens are divergent and require accommodative effort or a bifocal add to bring them into focus. If the child is aphakic or has little or no accommodation, he or she will need to use a bifocal spectacle prescription with the stand magnifier to adequately see the material.

CLINICAL PEARL

The stand magnifier is so manufactured that its lens is closer to the page than its focal length. This reduces peripheral distortion, but the light rays emerging from the lens are divergent and require accommodative effort or a bifocal add to bring them into focus.

For many visually handicapped children with motor impairments, telescopes provide a way to expand their knowledge of the world even though they are physically challenged. It is difficult for them to move closer to an object, but with the help of a telescope they can bring the object "closer to" them.

Most children are fascinated by hand-held telescopes and quickly learn to use them. If they cannot manipulate a telescope because of poor dexterity, a spectacle-mounted device may be tried. When a small refractive error exists, patients can easily use aids such as the

2.5× Selsi or the 3× Eschenbach sport glasses. If a significant refractive error exists, then a clip-on or flip-down telescope should be prescribed. Since custom spectacle-mounted telescopes are expensive, do not prescribe them until the patient has demonstrated that he can use one of the less expensive clip-on or flip-down systems.

CLINICAL PEARL

If a significant refractive error exists, a clip-on or flip-down telescope should be prescribed.

Nonoptical Aids

Nonoptical aids are as important as optical devices for many low vision patients. For individuals with more than one disability they may be even more important than optical devices. These aids can be used with, or in addition to, standard low vision aids.

Reading stands are especially helpful for the low vision patient with a motor impairment who is having difficulty holding a book or magazine. Stands are available that can clamp onto a wheelchair or rest in the patient's lap. Other accessory devices include large-print telephone dials, talking clocks and calculators, bold-lined paper, page turners, and large-print playing cards and games (Fig. 3-5).

Electronic Aids

When a multihandicapped child with low vision has a severe vision loss or a motor deficit prevents the child from manipulating a hand or stand magnifier, a closed-circuit television may be indicated. Magnification can be up to 60 times. When used with an electronic reading table, the patient may easily move the book while reading.

Additional electronic devices such as computers with large print, "talking" computers, and speech-recognition systems should also be considered. For many multihandicapped patients, computers represent the best method for learning about and communicating with the world around them. The visually handicapped child with motor impairment may also benefit from electronic page turners and other computer-assist devices (Fig. 3-6).

Training

If the multihandicapped patient is to successfully use the prescribed low vision aids, adequate training must be given. It may be tedious and difficult, so it is important that the teacher or rehabilitation

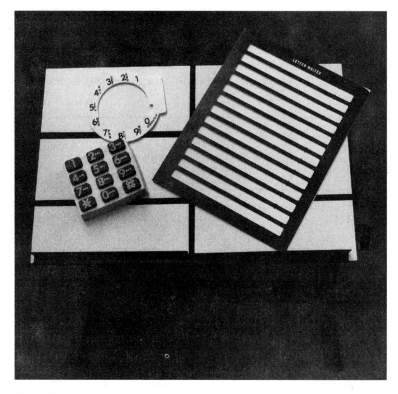

FIGURE 3-5 Nonoptical aids.

therapist keep the learning sessions short and stimulating. Studies[4] have shown that children who have attained the developmental level of a 2-year-old can learn to use simple magnifiers.

For a child to learn to use low vision aids, five basic skills need to be mastered. These are positioning, localizing, scanning, tracking, and focusing.[5] It is also necessary for the child to be able to position himself or herself comfortably, especially if motor control is a problem.

CLINICAL PEARL

Children must learn five basic skills to use low vision aids: positioning, localizing, scanning, tracking, and focusing.

Scanning and localizing are particularly important since the child must know how to find an object in which he is interested. For example, if he wants to use a telescope to read the clock on the classroom wall, he must know how to systematically search the wall until the clock is found. He must then be able to find the clock

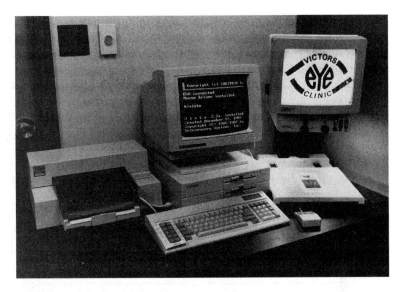

FIGURE 3-6 Computerized electronic aids can help many patients achieve a more independent way of life.

hands and read the numbers to determine whether it is time for lunch or recess. To follow an object as it moves or to read a series of words with a magnifier, he must develop tracking skills. Tracking may occur in more than one plane (for example, when a student uses a telescope to read the number on a bus as it approaches).

Although focusing the device should be one of the first learned skills, for many children it is the most difficult to master. The patient must learn how to hold the hand magnifier to produce maximum magnification with minimum distortion. It is important that the child understand the need to refocus the telescope when the object of interest changes position.

Follow-up

Once the initial low vision evaluation is completed, arrangements must be made to follow the child's progress. It is not uncommon to discover that a child has never received the prescribed low vision aids or that the low vision aid prescribed needs to be modified to better conform to the patient's requirements and abilities.

The initial follow-up can be a letter asking the patient's parents or rehabilitation teacher if the child received the aids and if there are any questions concerning their use. If all is going well, a follow-up appointment can be made in 1 to 3 months to determine whether the prescriptions need to be modified and to monitor the patient's progress.

CLINICAL PEARL

It is not uncommon to discover that a child never received the prescribed low vision aids or was never properly trained.

Summary

The three main goals for the rehabilitation of children with multiple disabilities are (1) determination of the correct refractive error, (2) prescription of task-specific simple low vision aids, and (3) provision of information to the child's caregiver concerning his visual status and abilities. Multiple visits and appropriate follow-ups are usually required to meet these goals.

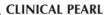

CLINICAL PEARL

The three main goals for rehabilitating multihandicapped children are determination of the correct refractive error, prescription of task-specific simple low vision aids, and provision of information to the child's caregiver concerning his visual status and abilities.

Techniques used to manage the multidisabled patient with low vision are similar to those used for many nondisabled individuals. For example, trial frame refraction is routinely employed in general low vision work, in patients with accommodative esotropia (who are prescribed bifocals set high to ensure that the child will use the add), and in vision therapy patients (who are followed to ensure that they are doing the training and to ascertain that their progress is according to expectation). By applying accepted optometric techniques to the visually impaired multidisabled population, we can make a substantial contribution to the development and rehabilitation of these special children.

REFERENCES

1. Landis SK, Dutson TD, Ludlum W: Vision examinations of handicapped children at the Oregon State School for the Blind. In Woo G (ed): *Low vision principles and applications,* New York, 1987, Springer, 419-424.
2. Meire F, DeLaey JJ: How do visually handicapped children use their low vision aids? *Bull Soc Belge Ophtalmol* 207:129-142, 1984.
3. Maino DM, Maino JH, Maino SA: Mental retardation syndromes with associated ocular defects, *J Am Optom Assoc* 9:707-716, 1990.

4. Ritchie JP, Sonksen PM, Gould E: Low vision aids for preschool children, *Dev Med Child Neurol* 4:509-519, 1989.
5. Cowan C, Shepler R: Techniques for teaching young children to use low vision devices, *Vis Impair* 84:419-421, 1990.
6. Maino JH: Ocular defects associated with cerebral palsy: a review, *Rev Optom* 10:69-72, 1979.
7. Ronis M: Optometric care for the handicapped, *Optom Vis Sci* 66:12-16, 1989.
8. Duckman RH: The incidence of visual anomalies in a population of cerebral palsied children, *J Am Optom Assoc* 50:1013-1016, 1979.
9. Lindstedt E: Accommodation in the visually impaired child. In Woo G (ed): *Low vision principles and applications*, New York, 1987, Springer, 425-435.
10. Lindstedt E: Failing accommodation in cases of Down's syndrome, *Ophthal Paediatr Genet* 3:191-194, 1983.
11. Maeda A: Trial frame refraction, *Optom Month* 10:122-126, 1979.
12. Brooks CW: Systematic method of subjective trial frame refraction, *Optom Month* 8:433-438, 1982.
13. Woodruff ME, Cleary TE, Bader D: Ocular findings in developmentally handicapped children, *J Pediatr Ophthalmol Strabismus* 9:162-167, 1972.
14. Faye EE: *Clinical low vision*, Boston, 1976, Little Brown, 338.
15. Leat SJ, Karadsheh S: Use and non-use of low vision aids by visually impaired children, *Ophthalmic Physiol Opt* 11:10-15, 1991.

Appendix 1: Simple Low Vision Prosthetic Devices

Hand Magnifiers

+ 5.00 D Bausch & Lomb Rectangular Magnifier
+11.00 D Bausch & Lomb Packette Magnifier
+12.00 D Eschenbach Hand Magnifier
+20.00 D Eschenbach Hand Magnifier
+20.00 D Coil Cataract Hand Reader
+20.00 D Bausch & Lomb Packette Magnifier

Stand Magnifiers

Eschenbach 1.5 (+2.00 D) Bar Magnifier
Bausch & Lomb +3.50 D Magna Rule
+8.00 D Eschenbach Illuminated Rectangular Stand Magnifier
+9.00 D Selsi Jupiter StandLupe
+17.6 D Coil Aspheric Stand Magnifier
+20.00 D Eschenbach Aspheric Illuminated Stand Magnifier
+24.00 D Eschenbach Aplanatic Illuminated Stand Magnifier
+33.00 D Agfa-fixed Focus Stand Magnifier

Telescopes

2.5 Selsi Monocular Telescope
2.8 Selsi Clip-on Monocular Telescope
2.5 Selsi Sport glasses
3 Eschenbach Binocular Sport glasses
4 Walters Monocular Telescope
6 16 Walters Monocular Telescope

Appendix 2: Low Vision Acuity Charts

Distance Charts

New York Lighthouse Distance Visual Acuity Chart (ETDRS): uses letters

Feinbloom Test Chart for the Partially Sighted: uses numbers

Allen cards: washable plastic with pictures of an apple, house, and umbrella

10 Foot Allen card chart: chart with apple, house, and umbrella symbols

Near Charts

Lighthouse near acuity test
Lighthouse continuous text card for children

Appendix 3: Suppliers

ABLEDATA (product database for commercially available
   rehabilitation aids)
4407 Eighth Street, NW
Washington, DC 20017
(202) 635-5826

Closing the Gap (information on computers and the disabled)
Rt 2, Box 39
Henderson, MN 56004

Eschenbach (low vision aids)
904 Ethan Allan Highway
Richfield, CT 06877
(203) 438-7471
Fax (203) 761-9791

Lighthouse Low Vision Products (low vision aids and testing
   equipment)
36-02 Northern Boulevard
Long Island City, NY 11101
(800) 435-4923
(718) 937-6959
Fax (718) 786-0437

Mattingly International (low vision aids)
938-K Andreasen Drive
Escondido, CA 92029
(800) 826-4200
(619) 741-0767
Fax (800) 368-4111

NolR Medical Technologies (light filters)
PO Box 159
South Lyon, MI 48178
(800) 521-9746
(313) 679-5565

Selsi (low vision aids)
40 Veterans Boulevard
Carlstadt, NJ 07072

Telesensory (CCTVs, computers)
PO Box 7455
Mountain View, CA 94039

4

Diagnosis and Management of Visual Dysfunction in Cerebral Injury

Michael G. Zost

Key Terms

Trauma	Head injury	Visual imperception
Cerebrovascular accidents	Stroke	Selective occlusion
Neuroplasticity	Neuropsychology	Optometric evaluation
Hemispheric specialization	Rehabilitation	Prisms
Field awareness	Transient ischemic attack (TIA)	Vision enhancement therapy
Neurological disorders	Focal ambient visual system	

Optometry's knowledge base and responsibility for the detection and management of various health/vision disorders continues to expand rapidly. We are being asked with increasing frequency to act as consultants or to provide services for persons with numerous unique visual conditions and demands. Patients who have survived cerebral injury are one such population. Cerebral injury results from many factors, including trauma, cerebrovascular accidents, space-occupying masses, infection, toxic encephalopathy, degenerative neurologic disorders, or other neurologic disease processes.[1]

It has been noted[2-4] that 100,000 deaths per year in the United States result from head injury, with 400,000 to 700,000 nonfatal head injuries being severe enough to require hospitalization. Head injury is the fourth leading cause of death in this country (1 in 16 deaths attributable to head trauma alone.[5] In addition, some 50,000 to 70,000 of these patients will retain varying levels of impairment. Only 20% of patients who survive head trauma regain enough function to return to some form of work. Approximately 60% do not return to the competitive work force, and 5% do not recover from coma.[4] The economic loss from this has been estimated to be $4 billion per year.[6] Perhaps more devastating is the loss of personal productivity and the disruption of lives of family and friends of the patient with a cerebral injury.

For cerebrovascular disorder, the morbidity statistics are based on stenoses and occlusions of blood vessels, in addition to hemorrhagic diseases of the brain. Thrombi and emboli cause 65% to 80% of strokes, and hemorrhages and hemorrhagic diseases cause 20% to 35%. Stroke is the third leading cause of death in the United States (1 in 10 deaths is attributable to stroke).[5] Of those who survive, the following summary details their outcome:

10% will return to work unimpaired.

40% will have a mild residual disability.

40% will need special rehabilitative services.

10% will require permanent or long-term institutionalization.

Stroke affects about 2500 people per million every year. Of that number, some 47% will die within the first month as a result.[7] In 1982, for example, a million deaths in the United States were due to vascular disease.

The prognosis for survival with or without impairment after cerebral injury varies depending on several factors—age of the patient at the time of injury being the primary one. Children tend to have a better prognosis than adults, although functional recovery may be less successful as a result of the disrupted development of the visual system.[8] Adolescent and young adult populations (15 to 24 years of age) are the most at risk of cerebral injury from vehicular accidents whereas older adults are more susceptible to vascular insult.[9] The type, extent, and location of the injury as well as any secondary complication (cerebral edema or infection) influence the degree to which the patient will ultimately be impaired.

The diversity of cognitive, behavioral, and sensory changes that occur is determined by the interaction of several variables—the etiology, the site(s) of insult, the diffuse or focal nature of the deficit, the acuteness of onset, the patient's age, handedness and cerebral dominance, and the preinjury intellectual, social, and emotional functioning of the patient. Behavioral and psychological disorders (such as severe depression, anger, frustration, and feelings of helplessness) all further complicate the prognosis, especially with regard to rehabilitation.

It is not uncommon for survivors of cerebral injury to be discharged from a hospital or even a rehabilitative program with unsolved deficits of cognitive, emotional, and social functioning. This may be due in part to the lack of an understanding and systematic approach by which to manage this population.[10] In the case of vision, Gianutsos et al.[11] state that patients may not exhibit symptoms of a compromised visual system because of other coexisting systemic disorders that threaten survival; and, in addition, there may be impaired cognition or altered subjective experiences.[12] For the patient and family, adjusting to these alterations can be difficult and confusing. Changes may be severe, varying from deep coma to multiple problems with speech, motor function (hemiplegia), emotional behavior, and cognition. Loss of sensation, movement confusion, restlessness, delirium, or unconsciousness may also develop, as may severe headaches, paralysis, or seizures.[13]

A patient's or family's concern for a specific deficit, such as memory, may not be the real problem. The real problem may be in the area of attention and concentration, which are required for accurate retention.[14] Deficits of cognitive function may include sensation and perception as well as attention and concentration, learning and memory, language skills, visual/spatial and manipulative skills, planning ability and judgment, initiating and performing goal-oriented activities, speed and efficiency of information processing, and quickness of response.

Perceptual deficits induced by cerebral injury are often layered. This means that it is not uncommon to treat one defective skill and then uncover another. For example, a patient may be retrained to read but may not remember what was read. You would now need to address this new problem as well.[15,16] Perceptual deficits may affect the skills needed for copying designs, completing models or puzzles, carrying numbers in arithmetic, or recognizing details in a picture.[14]

Pathophysiology of Head Trauma

The brain is often viewed as a rigid mass, when in fact it is more a firm jellylike substance. It floats within the hard bony skull completely enveloped by the cerebrospinal fluid. Closed head trauma (the most common form of head injury) leaves the dura intact. However, cranial bones may be fractured; and forces sufficient to fracture the skull are likely to cause brain injury as well.

Not all cerebral injury results in the same type of deficit. Traumatic brain-injured patients tend to exhibit multiple deficits whereas stroke survivors usually have cerebral lesions whose deficits are more discrete.[17] Patients with direct penetration of the brain stem generally do not survive to be seen for rehabilitative services.

The results of impact (for example, compression, stretching or tearing of nerve fibers, tension, shearing, and pressure gradients)[13,18] can cause primary lesions that lead to disruption of cognitive function. Secondary lesions may originate any time after impact and are generally due to circulatory disorders with or without edema, epidural, subdural, or intracerebral hematoma, brain stem injury from rotational forces, necrosis, elevated intracranial pressure,[19] herniation,[20] or cerebral ischemia. Compared to open head injury, closed head injury results in greater cortical damage.[3]

Disruption of the visual system results from injury to the optic nerves, chiasm, tracts, radiations, or primary and associated visual cortical areas. Optic nerve injury alone occurs in 1% to 2% of all closed head trauma cases. Complete optic nerve dysfunction occurs in 0.5%. The presence of unilateral or bilateral nerve injury is highly correlated with the site of impact. In 88% of cases the deficit is ipsilateral to the impact. Supraorbital and frontal head injuries are most likely to cause optic nerve dysfunction; injury to the temporal, parietal, and occipital regions is less likely to damage the nerve. In all cases, however, it is important to remember that even minor head injuries are capable of causing severe vision loss.[20]

A concussion (loss of consciousness), sometimes referred to as diffuse axonal injury or a mild head injury, is the result of a sudden acceleration/deceleration of the brain. It may be equated with a "short-circuiting" of the brain due to stretching, tearing, or compression of neural fibers (axons) and cells.[21,22] In most instances it causes the greatest damage at the surface of the cortex, varying from destruction of nerve cells to a simple electrochemical disruption of the cells. Neurological changes may not be apparent unless significant damage occurs.

Besides an immediate loss of consciousness, other changes due to concussion are noted in brain stem function—the development of macroscopic lesions, an alteration in cerebrospinal fluid flow, and the presence of electroencephalographic abnormalities. The severity of damage strongly correlates with the amount of movement of the brain: the greater the movement, the higher the potential for significant damage.[23]

With acceleration/deceleration and rotational forces no area of the brain is immune to injury. Sensory/motor impairments of the right or left hemisphere are the most reliable indicator of localized injury. Left hemisphere insult will routinely yield language deficits whereas right hemisphere insult causes visual/spatial and manipulative difficulties. The left temporal lobe houses verbal abilities, the right lobe nonverbal abilities. In addition to aphasia assessment of the patient with left cerebral injury, careful examination of visual constructive abilities is suggested. Even if only the highest cognitive functions (planning, initiating, and performing goal-oriented activities) are affected, a patient's ability to continue the pursuit of academic, management, or professional endeavors may be severely hindered.[14]

Contusions of the cortex are commonly encountered in individuals who have fallen and suffered a blow to the head. They are closely associated with impacts of short duration whereas concussions are associated with impacts of longer duration. Contusions are usually bilateral but asymmetrical. The original point of injury is referred to as the coup lesion, the point opposite as the contrecoup lesion (Fig. 4-1). The latter location of damage is due to the translational force of the blow, which may cause the brain to bounce off the bony wall opposite the impact site, leaving it bruised.[24] The areas most affected by this type of head trauma are the anterior temporal lobes and the orbitofrontal cortex.

Involvement of the brain stem (subthalamic nucleus, midbrain, pons, and medulla) will produce horizontal and vertical nystagmus, bilateral pupillary paralysis, gaze paralysis, and defects in articulation, phonation, vocalization, swallowing, and tongue movement. "Crossed syndromes" may result in paralysis of the eyes, face, and tongue, along with sensory/motor deficits on the opposite side of the body. Other disorders involve asynergy (poor coordination of organs or muscles), ataxia, and dysdiadochokineasia (the inability to stop one motor impulse and substitute another for it that is opposite).

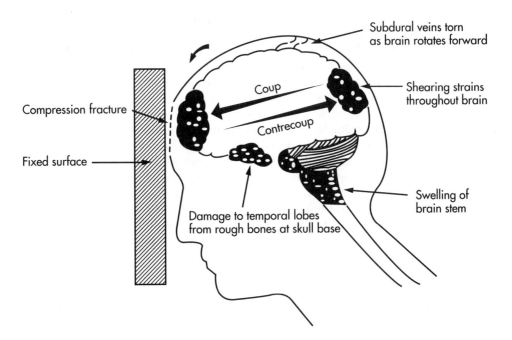

FIGURE 4-1 Closed head trauma caused by deceleration.

CLINICAL PEARL

Patients with a recent cerebral injury required 142% more time for the perception of a three-digit number. Patients with chronic impairments required 33% more time.

Compromised transmission between various cerebral structures occurs with diffuse white matter shearing, which is also responsible for many cognitive and behavioral disturbances. The effect on vision of white matter damage has been researched by Ruesch,[25] who determined that an effect occurs on the speed of visual processing of information that can be detected tachistoscopically. He found that, compared to normals, patients suffering from a recent cerebral injury required 142% more time for the perception of a three-digit number. Patients with chronic impairments required 33% more time.[26]

Cerebrovascular Accidents

Damage as a result of cerebrovascular involvement may include hemorrhage, thrombosis (clot formation), embolism (blockage of a vessel), compression of a vessel due to a tumor, or spasm of an artery. Cerebrovascular accidents (CVAs) result in deficits of varying severity. The presentation of cerebral ischemia with signs and symptoms that pass in 24 hours is considered a transient ischemic attack (TIA). Signs and symptoms that last over 24 hours but are resolved by 3 weeks are classified as a reversible ischemic neurological deficit (RIND). CVAs with lingering involvement (past 3 weeks) are a result of irreversible brain damage and are then considered a stroke.[27]

Strokes will occur with a thrombosis of or embolus in a cerebral artery, a cerebral arteritis or dissection, or a cerebral hemorrhage (Fig. 4-2). Strokes due to a thrombus or embolus cause some 65% to 80% of all CVAs and are considered primary *ischemic* events. The remaining 20% to 35% are considered primary *hemorrhagic* events. These can be caused by spontaneous subarachnoid hemorrhage (SAH), spontaneous intracerebral hemorrhage (ICH), or an arteriovenous malformation (AVM). SAH will occur most frequently in persons aged 35 to 65 years. ICH occurs most often in older adults with a history of hypertension. AVMs are frequently seen in young adults between the ages of 20 and 30 years.

A thrombus occurs when a blood vessel narrows due to an accumulation of material. An embolus is a piece of a thrombus that has broken off (a plaque) or some other foreign material that is floating freely in the bloodstream, with the potential to block off the vessel. A microaneurysm is a thinning of the arterial wall (commonly seen with increasing age). Symptoms of impaired circulation of the

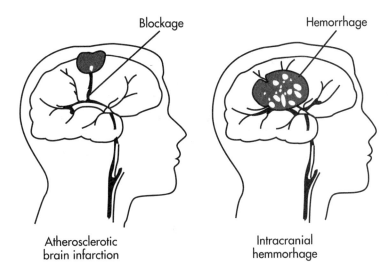

Blockage   Hemorrhage

Atherosclerotic   Intracranial
brain infarction   hemmorhage

FIGURE 4-2 Cerebrovascular accident.

carotid arterial system cause the patient to be aphasic and confused.[29] They may also cause transient monocular blindness (amaurosis fugax). Involvement of the vertebrobasilar system results in bilateral vision loss.[27]

Most strokes have effects that are manifested in the areas supplied by the middle cerebral artery. The result is a hemiparesis affecting the upper extremities more than the lower. Accompanying the hemiparesis is reduced postural control, which affects the ability to sit, stand, be mobile, and carry on normal daily functions.[30] If the anterior cerebral artery supply (Fig. 4-3) is involved, eye movement control, memory, and consciousness will be affected. These vessels serve the frontal lobes, upper portion of the chiasm, and intracranial portions of the optic nerve.[31] The posterior cerebral arteries (Fig. 4-4) supply part of the lateral geniculate body, optic tracts and radiations, portions of the midbrain, and the parietal and occipital lobes (primary visual cortex). Infarcts of the posterior cerebral arteries result in color anomia,[32] sensory aphasia, and visual field deficits (homonymous hemaniopia with macular sparing).[31,33] The vertebrobasilar system (Fig. 4-5) supplies sections of the temporal lobes, the cerebellum, significant portions of the brain stem, and the optic radiations. Obstruction of this system will lead to dysfunctions of the eye muscles, balance, and vision.

Mechanisms of Recovery from Cerebral Injury

The brain is significantly limited in its repair mechanisms. Not only is it incapable of regeneration by mitotic duplication (as seen in other tissues), it is unable to show regrowth (as seen with severed axons of

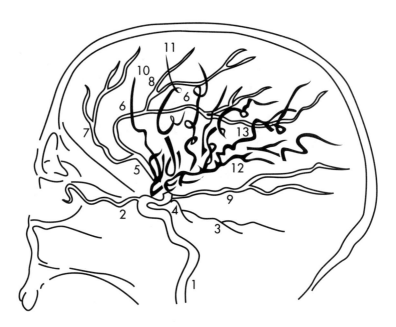

FIGURE 4-3 Normal course of the cerebral arteries at carotid arteriography. The middle cerebral artery is shown in *heavy black lines;* the anterior cerebral artery is shown in *open (white) lines. 1,* Internal carotid artery; *2,* ophthalmic artery; *3,* petrosal bone; *4,* dorsum sellae; *5,* anterior cerebral artery; *6,* pericallosal artery; *7,* frontopolar artery; *8,* callosomarginal artery; *9,* anterior choroidal artery; *10,* orbitofrontal artery; *11,* prerolandic artery; *12,* temporal arteries; *13,* posterior parietal artery. (From Martinez-Martinez PFA: *Neuroanatomy: development and structure of the central nervous system,* Philadelphia, 1982, WB Saunders.)

peripheral nerve tissue). Realistically speaking, it is obvious that recovery of actual function varies with the nature of the function, the complexity of the task, and the severity of the injury. Recovery speed may be delayed by edema, resorption of damaged tissue, and impairment of the circulation. The process of recovery can go on for months or years. The greatest recovery generally occurs in the first 6 months, with slow progress thereafter.[34] The most improvement is seen in expressive and receptive language skills and in memory tasks during the first month.

Four explanations for recovery from cerebral injury have been cited by Stein et al.[35]:

Hierarchical compensation. Particular functions are made up of contributions from various levels of cognitive function. The highest level is responsible for the most predominant and distinct contribution as long as there is not impairment. When injury

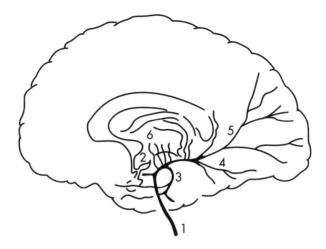

FIGURE 4-4 Pathway of the posterior cerebral artery. *1,* Basilar artery; *2,* posterior communicating artery; *3,* anterior temporal artery; *4,* lateral branch of posterior cerebral artery; *5,* medial branch of posterior cerebral artery; *6,* interpeduncular arteries. (From Martinez-Martinez PFA: *Neuroanatomy: development and structure of the central nervous system,* Philadelphia, 1982, WB Saunders.)

affects the highest level, the next higher level takes over and attempts to carry out the function.

Substitution. This is when other areas of the brain take over for the damaged area. Improvement results from reorganization or compensation of the brain through other areas (which may or may not be adjacent to the site of damage). The term *restitution* (restoration), which is another recovery mechanism, implies that improvement in function results from the increased integrity of the damaged system. It should not be considered which of these two processes (hierarchical compensation or substitution) is preferred, because both take place throughout recovery.[36,37]

Diaschisis. This is a form of shock that affects not only the lesion area but also adjacent areas. It is a state of depressed or lost function between cerebral centers or neural tracts.[38,39] Once the patient comes out of diaschisis, the function can be regained.

Dynamic reorganization. This is the rearrangement of cerebral function through the use of alternate routes (such as retraining or reeducation).

Neuroplasticity

Two mechanisms of neuroplasticity have been studied that may play a role in the recovery from cerebral injury. The first is the forming of *collateral sprouts* from adjacent intact cells to the damaged area.

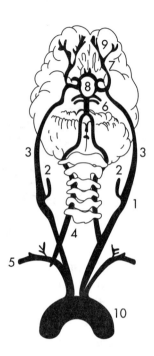

FIGURE 4-5 Vascularization of the brain from the aortic arch and the subclavian artery. *1,* Carotid sinus; *2,* external carotid artery; *3,* internal carotid artery; *4,* vertebral artery; *5,* subclavian artery; *6,* basilar artery; *7,* ophthalmic artery; *8,* posterior cerebral artery; *9,* eyeball, *10,* aortic arch. (From Martinez-Martinez PFA: *Neuroanatomy: development and structure of the central nervous sytem,* Philadelphia, 1982, WB Saunders.)

Collateral sprouting may contribute to recovery in both beneficial and maladaptive ways depending on the previous associated function of the intact cells. The second mechanism is the *unmasking and reprogramming of neural pathways* that were not predominantly involved in the functioning of the damaged area. The unmasked pathways are asked now to perform the function of the damaged site. With repeated use they may reach significant levels of function, but they almost never attain the level of efficiency of the original pathways. They are selected only if the demand for function is sufficiently high. Another possibility with unmasking is that the remaining intact fibers may strengthen their synaptic access within the pathway, giving them greater input and function.[39]

Neuroanatomy Review

The brain is divided into lobes, each within a hemisphere receiving and influencing specific functions. Beginning anteriorly are the *frontal lobes,* which are responsible for intellectual activities, abstract thinking, planning, and carrying out intentions. Immediately behind them and in front of the motor area is the *prefrontal cortex,* which is involved in organizing and sequencing complex motor behavior.

The *temporal lobes* are associated primarily with hearing, but they also provide some contribution to vision. Lesions in the left temporal lobe cause disturbances in understanding and recalling verbal material. The *inferior temporal cortex* plays a significant role in global visual processing. Patients with a lesion in the right temporal lobe exhibit greater difficulty (and at times an inability) to take discrete parts and make a meaningful whole—such as integrating fragmented visual information.

The *parietal lobes* are responsible for tactile recognition. A lesion in this area can cause inability to recognize numbers when traced with the finger, poor ability to recognize objects by touch, and poor ability to remember objects in space. Parietal lobe injury commonly results in perceptual deficits that disrupt ambulation and self-care activities. Specifically a lesion in the left posterior parietal cortex will affect both spatial perception and language skills.[40] Hemisensory neglect and an impaired sense of verticality are two of the most common alterations in patients with a lesion of the posterior parietal cortex.[30]

From the visual cortex in the *occipital lobe,* nerve pathways lead to higher centers in the parietal and temporal lobes, where visual sensations acquire meaning. Lesions in the visual cortex and in associated areas in the parietal lobes can produce visual/perceptual deficiencies. Spatial information (location and motion of stimuli) follows an upper pathway from the visual cortex to the posterior parietal cortex. Recognition of form, color, and objects follows a lower pathway to the inferior temporal lobe.[23]

The *cerebellum* integrates the smooth coordination of muscular activity. If it is damaged, general motor clumsiness occurs. This may, in turn, interfere with manual dexterity, the perceiving of imbedded figures, writing, and other forms of fine muscular performance. Dysfunction within the cerebellum yields problems with equilibrium, motor control, body image, laterality, and sometimes reading and speech. The cerebellum controls the proprioceptive functions (deep sensitivity) and vestibular functions (balance) of the inner ear.

Neuropsychology

Alexander Luria, a Russian neuropsychologist, categorized the brain into three functional units.[112] *Unit one* was considered to be the brain stem and other subcortical areas that control levels of excitation and wakefulness (reticular formation). Injury to these tissues would affect performance in all the other cortical areas. *Unit two* was made up of the temporal, parietal, and occipital lobes. It would be involved in receiving, analyzing, and storing information. *Unit three*, the frontal lobe, was involved in the programming of actions and the regulation and verification of behaviors based on continuous incoming information. Each of these units consisted of a primary, a secondary, and a tertiary zone: the primary to receive information, the secondary to organize and process the information, and the tertiary to integrate the information from other sensory areas.

Input from the sensors was thought to travel to the primary sensory areas (central processing) in the temporal, parietal, and occipital lobes, which simple action would constitute a response cycle. The first step in central processing (the registration phase) consisted of alertness, attention, continued concentration, and the ability to screen incoming data in relation to prior experiences. If no defect was noted, the brain would process the information (verbal in the left hemisphere, visual/spatial in the right) and the impulses would proceed through to the highest level in central processing. Then, if abstraction, reasoning, concept formation, and logical analysis skills were intact, no impairment of behavior should be observed.[14]

Hemispheric Specialization

Areas within the brain are capable of processing, analyzing, synthesizing, and integrating sensory stimuli.[41] With continued sensory processing, lateralization increases, and there is integration between the subcortical areas (Fig. 4-6). The left hemisphere (dominant in 98% of right-handed individuals and 66% of left-handers) takes care of verbal behavior and processing. It specializes in patterns that are propositional, analytical, sequential, time oriented, serial, and organizational. Being well adapted to learning and remembering verbal information, it is responsible for the processing of visual information (such as letters, words, and common objects). The right hemisphere is involved in nonverbal behavior (sensing spatial relations and music). It occupies itself with auditory tasks that involve melodies and nonmeaningful human sounds (grunts, belches, sneezes, etc.), visual/spatial tasks, and other nonverbal activities. Visually, the right hemisphere is responsible for the processing of nonlinguistic functions (such as depth, color, and shape discrimination).

Communication of information between the hemispheres occurs via axons (the white matter)[42] (Fig. 4-7), made up of association, commissural, and projection fibers. The association fibers link cortical areas within one hemisphere. Commissural fibers link the two hemispheres (as in the corpus callosum). The projection fibers travel vertically, communicating in both ascending and descending fashion as they link subcortical areas.

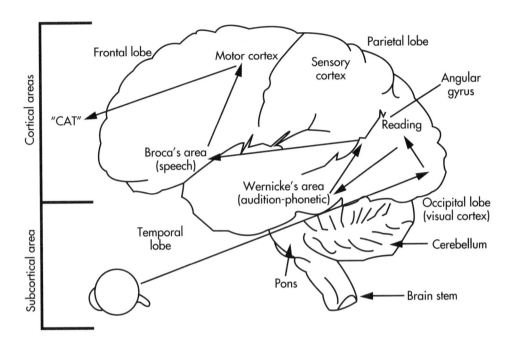

FIGURE 4-6 With continued sensory processing in the brain, lateralization increases, as does the integration between subcortical areas.

Transfer of interhemispheric information ceases with transection of the corpus callosum but appears to remain between the subcortical and cortical vision areas. This may be explained by the superior colliculi and their associated pathways, which act as subcortical pathways for the communication of information between cortical visual areas.

Vision Areas of the Brain

About a million nerve fibers leave each eye and transmit information to the central nervous system. This represents 70% of all afferent sensory fibers in the body.[43] At birth all retinal fibers are present. However, macular fibers are not yet myelinated so impulses are not conducted as fast or as strongly. With myelination the impulses become more distinct. The fibers responsible for peripheral vision are myelinated at birth and do perform normally. This is the only time when the peripheral visual system dominates the central.

A cross section of the optic pathway reveals that macular fibers are located centrally within both the optic nerves and the optic tracts.

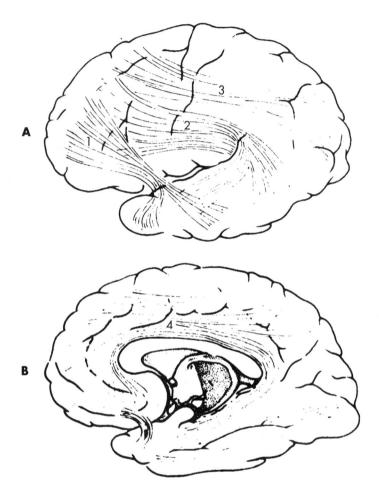

FIGURE 4-7 Communication via association, commissural, and projection fibers. **A,** The long association fibers of the white matter. *Upper,* Convex surface; *lower,* medial surface. *1,* uncinate bundle; *2,* arcuate bundle; *3,* frontooccipital bundle; *4,* cingulum. **B,** Principal corticothalamic connections. *1,* geniculocalcarine tract; *2,* geniculotemporal tract; *3,* cerebellothalamic fibers; *4,* medial lemniscus; *5,* thalamic fasciculus; *6,* mamillothalamic fasciculus; *7,* thalamocortical fibers; *VA,* ventral anterior nucleus; *VL,* ventral lateral nucleus; *VPL,* ventral posterolateral nucleus; *LGB,* lateral geniculate body; *P,* pulvinar; *DM,* dorsal medial nucleus. (From Martinez-Martinez PFA: *Neuroanatomy: development and structure of the central nervous system,* Philadelphia, 1982, WB Saunders.)

They end in the central area of the visual cortex. Around the central fibers wrap peripheral fibers. These end in the peripheral areas of the visual cortex.[43] In lower species, when the fibers from each nerve reach the chiasm, all decussate. In primates (including humans), however, only 50% decussate. Fibers from the optic nerve can be divided into three categories based on thickness. The thinnest fibers are W fibers, which travel exclusively to the superior colliculi. The remaining fibers are subdivided into X fibers, which synapse only with the lateral geniculate bodies, and Y fibers, which sometimes synapse with either the lateral geniculate bodies or the superior colliculi. The lateral geniculate bodies are composed of four upper layers containing small neurons (parvocellular layers) and two lower layers containing large neurons (magnocellular layers).[33] The parvocellular region is thought to be a more slow-acting conscious-processing system involved in object recognition. The magnocellular region processes faster and more unconsciously and is responsible for transmitting the functions of general awareness, posture, localization, and spatial orientation.

Some 80% of optic nerve fibers synapse with the lateral geniculate bodies; the remaining 20% course to the superior colliculi and pretectal area (Fig. 4-8). Many of these fibers end up in the midbrain and lower brain stem, linking with motor centers for balance, coordination, and movement.[43] Once fibers from the optic tracts reach the lateral geniculate bodies, they branch and course to synapse with one of three areas—two cortical and one subcortical.

The first of the cortical areas receives about 80% of the optic fibers from the lateral geniculate bodies. It provides functions like color vision, acuity, spatial analysis of the environment, and shape interpretation. The second cortical area is phylogenetically older in function. It involves the superior colliculi and contributes to motor functions like eye tracking skills. The third area is subcortical and contributes to functions like the light reflex.

At birth the occipital lobe is anatomically and functionally immature. Several weeks after birth the child develops the ability to fixate and by approximately 8 months of age is capable of seeing detail. Early development of the vestibuloocular system (cranial nerves III, IV, and VI [oculomotor, trochlear, and abducent]) assists subcortical eye movement adjustments. Cortical pathways, as transmitted through synapses in the superior colliculi, direct voluntary eye movements.[43] Padula and Shapiro[44] state that developmentally it appears that the infant brain's early primary duties are to organize motor function (such as developing control of limbs and head movements through the help of peripheral visual and vestibular systems).

As stated by Luria (Kreutzer et al.[113]), the sensory areas are organized into three zones—primary, secondary, and tertiary. Follow-

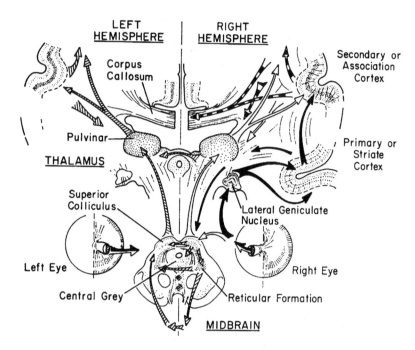

FIGURE 4-8 Communication within the midbrain, region.

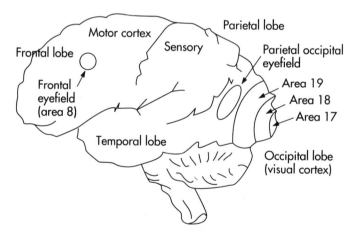

FIGURE 4-9 Vision-related areas of the brain.

ing is the description of these three zones and control centers, which are responsible for vision (Fig. 4-9):

Area 17 (primary visual cortex)

> The primary visual cortex, also called Brodmann area 17, receives visual information as a direct retinoscopic map. It

is made up of a disproportionately large number of macular fibers that end near the occipital pole. Afferent fibers from the superior macular quadrants terminate above the calcarine fissure whereas inferior macular quadrant fibers terminate below. Efferent fibers return to the lateral geniculate bodies, superior colliculi, and pretectal area. Area 17 is completely specific in its function, being involved only in visual reception. Damage to it results in compromised visual acuity and visual field defects. Because of its proximity to the base of the skull, it is more susceptible to the effects of trauma and subsequent edema than are the other areas in the visual cortex.[8]

Area 18 (visual association area)

Trauma to areas other than the occipital cortex can lead to visual sensory deficits. The secondary visual area, Brodmann area 18, interacts with the language centers of the left hemisphere and with spatial relations and other nonlanguage skills from the right hemisphere. It is critically involved in the interpretation of objects perceived, being the locale where visual perception and differentiation of shape, color, and size take place. Damage to it results in compromised word and letter recognition.

Area 19 (visual association area)

Brodmann area 19, known as the tertiary zone, is highly multifunctional, the site where visual information is decoded, coded, integrated, and stored. Normal function of this area is also critical to the interpretation of objects perceived. Disruptions here cause deficits in object recognition (agnosia). Efferent fibers from this area (and from area 18) course back to the lateral geniculate bodies, superior colliculi, and pretectal area. Area 19 is the visual association center responsible for associating and categorizing related visual messages; and, along with area 18, it contributes to saccadic eye movements.

In a young child, injury to area 17 will affect the development of areas 18 and 19; but if the visual system is allowed to follow its normal maturation course, the effect on the other two areas will not be critical. Lesions in the secondary and tertiary zones will result in perceptual deficits without affecting visual acuity.[45]

Area 8 (frontal eye field)

All voluntary eye movements are generated from this area. The extraocular muscles are controlled by both the frontal eye field (area 8) and the parietooccipital eye field (areas 17, 18, and 19). Area 8 is responsible for moving the foveas to an image (saccade), areas 17 to 19 for maintaining the foveas on the image (pursuit).

Five kinds of ocular movement require control by these centers[46]:
    Smooth pursuit
    Saccade
    Optokinetic nystagmus
    Vestibular reflex
    Convergence
Oculomotor dysfunctions will result from injury to these eye movement control centers or to the extraocular muscles themselves.[12]

Deficits in visual scanning (as from cerebral injury) will result in an inefficient gathering of visual information. They can also interfere with performance in the visual perceptual areas of closure, figure-ground detection, and visual memory. Therefore an accurate assessment of visual perceptual skills should not be undertaken without the prior knowledge of elementary oculomotor functioning obtained from observation of a patient's scanning movements.[47]

Visual Disturbances Following Cortical Insult

Patients surviving cerebral injury will often exhibit cognitive disturbance. The vision correlates accompanying such disturbances[48-50] are listed in Table 4-1.

Model of the Visual System Based on Two Pathways

The existence of a cortical and a subcortical visual system has long been a matter of debate. The control centers lie in the visual cortex and the superior colliculi. The cortical visual pathway is made up of the optic nerves, optic chiasm, optic tracts, optic radiations, and visual cortex. The subcortical visual pathway is thought to be made up of the superior colliculi, pulvinar, and parietal lobes. Holtzman[45] deter-

TABLE 4-1

Visual disturbances with cortical insult

Agnosia	Inability to understand or interpret what is seen
Alexia	Inability to recognize or comprehend written or printed words
Aphasia	Inability to recognize, comprehend, or express written or spoken words
Color anomia	Inability to name or recognize colors
Color dyschromatopsia or achromatopsia	Inability to see colors
Prosopagnosia	Inability to recognize a familiar face (complex nonverbal stimuli)
Simultanagnosia	Inability to recognize more than one element at a time
Optic ataxia	Mislocalization when reaching for or pointing at objects

mined that neither the cortical nor the subcortical visual system functions well in isolation. Interaction is critical for optimum performance with regard to stimulus recognition and orientation. The retinal information to the visual cortex involves more conscious perception (such as detailed analysis of visual stimuli). Retinal information received by the superior colliculi is used for unconscious functions (such as visual/motor control and spatial recognition).[51,52]

The superior colliculi (in the tectum of the midbrain) play an important role in coordinating eye and head movements. They are at times referred to as the secondary visual pathway, since the visual information that travels via them to the midbrain is important for oculomotor reflexes and orientation of the head and body.[33] Cortical lesions will impair the ability to discriminate form whereas superior collicular lesions will impair the ability to localize spatially.[53] Minimum disruption of visual/motor control is seen with lesions of the secondary visual pathway, although minor deficits in localization or increased response times may be seen.[54]

Model of the Visual System Based on Function

Vision can be broken down into two functional modes of processing—focal and ambient. Focal vision (made up of foveal, parafoveal, and primary visual cortical inputs) selects areas in the environment to which attention needs to be directed. The focal mode contributes in answering the "what" of vision (object recognition and identification). Information such as the shape and color of objects is transmitted via this pathway to the inferior temporal cortex. It is here that this information is matched against stored visual templates to correctly identify the object. The focal mode is attention oriented and centers on detail in small areas of space.[52] It performs adequately when simply receiving information. Whereas the ambient mode functions without awareness, the focal mode is bound up with consciousness. This is not to say, however, that humans are incapable of shifting attention from the focal mode to the ambient mode.

The ambient mode (more midbrain in location) is concerned with the question of "where" or the location of objects. Data about the movement and position of objects are transmitted via this pathway to the posterior parietal cortex, which provides a reference of where objects of interest are located in the environment.[55] The ambient mode mediates posture, motion, and spatial orientation and interpretation. It is more peripheral in nature, expansive, and involved in object localization and mobility. It relates increasingly to the motor system and to space around the body. It is thought to assist visually with peripheral fusion.[56] Ambient visual performance helps to coordinate motor activity. It receives input from the other sensory systems, especially that of kinesthesia. Routinely, the ambient mode functions as if without effort.

In any injury that has the potential to affect both the central and the autonomic nervous system, vision effects are often what disrupt ambient function. It is thought that this takes place at the level of the midbrain, which is where vision is integrated with vestibular, kinesthetic, and proprioceptive functions. In the case of traumatic injury, Padula et al.[56] termed the condition *posttraumatic vision syndrome.* Table 4-2 presents the signs and symptoms commonly seen with this syndrome.

CLINICAL PEARL

When assessing vision, perimetry evaluates only the focal mode.

In an attempt to evaluate the focal and ambient systems, current optometric techniques must be carefully assessed and chosen for their ability to adequately quantify and qualify each mode. There is little argument with the diagnostic value of classical perimetry. However, in assessing vision, it evaluates only the focal mode. In addition, it uses shapes that are too small and movement that is too slow for ambient vision to be sufficiently stimulated. The natural environment contains shapes with larger dimensions, more movement, and relatively greater velocities that better arouse the ambient visual system.[53] Therefore, classical perimetry is insensitive to assessing the ambient mode. Other tests (such as visual acuity and contrast sensitivity function) are better. Unfortunately, the results of these have been extrapolated to interpret the status of ambient vision, which has led clinicians to underestimate or overestimate a patient's true function.[53] Assessment of ambient function is presently limited to observations of how the patient moves about a room and around obstacles.[53]

TABLE 4-2

Posttraumatic vision syndrome

Characteristics	Symptoms	Additional signs
Accommodative dysfunction	Altered coordination and mobility	Field defects
Balance and posture difficulties	Asthenopia	Lagophthalmus
Convergence insufficiency	Diplopia	Nystagmus
Exophoria	Objects appear to move	
Exotropia	Poor tracking abilities	
Lowered blink rate	Staring behavior	
Spatial disorientation	Visual memory problems	

Adapted from Padula and Shapiro.[44]

CLINICAL PEARL

Clinical perimetry is insensitive to assessment of the ambient mode.

Some individuals with substantial field loss as measured by conventional perimetric standards have reported actually being aware of motion when large shapes are moved into the area of their field loss. Experimentally, ambient vision continues to function normally in patients after hemisphere commissurotomy (severing fibers in the corpus callosum). However, focal vision is divided and separated along a vertical midline,[57] and patients with peripheral vision loss typically exhibit additional eye and head movements as well as move more cautiously, especially when walking.[58]

CLINICAL PEARL

Assessment of ambient function is presently limited to observations of how the patient moves about a room and around obstacles.

Clinical Effects of Cerebral Injury on Visual Function

The clinical manifestations of cerebral trauma can present under either monocular or binocular conditions with resultant acuity reduction, field loss, or even complete blindness. Survivors will often have binocular vision disorders such as strabismus (horizontal/vertical), shifts in their phoric posture, oculomotor dysfunction, and convergence and accommodation deficiencies (insufficiency/infacility). The severity of these may vary from a slight increase in exophoria to a noncomitant strabismus with intractable diplopia. Other visual signs and symptoms commonly associated[12,19,37] are reduced visual acuity at distance and/or near, visual field defects, diplopia, diminished stereopsis, increased exophoria and at times exotropia, reduced reaction time, reduced accommodative ability and flexibility, eyestrain, dry eye symptoms from a decreased blink rate and reduced eye-hand coordination.

In the study by Gianutos et al.,[11] 90% or greater of the cerebral-injured patients optometrically screened were referred because of inadequately corrected distance acuity alone (less than 20/40 best corrected). Binocular dysfunction and accommodative insufficiency noted 73% and 69% referal rates. Perceptual abilities were sometimes altered, resulting in deficits of visual memory and discrimination, size and shape constancy, visual matching and closure abilities,[12] and object localization.

Integration of inaccurate visual information with information from the kinesthetic, proprioceptive, and vestibular centers will affect the efficiency and accuracy of balance mechanisms, coordinated movements, fusion, cognitive function, and previously established pathways for sensory/motor matches. Patients exhibiting these effects may show increased muscle tonus in the head, neck, and shoulders with notable head and neck extension.[56]

Visual field defects can present with great variability depending on the location and severity of the insult. Their classification and description are based on several factors[59]—whether the loss is relative or absolute, the area involved (total, sector, central, peripheral, altitudinal, hemianopic), and the symmetry (congruous, incongruous, homonymous).

Interestingly enough, asymptomatic defects are reported in 29% of patients with transient ischemic attacks and in 57% of those with minor strokes. The most commonly exhibited defect is scotoma located solely or predominantly in the upper visual field (85% of cases[60]).

One frequently observed change in vision with cerebral injury involves convergence. Convergence depends on the integrative functions of both cortical and subcortical areas. The shift with insult is predominantly toward a greater exo-posture, and the result is convergence insufficiency. However, research by Krohel et al.[61] has found that the severity of convergence insufficiency does not correlate positively with the severity of cerebral injury.

Anatomically, convergence is diffusely organized over the pretectal region (brain stem), as are accommodation and pupillary reactions. A unilateral lesion in this area will symmetrically affect both functions.[62] Convergence, which is an essential part of the near vision complex,[63] consists of both reflexive (tonic, proximal, accommodative, and fusional vergences) and voluntary components. Accommodative and fusional vergences are usually affected by cerebral injury—the former being responsible for general alignment of the visual axes, the latter for fine-tuning this alignment. Fusion as achieved by fusional vergence depends on the magnitude of the deviation, status of the sensory fusion system, and amount of fusional vergence available.[64] Patients manifesting a convergence insufficiency often complain of difficulty with reading and diplopia at near. Lesions in both the occipital lobe and the upper midbrain appear capable of generating this defect.[61]

CLINICAL PEARL

Accommodative convergence is responsible for the general alignment of the visual axes; fusional convergence fine-tunes this alignment.

Visually mature individuals may develop strabismus as a result of pathology, injury, or decompensation of a latent deviation. Noncomitant strabismus of recent origin is often the result of a car accident but can also be caused by CVAs, cerebral tumors, or aneurysms.[65] A noncomitant strabismus would be observed during version testing. The centers for motor fusion are responsible for this disruption.[66]

Midbrain lesions that are acquired after the age of 10 years can cause a disruption of fusion without suppression, resulting in an intractable diplopia.[67] If diplopia occurs in juvenile cerebral-injured patients, a common adaptation is for the brain to suppress a portion of the input to one eye. Adolescent and adult patients will not adapt to diplopia as readily, if at all. They may be observed to exhibit abnormal head postures and motor responses to aid in fusion or to occlude/degrade vision in one eye. Surprisingly, even with today's technology, patients with any of the above-mentioned visual dysfunctions are routinely instructed to patch an eye or avoid any of the factors that might heighten their awareness of the problem (near-point tasks especially). Emotional depression has resulted from the limitations or lack of ability to perform normal everyday activities as a result of these impaired abilities.[68]

With the significant contribution that vision has to routine cognitive and motor function, it is not difficult to appreciate the devastation a person with cerebral injury feels when visual function is even slightly impaired. It is important to realize that addressing the quality of visual functioning early as well as throughout the rehabilitation program is essential.[56]

Visual Imperception

A commonly seen and frequently confusing disorder attributable to cerebral injury is visual imperception. It occurs not only in adults but also in children,[69] not a congenital or learned condition but an acquired disability,[49] and is often referred to as hemispatial neglect, visual/spatial neglect, hemispatial agnosia, hemiinattention, unilateral visual neglect,[70] and hemiimperception.[11] Researchers and clinicians have differed with regard to which is the best description (neglect, inattention, or imperception). Since the terms *neglect* and *inattention* imply a degree of conscious ignoring or avoidance of something, they will not be used here. *Imperception* expresses that little or no perception is available. It is passive, unconscious, and a truly diminished awareness, not an avoidance, which agrees with what current research has confirmed is the case. Therefore, for the sake of continuity, "imperception" will be used throughout the remainder of this chapter.

Gianutsos et al.[11] noted that visual imperception causes a significant hindrance in the rehabilitation program. It leads to deficits in localization, scanning (saccades), fixation, and orientation responses.[12] Patients with visual imperception routinely exhibit visual field defects.[71]

Visual imperception can be separated into two subgroups. The more severe variation, characterized by the total absence of response to a stimulus, is an inability to appreciate objects (complete unawareness) in the hemifield contralateral to the cerebral injury. It is often referred to as contralateral imperception, and patients with it show demonstrable visual field defects. The milder variation, commonly called visual extinction, occurs when two symmetrically placed stimuli (with respect to the patient's midline) are presented. The patient will exhibit a tendency to ignore only the stimulus opposite the side of injury.[72] There will be no gross clinical signs of disturbance, but signs will appear during testing, with an increased number of omissions occurring on the side opposite the injury. Thus a patient without field defects may require a more refined testing technique to elicit the imperception. Although both imperception and hemianopia may be present, it is not uncommon for one to occur without the other.[40] Also, visual field defects have not been shown to exacerbate imperception.[73]

Hemianopias are usually described as an opaque curtain covering half of what is seen. This is also true of areas affected by visual imperception. The regions involved may vary as to the density of imperceived areas; and, in fact, the patient may be completely unaware of any change in vision, which is significant to the ability to function normally.

Imperception can be caused by lesions at different cortical sites. The most common location is the right parietal lobe,[75] but a high frequency also exists for anterior (frontal lobe cortex) and posterior (temporal, parietal, and occipital lobe cortical) lesions in either hemisphere. A study by Albert[76] showed that visual imperception occurred in 37% of patients with right brain damage and in 30% of those with left brain damage. So, right hemispheric involvement is only slightly more frequent in occurrence. However, the severity of the imperception varied significantly. Left hemisphere damage produced a milder imperception whereas right hemisphere lesions produced a more pronounced effect. Comparing the severity within each hemisphere shows posterior damage yielding a more pronounced effect (more severe imperception) than anterior damage. Imperception as a result of insult to deep structures occurs when gray matter of the thalamus and basal ganglia is injured. Lesions involving subcortical white matter rarely cause imperception.[77]

Imperception and Attention

Hemiimperception is considered to be an attentional defect. Cubelli et al.[75] concluded that it could not be interpreted as a disruption of one individual mechanism; rather it encompassed several mechanisms involving several levels of cognitive processing. With continued research it has come to be recognized as occurring with greater variation than in just a left-right, hemifield, horizontal plane. This has been confirmed by Shelton et al.[78] in 1990, who found that attention may be directed in isolation or in any variation and combination of three orientations (vertical, horizontal, and radial). Imperception may affect peripersonal space (that is, near or on the body) and extrapersonal space (off the body).[16,79]

Functional Signs and Symptoms of Visual Imperception

Visual imperception can occur without clinical signs of field loss or dysfunction of the oculomotor system. With right brain damage there is a significant correlation between reduced abilities of visual/spatial organization and dressing apraxia. The location of visual imperception will include the middle of the field of vision and both sides to varying degrees. This occurs more often than just in the hemifield contralateral to the lesion. Diagrammatically, imperception and hemisphere damage can be viewed as in Figure 4-10.

RIGHT HEMISPHERE DAMAGE

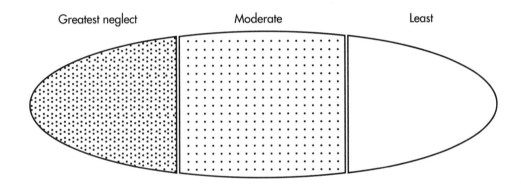

LEFT HEMISPHERE DAMAGE

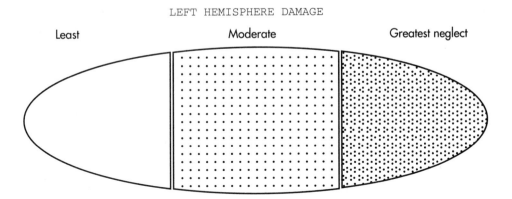

FIGURE 4-10 Imperception with respect to hemispheric damage.

Other functional observations seen with imperception include routine daily activities (such as when a man will shave only half his face or a woman will apply makeup to only one side of her face), difficulty telling time from a clock, eating food from only one side of the plate, and misjudging distances.[70,80] Severe damage will affect reading, writing, drawing, and communication. Mild impairments may show only minimum effects on daily activities (such as clerical work or driving). In general, patients with cerebral injury exhibit a longer mean response time than do those without. Patients with right side lesions and visual imperception have slower response times than do patients whose lesions are on the left side and who may or may not have visual imperception.[81]

Testing of Visual Imperception

Many tests (Fig. 4-11) have been devised to assess the various aspects of imperception—three-dimensional constructions, line cancellations, copying of standardized figures or drawings, routine behavioral daily activities, and computer programs (Fig. 4-12). Currently there are test batteries with combinations of these available and in use.[82]

Tests to assess for imperception (such as the Imperception Test Batteries) have been developed by Stone et al.[83] The ITB is an evaluation with two 10-minute parts of seven items each. One part is

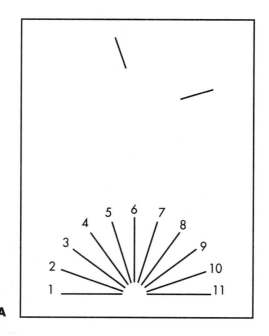

A

FIGURE 4-11   Tests of hemiimperception. **A,** Standard line orientation task.   *continued*

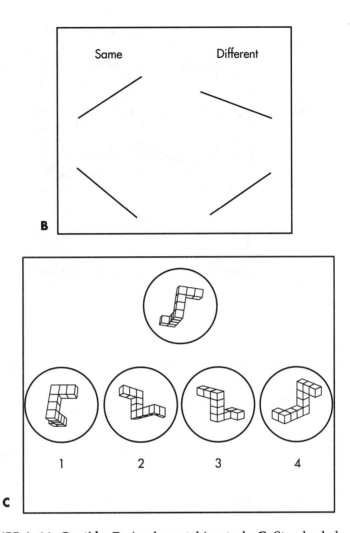

FIGURE 4-11, Cont'd. B, Angle-matching task. **C,** Standard shape rotation task. (From Wallock EM: *Cogn Rehabil* 35:28-29, 1987.)

sensitive to right visual/spatial imperception, the other to left imperception. The test is constructed using relevant daily activities such as reading the newspaper, eating a meal, and sorting through coins.

The Rivermead Behavioral Attention Test (Table 4-3) consists of nine items that simulate routine daily activities.[70,84] It takes 10 to 15 minutes to administer[70] and is usually given with six additional subtests from the BIT (Behavioral Inattention Test).

The BIT, developed by Wilson, Cockburn, and Halligan,[70] consists of six conventional subtests (Table 4-4), including line bisection and cancellation exercises. Of the six subtests, letter and star cancellation[85] (Fig. 4-13) has been found to be the most sensitive for detecting imperception by identifying 74% of patients with no false-positives.

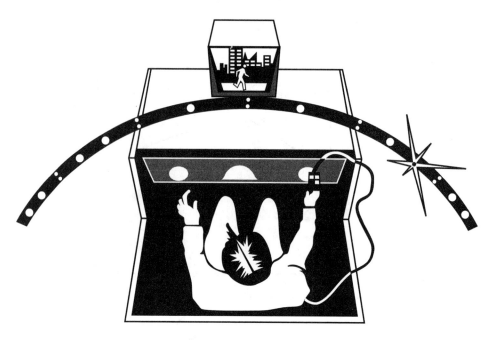

FIGURE 4-12 Tests devised to assess the various aspects of imperception include computer programs.

TABLE 4-3
Rivermead Behavioral Attention Test

Eating a meal (simulation)   Setting the table
Dialing a telephone   Sorting coins
Reading a menu   Copying an address
Telling the time (digital)   Following a map
Telling the time (analog)

TABLE 4-4
Behavioral Inattention Test

BIT Subtest	Goal
Line cancellation	Cross out each of 40 randomly arranged lines
Letter cancellation	Cross out 40 stimulus targets scattered among 170 upper case letters
Star cancellation	Cross out 56 small stars interspersed with 52 large stars, 10 words, and 13 letters
Figure copying	Copy three outline drawings of a four-pointed star, a cube, a daisy, and three simple geometric shapes
Line bisection	Bisect three black lines (204 mm) arranged in stepwise fashion across a page
Representational drawing	Draw from memory a clock face, a man or woman, and a butterfly

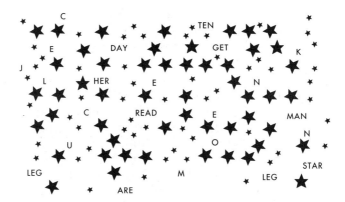

FIGURE 4-13 Star cancellation test. Dimensions of the original are 298 × 208 cm. (From Halligan PW, et al. *Lancet* 2:909-911, 1989.)

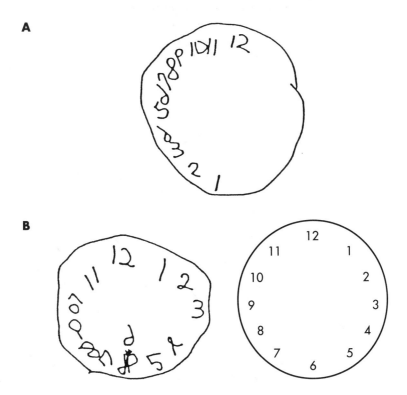

FIGURE 4-14 Drawing a clock dial with and without a model. **A,** The patient drew the dial plate without a model. **B,** The copy of the model (*left*) of a dial plate (*right*).

Imperception may be elicited when a patient is asked to draw a clock (Fig. 4-14), a stick figure, or a rectangle. Positive signs would be interpreted if details from half the drawings are missing. Imperception may also be inferred if items drawn are rotated around the vertical axis, causing a distorted sense of verticality.[30]

Most traditional imperception assessments include line bisection and cancellation exercises (for example, Albert's test of line cancellation)[76] (Fig. 4-15). When asked to bisect a horizontal line, patients who exhibit left visual imperception may draw the bisecting line significantly to the right of center.[86] Patients with altitudinal imperception will bisect a vertical line above or below its true center.[87] Patients with altitudinal imperception in the lower field will make spatial judgments higher than normal, as in the case of bisecting a line at a point higher than center. These individuals show deficits in attending to stimuli in the inferior field.[88] Bilateral lesions of the parietooccipital region[89] or dorsal portions of the occipital lobes are the cause (Fig. 4-16), but lesions of the inferior temporal lobes or occipital lobes[78,90] also force patients to make spatial judgments lower than normal, as with bisecting a line below the center point.

Patients with both a hemianopia and a hemiimperception will bisect only the portion of the line that they perceive. They will not scan for the missing portion. Hemianopic patients without hemiimper-

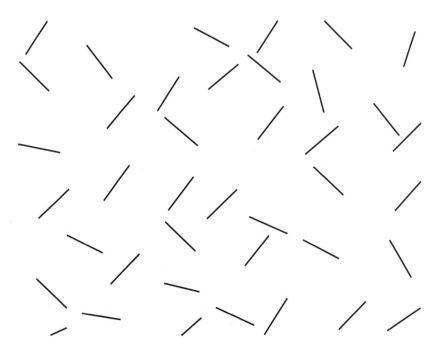

FIGURE 4-15 Albert's test of line cancellation (for visual imperception). (From Albert ML: *Neurology*, 23:658-664, 1973.)

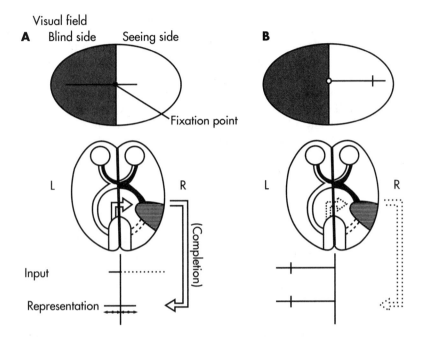

FIGURE 4-16 Anatomy of imperception. **A,** The mechanism underlying unilateral spatial neglect in the line bisection test. **B,** Recognition of rightward deviation of the subjective midpoint in the seeing right visual field. The patient is forced to maintain fixation of the left end point of the line. (From Ishiai S, et al: *Brain,* 112:1485-1502, 1989.)

ception will see the entire line and bisect it correctly because they scan for the end points of the absent portion. In other words, they use a strategy wherein they look at the missing side to compensate for their field defect. They have been found, in one study,[91] to fixate a point in the right portion of the line and mentally construct a complete line around this point. Patients with both conditions (hemianopia and hemiimperception) lack such a fixation pattern for compensation.[91]

Computer tests have also been developed to assess visual imperception. They appear to be more sensitive in detecting visual imperception than conventional occupational therapy and bedside tests.[92] Two such programs are the MATCH and the FASTREAD, tachistoscopic reading tests that are sensitive to central field hemiimperception.[74]

Management of Visual Imperception

The lack of treatment techniques for visual imperception has, in part, been a result of the inadequate understanding and evaluation of it.[70] There are differing approaches or philosophies as to how best to address visual imperception. One is to encourage the patient to attend visually to the imperceived[30] or absent side. With patients who show a constant deviation to the right (as in gait), conventionally therapists attempt to make them aware of their tendency and teach them to compensate.[93] The thought is that patients who become aware of an imperception will gain the insight that may positively affect their rehabilitation. Treatment then should be directed to aiding them in understanding their condition, if not also helping them to "see" it.[74]

A study by Riddoch and Humphreys[94] found that imperception appears to lessen if patients are cued and forced to attend to stimuli in their imperceived field, even with competing stimuli from the non-competing field. Once the patient is no longer compelled to attend to the field of imperception, he or she can be reoriented to stimuli in the nonimperceived field. The authors[94] concluded that these patients lose the ability to automatically orient themselves to the space contralateral to the injury, even though the process regulating this function remains intact.

Ishiai et al.[93] noted that treatment of hemiimperception by means of line cancellation can be improved through modification (that is, numbering the middle of the line as opposed to simple bisection) (Fig. 4-17). This appears to increase the patient's motivation.[93] Hyper-threshold stimuli or increased attention to the affected field may also be necessary to provide a solution for this problem.[74]

Exercises in reading, drawing, and visual/spatial concepts should be performed in a systematic fashion. Improvements in scanning can be achieved through gaze-direction exercises. During these sessions, extraneous information (visual noise) should be kept to a minimum.[95]

A perceptual treatment program for right brain injury consists of basic visual scanning, somatosensory awareness and size-estimation training, and complex visual organization tasks.[80] Scanning therapy should include the following[96]:

1. The patient should be presented with a sufficiently interesting task to cause head turning.
2. An initial cue stimulus should be presented on the left side to serve as an anchor.
3. The density of the stimuli should be minimized to enhance the treatment process in patients with right cerebral injury.[97]
4. Patients tend to move too rapidly to the right (tracking) and will benefit from pacing to help them slow down.

What may also be of help is the use of bilateral simultaneous sensory stimulation. It should include the side of the body where impairment of stimulation occurs, which is controlled by the contralateral damaged cerebral hemisphere.[98] Treatment should encompass exercises that provide awareness through more than one sense—for example, tactile stimulation of both hands at the same time, to provide simultaneous input and confirmation.

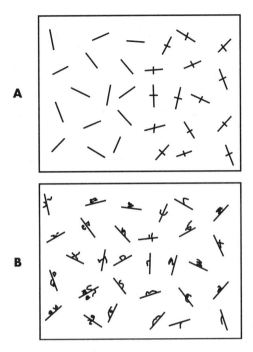

FIGURE 4-17 Numbering of lines during a line cancellation test. **A,** First trial, in which patient was asked to cross out lines. **B,** Second trial, in which the patient was asked to number the lines. (From Ishiai S, et al: *Neurology* 40:1395-1398, 1990.)

One home technique similar to Michigan Tracking (a vision therapy strategy) is visual cancellation. It utilizes a variety of symbols: letters, words, pictures, shapes. The level of difficulty increases with added stimulus characters and a greater density of extraneous stimuli. At the onset of therapy a task may need to be designed with boundaries or guidelines. This will act as an anchor or cue for the beginning and ending of lines. Such aids can be eliminated with improvements in performance. Regular newspaper text can be used instead of the symbols.

Patients with disrupted spatial organization and sensory awareness will exhibit abnormalities in localizing the body's midline. This involves discerning distances between stimuli both on and off their body. Spatial organization is improved through the use of visual comparisons of shape, size, and distances between various objects. Training can utilize blocks or Plexiglas rods of various lengths for size estimation. Tasks should be performed directly in front of the patient on both the impaired and the unimpaired side. Areas of somatosensory awareness, size-estimation training, and complex visual organization will follow a normal hierarchical sequence, from simple tasks to more complex ones. Feedback should always be provided with respect to overestimation or underestimation. Compensating strategies are used to improve efficiency.[99] Training programs that incorporate spatial organization and sensory awareness, in addition to scanning training, are found to be more effective than ones that address only scanning. Even with scanning training that did improve some visual perceptual disorders, however, several areas (such as line cancellation and location of body midline) were not improved.

Diagnostic Tests

Current techniques used for systemic medical diagnosis have become highly sophisticated. The results provide a clearer picture of the extent of cerebral injury and help guide the medical team toward prompt intervention. However, even with the improved accuracy and validity of these procedures, no test results should be used in isolation. They should all be correlated with the patient's history and physical evaluation. Some of the more commonly performed medical procedures[27,100,101] used with this population are described in Table 4-5.

Neuropsychological Evaluation

Disruption and alteration of cognitive, emotional, and behavioral functions as a result of cerebral injury can lead to an evaluation with one of several neuropsychological test batteries.[14,37,98,102] A well-known assessment tool is the LNNB (Luria Nebraska Neuropsychological Battery). This standardized test assesses the quantitative and qualitative aspects of basic function of the major voluntary systems of the brain. It uses both quantitative and qualitative methods and is routinely administered by neuropsychologists. Quantitative methods are based on the counting of errors and the length of time it takes to perform a given task. This approach has proven to be valuable in evaluating the extent of damage in a brain-injured patient. Qualitative methods are based on the examiner's observations of how and why the patient makes the errors and takes the time he does. The areas explored are listed in Table 4-6. The LNNB uses fewer items per area but assesses a wider range of skills in a relatively short time frame compared with other assessment vehicles. Within the visual scale, a patient's ability to analyze pictures and drawings of varying detail and quality is explored. The other scales also require visual input to yield adequate evaluations of performance. For instance, it is not uncommon for a patient with basic cognitive deficits to be unable to perform certain components of the evaluation that require prolonged attention or supervision. Therefore the evaluation may need to be broken down into periods of 15, 20, or 30 minutes over several days.

TABLE 4-5
Diagnostic Procedures

Computed tomographic scanning	Painless three-dimensional x-rays that provide details of cerebral structure with little or no risk to the patient; used to detect tumors, cysts, strokes, hemorrhages, or other alterations in brain tissue
Magnetic resonance imaging (MRI)	Provides detailed images of brain tissue through the use of a large magnetic field and a radiofrequency signal; a different way of imaging brain tissue that does not, however, eliminate the need for CT scans
Cerebral and carotid angiograms	Performed to visualize arteries of the head and neck that transport blood from the heart to the brain; x-ray pictures of vessels can be seen with the help of dyes; extremely helpful in providing insight into arterial disorders such as vessel malformations, aneurysms, and strokes; also aids in providing information as to the location and severity of arterial blockage; can assist in the selection of treatment regimens
Electroencephalography (EEG)	Test of cerebral function; it records normal and abnormal electrical activity of the brain, helping to diagnose or rule out cerebral conditions that may produce irregular brain waves (as in epilepsy, degenerative disorders, or conditions that result in alterations or loss of consciousness); is not used to treat illness or measure intelligence
Electromyography (EMG)	Records the electrical activity from skeletal muscles; only assists in clarification of disorders of muscles and nerves, is nonspecific for any particular condition
Nerve conduction velocities (NCV)	Determines the velocity and characteristics of electrical impulses traveling through the limbs and face; velocities for a given patient can be compared with known standard values; the speed of conduction may be slowed in various disorders
Complete blood count (CBC)	Evaluates the blood for possible factors that might predispose to a CVA (increased blood viscosity from polycythemia [ischemic stroke], decreased coagulating blood factor as seen in blood disorders [hemorrhagic stroke], elevated erythrocyte sedimentation rate as in connective tissue disorders or white blood cell count from bacterial endocarditis [ischemic stroke])
Auscultation	Noninvasive procedure that can be performed by the optometrist; the bell of a stethescope is placed at the bifurcation of the common carotid artery; 8 out of 10 patients with more than 50% blockage of the internal carotid artery will have bruits

TABLE 4-6

Luria Nebraska Neuropsychological Battery (LNNB)

Motor behavior	Perception and production of verbal and nonverbal auditory stimuli
Analysis of tactile feedback	Visual analysis of verbal and nonverbal stimuli
Reading	Short- and long-term memory
Writing	Verbal intellectual functions
Arithmetic	Nonverbal intellectual functions

When a deficit is indicated by any part of the evaluation, additional testing may be used to provide a more in-depth view of the problem.

Another frequently used assessment is the HRB (Halstead-Reitan Neuropsychological Test Battery), the most widely used instrument in the United States and Canada for assessing brain-behavior relationships. It is directly related to prescribing and implementing a cognitive rehabilitation program for the patient with cognitive impairment and can be used to evaluate visual/spatial skills in relation to simple and complex tasks[14] (Table 4-7). A program specifically designed to treat these neuropsychological deficits, as determined by the results obtained from the HRB, is called the REHABIT[98] (Reitan Evaluation of Hemispheric Abilities and Brain Improvement Training) (Table 4-8).

Optometric Evaluation

Studies of cerebral-injured patients are seriously lacking in data on the visual system.[37] There is a real need for practical functional assessment that would be appropriate to evaluate the needs of patients with cerebral injury.[74] Such a vehicle would help all members of the rehabilitation team serve the patient's goal of regaining his or her full potential. Early recognition of the signs and symptoms (Table 4-9) would minimize the morbidity rates in patients who have survived a serious head injury.[8]

Several studies have actually addressed ocular function, visual acuity (occasionally), and visual fields (as generally determined by confrontation fields); however, tests of binocularity are routinely

TABLE 4-7

Halstead-Reitan Behavior Tests

Sensory input	Language
Spatial and manipulatory abilities	Motor output
Attention and concentration	Learning and memory
Executive functions—logical analysis, conceptualization, reasoning, planning, and flexibility of thinking	

TABLE 4-8

Five tracks of training for the REHABIT

Track A	Equipment and procedures for developing expressive and receptive language and verbal skills and related academic abilities
Track B	Abstract reasoning, logical analysis, and organization in language and verbal areas
Track C	Reasoning, organization, planning, and abstraction skills without particular regard to content
Track D	Abstraction with relation to visual/spatial and manipulatory skills
Track E	Fundamental aspects of visual/spatial and manipulatory skills

TABLE 4-9

Patient Symptoms: Professional Observations and Possible Area of Visual Dysfunction

Convergence Problems
(Pointing System)
- closing one eye
- double vision
- muscle palsy
- headaches
- pain
- reading problems
- print blurry
- ocular discomfort

Strabismus
(Eye-turn)
- closing of one eye
- double vision
- head tilts or head turns
- sudden onset of eye turn
- muscle palsy
- difficult judging depth and three dimensional viewing

Accommodations Problems
(Focusing System)
- focusing problems
- headaches
- pain
- double vision
- squinting
- closing one eye
- reading problems
- ocular discomfort

Visual-Perceptual
- problem judging size
- problem judging distances
- coordination problems
- left-right confusion

Motilities
(Tracking System)
- inability to follow objects smoothly
- reading problems
  - skipping words
  - re-reading words
  - reversals
- nystagmus involuntary movement or rotation of the eyes

Field Defects
- bumping into chairs, objects, etc.
- difficulty seeing at night
- tunnel vision
- holding on to walls, other people, etc.

From Cohen AH, Soden R. An optometric approach to the rehabilitation of the stroke patient. J *Am Optom Assoc,* 52:795-800, 1981.

omitted, even though disorders involving binocularity (that is, convergence insufficiency) are cited with significant regularity.[11] It has also been noted[84] that disorders of visual/spatial processing are commonly overlooked or misdiagnosed during routine clinical and neurological evaluation. Patients with visual/perceptual deficits easily pass routine ophthalmological evaluations, and yet their symptoms and complaints continue, which points essentially to visual/perceptual and binocular vision disturbances. Deficits in visual scanning alone can lead to an inefficient gathering of information, which can then interfere with performance in the areas of closure, figure-ground detection, and visual memory. Therefore an accurate assessment of visual/perceptual skills should not be performed without the prior knowledge of elementary oculomotor function (as by scanning).[47]

A thorough visual assessment should include tests of binocular function, visual perception, oculomotor function, visual fields, refractive analysis, and ocular health. Diagnostically Krasnow[104] has noted that there must be inclusion of sufficient fusional vergence testing with cerebral-injured patients to accurately determine the diagnosis. The optometric assessment* should consist of the areas listed in Table 4-10 and, in addition, should include having the patient do the following:

1. Read a paragraph of text; this will pick up most cases of alexia
2. Copy a line drawing; this will disclose most perceptual disorders
3. Describe in detail what is seen in a photograph
4. Look at photographs of famous personalities and identify them; this will pick up most prosopagnosia cases
5. Reach for objects in space in each hemifield; misreaching may mean optic ataxia
6. Name and sort colors; misnaming is color anomia, missorting (such as on the Farnsworth D15) central achromatopsia

Because of the concentration and fixation required, conventional diagnostic testing involving quantitative perimetry may be difficult for this population. Most automated perimeters offer "central 30°" programs, which again assess only focal visual integrity or near peripheral integrity. There are no standard optometric tests to evaluate ambient visual integrity. Questionability of the accuracy and reliability of peripheral visual field assessments has led to hesitancy in accepting them. Also in question has been the influence of relative field losses versus absolute hemianopic defects on these tests when applied to this population.[74]

CLINICAL PEARL

Palsies of the third (oculomotor) and sixth (abducent) nerves are usually detected early. However, fourth nerve (trochlear) palsy is commonly missed. The usual cause of fourth nerve palsy is trauma.

---

*References 49, 56, 65, 66, 105, 106.

TABLE 4-10
The optometric assessment

Case history	Includes observations by family and friends; descriptions of the patient's preinjury and present cognitive, physical, and visual status are also of importance
Professional observation	Noncomitant deviations can result in the patient's making compensatory head turns, tips, and tilts to maintain single binocular vision; a previous binocular now monocular visual system may manifest alterations of midline constancies with potential distortions in balance and posture
Extraocular muscle assessment	Including pursuits, saccades (King-Devick or Developmental Eye Movement Test), ductions, versions, cover test at distance and near (may need to be assessed in the nine positions of gaze), and pupillary reflexes; a handy tool to use with non-comitant deviations is a hand-held Maddox Rod/Risley Prism; it allows free space measurement of the angle in all nine positions of gaze and at any distance; red lens testing or Hess-Lancaster tests in the nine cardinal positions may also be used
Refractive and binocular vision analysis	Includes refraction to subjective binocular vision assessment at distance; a thorough evaluation of general binocular vision skills (phorias and forced vergences) at both distance and near is essential; near point retinoscopy of each eye should be performed to ensure balanced input for more efficient visual information processing between eyes; assessment of accommodative function is critical with this population, evaluating amplitude, lag, and facility of accommodation will aid in determining an appropriate near-point prescription if needed Assessment of high level binocular skills (sensory fusion) such as peripheral and central second- and third-degree fusion as well as luster is also important; when with vision therapy and/or surgery the offending pathology subsides, the emphasis of sensory fusion alone may improve the ability to maintain single binocular vision
Ocular health assessment	Including color vision testing and tear quality assessment with observations of blink rate, tonometry, and dilated fundus evaluation
Visual field assessment	1. Central fields—Amsler grid and automated perimetry 2. Peripheral fields—Goldmann or automated perimeter 3. Binocular fusion fields and monocular field of fixation—It is important to know whether single vision is achieved by fusion or through suppression; even if it occurs as a result of suppression, it is not always considered detrimental with this population

---

TABLE 4-10
continued

	Binocular fields of fixation (diplopia fields) is the area of visual space in which the patient can move his eye to the various positions of gaze without experiencing diplopia; a perimeter capable of allowing a kinetic visual field to be plotted (such as the B&L Autoplot or an arc perimeter) is an excellent means of obtaining binocular fields of fixation; the test can be done with Anaglyphs glasses; the Autoplot allows the field to be plotted immediately
	Monocular and binocular fields of fixation should be performed before beginning vision therapy; an appropriate response with the monocular field of fixation test is when a small letter can no longer be discerned
	The three possible responses to binocular field of fixation are
	a. Luster (indicates fusion)
	b. Two lights (indicates diplopia)
	c. One red or one green light (indicates suppression)
	This test can also be used to monitor the progression of vision therapy treatment
	4. Single and double simultaneous stimulation test—involves competitive stimulation conditions such as two simultaneously presented visual stimuli with mirror symmetry to the vertical midline
	5. Confrontation fields—can be performed when patients are nonmobile
Electrodiagnostic testing (when applicable)	Visual evoked potential
Visual perceptual assessment	All visual materials are presented at the midline of the patient's body, since drawing and reading require a symmetrical exploration of space; the patient should be assessed with tests that measure both motor and nonmotor demands
	1. Copying of forms
	2. Reading
	3. Pegboard
	4. Circus Puzzle
	5. Laterality/directionality—Jordan Left Right Reversal Test and/or Reversal Frequency Test
	6. Perceptual screening—Motor Free Visual Perception Test or the Test of Visual Perceptual Skills—assess visual memory, spatial relationships, figure-ground, and closure

---

In the general population, palsies of the third and sixth cranial nerves (oculomotor and abducent) are usually detected early; but fourth nerve (trochlear) palsies are often missed. The most common cause of a fourth nerve palsy is trauma. Even a minor head injury can affect this nerve, because of its long pathway and thin attachment at the brain stem. Assessment may be done by means of the head tilt test of Bielschowsky. In general, surgery for a fourth nerve palsy is postponed at least 6 months to allow for spontaneous recovery. Prompt diagnosis and referral for a palsy of this nerve will usually avoid unnecessary testing, treatment, and costs.[107]

Computer Diagnostics

Because of today's advanced technology, computers have succeeded in making inroads into the health care system. Gianutsos[74] has developed software programs (REACT, SDSST, SEARCH) that may be used on an IBM or Apple computer for the functional assessment of visual fields, with emphasis on the cerebral-injured population. These include the reaction time measure of visual fields (REACT), the single and double simultaneous stimulation test (SDSST), and the shape/inspection matching inventory (SEARCH).

Management of Cerebral Injury

With cerebral injury the emergency medical needs of the individual are of urgent primary concern. The medical team's goals are to help the patient survive and to identify the cause and possible sequelae of the injury so damage to the brain and surrounding tissues will be minimized. During the acute phase, treatment focuses on managing life-threatening conditions and physical injuries. If there is an ocular concern (that is, damage to the globe, optic nerve, orbit, or oculomotor system) at the time of evaluation, an ophthalmologist will routinely be called in to provide diagnostic and therapeutic care. The role of this professional is to determine the physiological state of the eye and provide treatment of ocular structures through surgical or medical means to minimize any loss of sight.

Rehabilitation facilities are commonly located in or affiliated with medical facilities. Because of the influence of a more "medical" model, it is not uncommon for survivors of cerebral injury to be referred to an ophthalmologist. This is not to diminish the importance of healthy end organs and pathways; however, functional aspects of vision beyond the anatomy (such as information processing) are routinely overlooked more often than not[56] and would be more appropriately addressed through the expertise of a functional optometrist.

Of significance, Gianutsos and Ramsey[108] state that few facilities utilize rehabilitative optometric services on a regular basis. However, the high incidence of visual system dysfunction should provide compelling evidence for rehabilitative optometric assessment and management.[12]

Rehabilitation programs in general are oriented toward the recovery of physical disabilities, which often results in the overlooking of cognitive problems and visual imperception.[109] At times, patients are unaware of these deficits or refuse to acknowledge their existence. However, the greatest restoration of preinjury function may ultimately occur if these skills (visual) are remedied.[11]

A significant concern today is the real scarcity of rehabilitation programs to treat this population.[2] Even if a patient manages to become involved in a program, the skills needed for daily living involving cognitive, emotional, and social functions may not be adequately considered if, indeed, they are considered at all.[11]

Hayden and Hart[26] state that, until recently, the "rehabilitation of head injury meant remediating as many of the physical problems as possible, and then discharging the patient. Statistics clearly show that outcome after such treatment is bleak." Extensive studies[26,40] have shown that the reeducation of visual/perceptual skills in patients with left hemiimperception as a result of right hemisphere damage has shown improvement as a result of the practice of specifically designed exercises.

Studies even indicate that early intervention results in faster progress with therapy.[18] It has been shown that late admission of patients to a rehabilitation program (more than 35 days after injury) led to their requiring twice as much treatment as was required by patients admitted earlier. Potential cost savings of an average $40,000 could be realized per patient for acute hospital care through the prevention of secondary complications or improved neurological outcome alone.[9]

The Rehabilitation Program

If cerebral injury occurs, a comprehensive rehabilitation program should be recommended that will provide for evaluation, training, and interaction in all routine activities of daily life.[2] A thorough assessment of each area is imperative. Any problem that is not observed or diagnosed before the rehabilitation program will surely alter the design and potential outcome.[11] It will be most difficult, then, for a patient to compensate for a deficit if there is a lack of awareness of it because of the lack of diagnosis.

The initiation and subsequent modification of a cognitive rehabilitative program can depend on many factors—the prescribed medications (or nonprescribed substances), the emotional lability of the patient, the severity of the impairment and its stability, any developing conditions, the mental aptitude of the patient, and the possibility of litigation.[110] Therefore, what should be the approach of the rehabilitation program? Should it be to optimize residual function through visual strategies or explore other alternatives through nonvisual strategies? Should the intact areas of the brain be asked to take over for the injured ones?[103] Should we be trying to improve defective skills or training new ones?

Gresham[17] states that an essential goal of rehabilitation is to preserve as much prestroke function as possible. Then reeducating the patient[104] in those remaining deficits that are of greatest functional need must follow. Rehabilitation may use approaches such as redevelopment of lost functions or reeducation of the patient to adapt existing functions to achieve a greater degree of independence. Traditional cognitive rehabilitation methods attempt to direct treatment toward the altered behavior or process. However, Stern and Stern[111] suggest using the principle of compensation. Their premise is not to enhance an already intact area (direct approach) but rather to utilize undamaged areas to reach or bypass the damaged connection (indirect approach). Their focus is on abilities already used by the patient.

Luria (as reported by Bracy[112]) felt that basic processes make up complex function systems that yield observable behaviors and the regaining of complex behaviors would be more easily attained through the treatment of basic processes. Rehabilitation attempts to retrain an existing process, or teach a new one if the existing process is untrainable. The retraining involves using repetitive exercises for skills that are impaired. It is crucial that the impaired skill be adequately pinpointed with selected exercises that progress in a sequential fashion. Hierarchy of progression is key. Theories concerned with the development of human cognition and behavior have evolved as a result of the work of Piaget (cited by Bracy[112]). However, it cannot be assumed that the pathological regression of behavior as seen with cerebral injury is a reverse of Piaget's cognitive developmental model. It may be difficult or even impossible to access a compromised function; and in these cases (such as with right hemisphere injury) it may be necessary to develop strategies that utilize left brain function to compensate for the impairment. Because the left brain region is more analytical and language oriented in nature,[95] research into methods of enhancing the rehabilitation process has been looking at ways to use parallel processes in reciprocal directions. An example of a parallel process would be the verbal/visual pathway, and a goal would be to reeducate the patient to visualize something through verbal description of it.

Success throughout the rehabilitation program should be in terms not of full restoration of function but of the progress a patient has made toward achieving his or her full potential.

The Rehabilitation Team

Because of the specificity of the brain, many professions have evolved subspecialty areas to handle its care. It is not uncommon for these professions to exhibit a great deal of overlap of duties and services. The rehabilitation team is generally medically based in nature, consisting of physicians, psychologists, neurologists, and neuropsychologists; but it also contains cognitive rehabilitation specialists, physical therapists, occupational therapists, speech pathologists, and several other disciplines. Duties specific to each member of the team[103] are listed in Table 4-11.

TABLE 4-11
The Rehabilitation Team

Neurologist	Evaluates the medical integrity of the body's neurological systems
Neuropsychologist	Evaluates behavior and higher cognitive functions of the body's neurological systems; this is a relatively new field that tends to approach the brain and cerebral function as a whole and not as separate systems; neuropsychologists routinely provide evaluations for children and adults with impairments as a result of head trauma, stroke, brain tumors, cerebrovascular accidents, chronic psychological disorders, and chemical poisoning or toxicity; also children who suffer from oxygen deprivation at birth, learning disabilities, mental retardation, and genetic disorders would benefit from a neuropsychological evaluation
Physician	Evaluates and manages systemic disease or disorders that have led to and or resulted from the cerebral injury
Cognitive rehabilitation therapist	Provides treatment designed to remedy disorders of perception, memory, and language in cerebral-injured patients
Physical therapist	Treats physical disabilities by the use of natural forces (electrical, hydrodynamic, pneumatic, mechanical, and light therapy), massage, and regulated therapeutic exercises
Occupational therapist	Provides training and rehabilitation of physical disability through the use of creative avocational or vocational activities involving both mental and physical capabilities
Psychologist	Assesses and treats disturbances of mental, emotional, and behavioral function as well as those due to cerebral injury
Speech pathologist	Assesses and treats speech mechanics and basic organization
Optometrist	Primary role is vision care; purpose on the rehabilitation team is to provide the other disciplines with a baseline status of visual system function; prescribes and monitors all optical devices, integrating visual efficiency and perceptual enhancement programs with programs developed by the occupational therapist, physical therapist, speech pathologist, and cognitive rehabilitation therapist

A 1984 survey by *Cognitive Rehabilitation* noted that the percentages of rehabilitation facilities employing psychologists, occupational therapists, speech pathologists, and recreational therapists were 85, 80, 78, and 57, respectively. Cognitive rehabilitation is the interdisciplinary or multidisciplinary use of physicians, physical therapists, occupational therapists, recreational therapists, psychologists, neurologists, cognitive rehabilitation specialists, speech pathologists, audiologists, psychosocial counselors, and professionals from several other disciplines.[113]

The content of the programs offered can differ in scope—from simple body stimulation[44] to computerized treatment exercises.[72,112] The program can be administered at independent rehabilitation centers, nursing homes, and intensive care wards and as home-based services.[17] With such variation it is not uncommon for a patient's needs to be overlooked or receive little attention with regard to cognitive therapy or counseling support for family members. Patients and their family often equate rehabilitation with *restoration* (as in cuts and bruises). However, cognitive rehabilitation should be viewed not as restoring but as retraining and relearning. Even with the most advanced of rehabilitation programs, many patients do not return to complete preinjury status.[112]

With visual disturbances as a result of cerebral injury, it can be difficult to use vision as the brain's principal sensory modality.[114] Traditional medical therapy for visual dysfunctions has generally been with one of four approaches[105]: surgery, spectacles with prism, total occlusion of one eye, or no treatment.

Many times patients with visual impairment are told that nothing more can be done. They are left to learn to live with their limitations.[68] Even with the minimum research that has been done in the visual treatment of cerebral-injured patients, however, we should not deprive them of a more independent existence.[105]

The optometric intervention should have as its goal to increase the clarity and brightness of visual acuity, eliminate diplopia, improve awareness and cognitive function,[12] and enhance performance of vision-related abilities so the highest quality of life and independent functioning will be maintained. This can be achieved with separate prescription eye wear for distance or near, prismatic correction or compensation, selective occlusion for specific distances, magnification or enhancement through low vision devices and techniques, vision therapy, impact-resistant lenses, or absorptive filters.[20]

In-office optometric management may at times be prohibitively difficult. Therefore, involvement with a rehabilitation facility can promote greater access for and to patients. In addition, it will provide the necessary interaction among all members of the rehabilitation team.

Treatment Options

Lenses

The providing of correction for refractive errors to improve acuity is always of significant concern, especially with this population. Patients who have been in automobile accidents may lose their prescription eye wear at the time of injury. Spectacles can be lost in a hospital stay, or the patient may have forgotten to wear his or her correction because of newly acquired cognitive deficits. Appropriate prescription lenses for the correction of distance vision are the foundation of therapy for these persons, with near-point needs assessed next. Special attention should be given to prescribing near-point lenses for people working with computers, which are routinely used in cognitive rehabilitation programs. Either bifocal or single-vision reading lenses should be fabricated of impact-resistant material such as polycarbonate, polystyrene, or CR-39. With ground-in prism above 2 prism diopters ($\triangle$) it is best to have the lenses made up in CR-39 since this is optically more stable than polycarbonate.[115]

It needs to be emphasized that lenses should not be prescribed based on acuity alone.[105] Padula et al.[56] noted that with the appropriate combination of lenses and/or prisms, muscle spasticity decreased and posture improved. The authors found that motor abilities also were positively affected. These observations necessitate a dynamic evaluation of the patient while sitting, standing, and moving.

Prisms: use of ground-in or Fresnel

Neutralizing prisms for patients with noncomitant strabismus can provide single binocular vision when the head is held straight; but as the eyes move from primary gaze, diplopia may occur because of underacting or overacting extraocular muscles. This will limit the field of single comfortable binocular vision. Even with a compensatory head tilt or turn, some prism may be needed to neutralize any residual deviation or provide additional comfort. It is not mandatory that spectacles correct for a deviation at all distances, however. Patients with a noncomitant deviation may require more than one pair of spectacles for different distances. Prismatic amounts generally not exceeding 8 to 10 $\triangle$ can be fabricated in the form of ground-in lenses. Fresnel prisms may be used in higher amounts. Sectors of Fresnel prism can be cut and placed to compensate for the varying deviations in different positions of gaze. Frequently both horizontal and vertical prisms, or even a resultant oblique neutralizing prism, will be prescribed.[65]

CLINICAL PEARL

Patients with a noncomitant deviation may require more than one pair of spectacles for different distances.

Neutralizing prisms may also be used with patient to compensate for an exo shift in their phoric posture. Customarily, small amounts of base-in prism (1, 2, or 3 △ per eye) are all that are needed to provide tremendous binocular relief. The amount of prism should not be considered part of the permanent correction. Rather it is used to relieve visual stress and facilitate performance in a vision therapy or cognitive rehabilitation program.

A study by Kohler[116] found the following to be true:

1. Acceptance improves with prisms worn for longer than for shorter periods.
2. Weak prism amounts allow for better acceptance than strong prism amounts.
3. Children are more accepting of prism correction than adults.

Prisms (Fig. 4-18) geometrically distort light more than any other lens form. Both glass and resin prisms produce nonuniform (asymmetrical) magnification throughout the visual field. The image is relatively larger toward the base than toward the apex. The apex and base, in particular, distort light more noticeably than the center. The apex of a prism shows a minus cylindrical effect, resulting in with-motion when rotated. It projects an image away and is said to contract space. The base shows a plus cylindrical effect, resulting in an against-motion when rotated and projects an image closer. It is said to expand space.[117] Straight lines bow toward the base and away from the apex, which effect can be reduced by fabricating prescriptions with a relatively steeper base curve (that is, +9.00 △).[118]

Yoked prisms (bases in the same direction—that is, base right, base left, base up, base down) may be used for several therapeutic purposes. They can shift the patient's visual environment toward the field of gaze where a deviation is least, as in a noncomitant strabismus[65]; they can also influence accommodative and convergence relationships along with ambient relationships. The amount of prism prescribed is based on the change in performance of visual/motor and peripheral awareness abilities.[105] Many times yoked prisms will improve accommodation and vergence abilities without needing any or as much vision therapy. This is due to the greater balance that is achieved within the visual system. Prisms used in this fashion will also present a unique set of perceptual distortions. Vertically yoked prisms have been said to either expand or contract one's perceptual environment. Base-up prisms make objects appear nearer and smaller; base-down prisms make them appear farther away and larger. Base-out prisms induce an increased curvature of the field (pin cushion); base-in prisms tend to reduce or flatten it (barrel).[119] Whenever prisms are used, the patient and others involved should be informed of the associated perceptual distortions that may be experienced.

Field awareness

Numerous optical devices can be utilized to assist the cerebral-injured patient manifesting a visual field loss. Fresnel prisms, mirrors attached

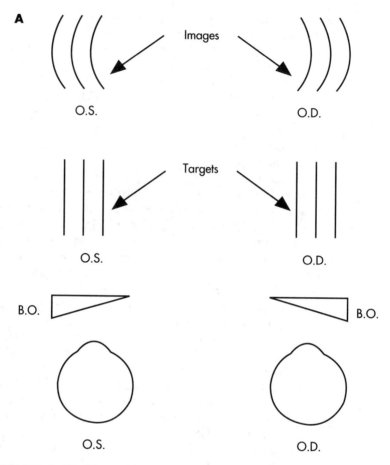

FIGURE 4-18 Nonuniform magnification. **A,** Images and targets.
Continued.

to the spectacle frame, wide-angle lenses, and reverse telescopes are commonly used to help achieve a greater awareness of the missing hemifield. Fresnel prisms act as simple alerting devises that compel the patient to explore the absent field. Placement begins by taking half a prism membrane and placing it temporally on the same side as the hemianopia, with the base toward the defect, approximately 2 mm from the center of the pupil.[120] This is to avoid interfering with macular vision. The patient is then instructed to scan into the prism, at which point a small portion of the missing hemifield will shift into view. The patient should not stare through the prism continuously, but should use it only as a spotting device.

Mirrors are sometimes used for field awareness on the blind side. The angle between the front surface of the lens and the mirror

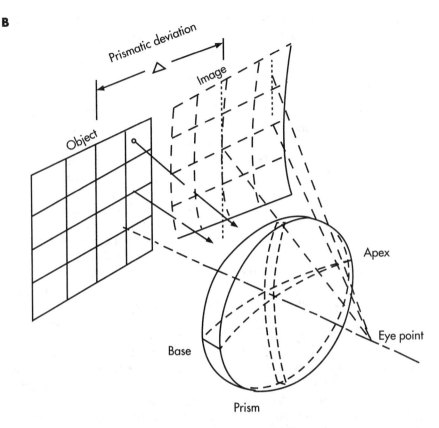

FIGURE 4-18, Cont'd. B, Distortion of the image of an extended object by an ophthalmic prism.

measures about 35°, depending on the severity of impairment. The mirror is utilized not for reading but for orientation and mobility.[50,121,122] A notable concern with it is that whatever is viewed will be reversed.

Patients who exhibit a homonymous hemianopia can improve their reading ability by simply rotating the material 45° to 90° and reading on a slant or vertically.[50] For the patient with a left hemianopia the most benefit can come from rotating the text leftward (reading down to up). Patients who have a right hemianopia will do better rotating the text to the right (reading up to down). In both situations the text that has already been read should be moved into the blind field; this will allow the deficit to act as a sort of typoscope.

Patients who experience central vision loss can benefit from low vision aids, to increase the angle that the image subtends. It is hoped that this larger image will stimulate intact neuroretinal tissue. Hand and stand magnifiers as well as high-plus spectacle lenses are recommended for near tasks whereas telescopic aids will assist with far and intermediate tasks. Nonoptical aids (such as a typoscope) will help the patient with pacing, which stabilizes tracking. It will also reduce the crowding effect of text by minimizing the extraneous "visual noise."

Occlusion: full, partial, or graded

Patching of an eye can provide immediate relief to the visual system hampered by diplopia or a binocular vision dysfunction. However, long-term use of total occlusion of an eye must be weighed against the costs of reduced binocular vision and peripheral information input. Additional considerations to be addressed are the reduction of visual field awareness and the disruption of spatial information. If diplopia cannot be eliminated with normal fusion, prisms, or the aid of vision therapy, then occlusion should be explored. However, the use of lens and/or prism combinations must be carefully weighed against total occlusion before any action is undertaken.[56] Cosmetically acceptable selective occlusion methods include transparent and stippled nail polish or a Bangerter Occlusion Foil or Clin Patch Occluder.[65] It would be preferable for the patient to use occlusion only as needed and not to embark on a full-time wearing schedule. Options for occlusion therapy are diagrammed in Figure 4-19.

Binasal tapes for occlusion are often used to encourage simultaneous peripheral awareness. They provide an orientation point that serves to anchor the visual system as the patient attempts to decipher an unstable visual environment.[105,123] They act similarly to yoked prisms, in that they force the patient to be more aware of and use the peripheral environment. With central fusion disrupted by a cerebral injury, it can be a relief to the visual system to be able to rely on peripheral vision for stability and fusion.[123,124]

Monovision contact lenses[125] can be used for minimizing diplopia. Traditional monovision techniques are utilized with one eye blurred for near and the other for far. The inequality in retinal image clarity is the factor that reduces the diplopia awareness by helping the patient learn to ignore the blurred image.

Cycloplegia, which is a modified form of the monovision technique, can be used on the distance eye of a prepresbyopic cerebral-injured patient to keep that eye from competing with the other for near tasks.

Instead of occlusion, if diplopia is present an inverse prism can be used to create a greater separation of the diplopic images, which will be more easily ignored.[125] Occlusion methods are listed in Table 4-12.

Dry eye therapy

For patients with reduced blink rates or lagophthalmos, artificial tears or ointments are routinely prescribed. For more involved cases, bandage contact lenses or punctal occlusion may be necessary to maintain comfort and optimum corneal integrity.

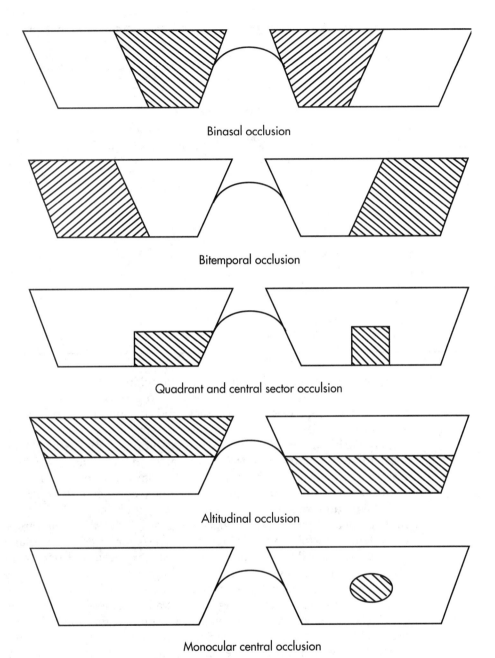

Binasal occlusion

Bitemporal occlusion

Quadrant and central sector occulsion

Altitudinal occlusion

Monocular central occlusion

FIGURE 4-19 Selective occlusion techniques.

Vision enhancement therapy

The modification of traditional vision therapy procedures or the design of new techniques is the goal in assisting cerebral-injured patients to better process visual information. It is not uncommon for

TABLE 4-12
Occlusion

Types
Full/partial
Opaque/graded (penalization)

Methods
Slip-over or strap style
Stick-on
Opticlude–Micropore—sticks best, with less irritation
Coverlet—cloth stick-on
Spectacle lens modification
Nail polish stippled on lens
Fine sand paper to lens surface
Scotch Magic Tape
Original Scotch Transparent Tape
Atropinization
Overcorrection—contact lens or spectacle lens
Filters/tints
Occluder foils
Binasal/bitemporal

progress and change to be slow in this population. Vision therapy is prescribed to reduce the effort necessary to process visual information; it also improves the accuracy and flexibility of the visual system.[106]

Large-angle monocular calisthenics (as proposed by Griffin[126]) are used to restore muscle action in the affected eye. They also help prevent secondary contracture or adhesions of a paretic muscle (noncomitant strabismus) acquired secondary to cerebral injury. They are designed to force the eye to move, with emphasis on the affected muscle's field of action. The unaffected eye is occluded while the paretic eye attempts to follow a moving object. All fields of gaze, especially those most affected by the paretic muscle, are explored. The documentation of results will aid in monitoring progress.[65]

Fusion therapy should be initiated in real space as opposed to instrumental space. The viewing distance and position of gaze where fusion meets the least resistance are the optimum beginning point and are established by having the patient turn toward the most affected action field, which moves the eyes away from the field where fusion exists. The goal is then to work toward the positions of gaze where fusion is least stable or absent. With the various techniques a patient can then move his head and thus force the eyes into different positions of gaze. The patient is asked to be aware of and to emphasize any changes other than the desired ones.[127] A realistic goal or end result for therapy may not be single clear, comfortable, binocular vision at all distances; rather, it may be fusion free of diplopia out of instrument yet with suppression or diplopia in instrument.

Vision therapy must also emphasize the need for adequate assessment and training of specifics within the fusional system. Higher fusional abilities (such as peripheral and central second- and third-degree fusion as well as luster) must be evaluated and emphasized with all fusional therapy. Sequencing should proceed from large peripheral objects (more easily fused) to smaller central ones. Large stereoscopic targets will provide a strong fusion lock, because they stimulate more peripheral retinal areas (paramacular and perimacular). This is generally better for initiating fusion therapy than would be the case using smaller stereoscopic targets (which stimulate only the central retina).[65] Feedback should always be provided to the patient. Since suppression is not usually present within this population, the diplopia that a patient experiences may at times actually prove to be a positive rehabilitation tool (awareness of when fusion is lost). Throughout the treatment program it is imperative that the patient be given constant error-correcting feedback.[80] All procedures should be performed with the patient wearing the proposed distance prescription.[65]

Cohen and Soden[68] advocate a five-phase fusion therapy regimen for patients with cerebral injury:

1. Bicircuit awareness
2. Controlled superimposition
3. Controlled fusional awareness
4. Fusional facility
5. Dynamic fusional development

These are also known as *monocular in a binocular field training,*[127] and they allow the patient to compare what each eye sees. Techniques utilize both eyes open and seeing one object. The object is so constructed that each eye shares some common details, but each eye also sees certain details visible only to it; thus better feedback is provided to the patient and clinician regarding whether and under what conditions the patient can use binocular vision.

The next skill area addressed is accommodation. It is not uncommon for both ocular motility and accommodation to proceed concurrently. Accommodation also progresses in sequence: monocular to biocular abilities. Later in therapy, accommodation is integrated with the vergence system during the integration phase. This involves using minus lenses while stimulating base-in vergence and plus lenses with base-out vergence (BIM/BOP). In each of the accommodation phases work begins by building maximum amplitudes while emphasizing speed, accuracy, stamina, and sustainability. It is only after completion of this that work on facility (flexibility) can begin. Emphasis to the patient should be on the importance of becoming aware of any associated feelings (that is, awareness of size and distance changes) throughout the program. For a patient to move on to the next level, it is necessary that the current technique be correctly demonstrated and its purpose and overall goals completely understood. Emphasis on the awareness of contrasting "feeling tones" experienced while performing the techniques provides feedback and aids in accelerating success in the program.

Vergence therapy has fewer phases, with only a binocular and an integration (BIM/BOP) phase. The sequence proceeds from using peripheral stereoscopic targets to using central stereoscopic targets to using peripheral flat fusion targets. Goals for the vergence system also begin with range extension (that is, building amplitudes first) while emphasizing perceptual awarenesses of silo, float, localization, parallax, and physiological diplopia during performance. It is not until these are attained that facility/flexibility (recoveries) through look-aways or jump vergences can begin.

Visual/perceptual therapy

Training of the integrative/analytical abilities of a patient begins with procedures that address body image and awareness (laterality/directionality). Next, visual/spatial orientations and, finally, object recognition and construction are explored. Therapy for the highest of cognitive functions involves abstraction skills. Survivors of cerebral injury have difficulty abstracting on either a verbal or a nonverbal level. This can be seriously disabling. Techniques to correct nonverbal abstraction involve the construction of block designs. Initial work begins with simple two-block two-dimensional designs and progresses to multiple-block three-dimensional patterns.[99] Sources of additional perceptual and cognitive therapy techniques and materials can be found in several texts.[102,128,129]

Computer-assisted cognitive rehabilitation (CACR)[130,131] utilizes specially designed software programs (SoftTools) that are compatible with Apple, Atari, and IBM computers or clones. This makes them suitable for use by cerebral-injured patients, who can participate in as much as 20 to 30 hours of self-directed or family-directed therapy per week (compared to 3 hours of patient/therapist therapy). The programs aid in reorganizing foundation skills and reeducating the patient in visual/spatial, conceptual, memory-retention, and problem-solving skills.[110]

Summary and Conclusions

The minimum that any optometrist can do for this population is provide appropriate prescriptions for distance and near and minimize if not correct diplopia.[11] Optometrists with the desire and ability to offer more should do so within the limits of their licensure. The value of the input that optometrists can provide patients, families, and other members of the rehabilitation team is immeasurable. Every effort should be made to inform all involved parties of these visual recommendations and prescription to optimize the benefits that can be gained.

REFERENCES

1. Engum ES, Lambert EW, Scott K: Criterion-related validity of the cognitive behavioral driver's inventory: brain-injured patients versus normal controls, *Cogn Rehabil* 2:20-26, 1990.
2. Direnfeld G: Traumatic brain injury and case management, *Cogn Rehabil* 5:20-24, 1990.
3. Baker R, Epstein A: Ocular motor abnormalities from head trauma, *Surv Ophthalmol* 35:245-267, 1991.
4. Zinman D: The dilemma of head injuries, *Newsday* March 18, 1986, 1-7.
5. Kent T, Hart M, Shries T: Introduction to human disease, New York, 1979, Appleton-Century-Crofts.
6. Report on national head and spinal surgery conducted for NINCDS, *J Neurosurg* (Suppl) S1-S43, 1980.
7. Alexander L: Pre-stroke signs and symptoms, *Rev Optom* 8:45-53, 1979.
8. Shokunbi T, Agbeja A: Ocular complications of head injury in children, *Child Nerv Syst* 7:147-149, 1991.
9. Cope DN, Hall K: Head injury rehabilitation: benefit of early intervention, *Arch Phys Med Rehabil* 63:433-437, 1982.
10. Ben-Yishay Y, Diller L: Rehabilitation of cognitive and perceptual defects in people with traumatic brain damage, *Int J Rehabil Res* 4:208-210, 1981.
11. Gianutsos R, Ramsey G, Perlin RR: Rehabilitative optometric services for survivors of acquired brain injury, *Arch Phys Med Rehabil* 69:573-578, 1988.
12. Kadet TS: Vision rehabilitation in traumatic brain injury. In *Essays on vision*, Santa Ana Calif, 1990, Optometric Extension Program Foundation, 13-20.
13. United States Department of Health and Human Services: Head injury: hope through research, Bethesda Md, 1984, National Institutes of Health.
14. Bennett T: Use of the Halstead-Reitan neuropsychological test battery in the assessment of head injury, *Cogn Rehabil* 3:18-24, 1988.
15. Weinber J, Diller L, Gordan WA: Training sensory awareness and spatial organization in people with right brain damage, *Arch Phys Med Rehabil* 60:491-496, 1979.
16. Savir H, Michelson I, David C, et al: Homonymous hemianopsia and rehabilitation in fifteen cases of C.C.I., *Scand J Rehabil Med* 9:151-153, 1977.
17. Gresham G: The rehabilitation of the stroke survivor. In Barnett H, et al (eds): *Stroke: pathophysiology*, diagnosis, and management, vol 2, New York, 1986, Churchill Livingstone, 1259-1274.
18. Mesalam L: The power of communication, *Cogn Rehabil* 3:32-36, 1988.
19. Freeman P, D'Elja D, Nepps P: Differential diagnosis and treatment of frank neurological damage: a case report, *J Am Optom Assoc* 53:905-907, 1982.
20. Tierney DW: Visual dysfunction in closed head injury, *J Am Optom Assoc* 59:614-622, 1988.
21. Gennarelli T: Mechanisms and pathophysiology of cerebral concussion, *J Head Trauma Rehabil* 1:23-29, 1968.
22. Symonds C: Concussion and its sequelae, *Lancet* 1:1-5, 1962.
23. Davidoff DA, Kessler HR, Laibstain DF, Mark VH: Neurobehavioral sequelae of minor head injury: a consideration of post-concussive syndrome versus post-traumatic stress disorder, *Cogn Rehabil* 2:8-13, 1988.

24. Begali V: *Head injury in children and adolescents: a resource and review for school and allied professionals,* Brandon, Vt, 1987, Clinical Psychological Publishing.
25. Ruesch J: Dark adaptation, negative after images, tachistoscopic examinations, and reaction time in head injuries, *J Neurosurg* 1:243-251, 1944.
26. Hayden M, Hart T: Rehabilitation of cognitive and behavioral dysfunction in head injury, *Adv Psychosom Med* 16:194-229, 1986.
27. Kelley R: Cerebrovascular disease. In Weiner W, Goetz C (eds): *Neurology for the non-neurologist,* ed 2, Philadelphia, 1989, JB Lippincott, 52-66.
28. Muir B: *Pathophysiology: an introduction to the mechanisms of disease,* New York, 1980, John Wiley & Sons.
29. Lyle WM, Williams TD: Clues to cerebrovascular insufficiencies, *J Am Optom Assoc* 52:809-811, 1981.
30. Kelly J, Hutner-Winograd C: A functional approach to stroke management in elderly patients, *J Am Geriatr Soc* 33:48-60, 1985.
31. Wolff E (ed): *Anatomy of the eye and orbit,* Philadelphia, 1976, WB Saunders, Chapter 8.
32. De Renzi E, Zambolin A, Crisi G: The pattern of neuropsychological impairment associated with left posterior cerebral artery infarcts, *Brain* 110:1099-1116, 1987.
33. Martin J: *Neuroanatomy: text and atlas,* New York, 1989, Elsevier Science Publishing.
34. Gruzzman M: Reversal operation after brain damage, *Brain Cogn* 1:331-354, 1982.
35. Stein DG, Rosen, JJ, Butter N: *Plasticity and recovery of function in the central nervous system,* New York, 1974, Academic Press.
36. Rothi LJ, Horner J: Restitution and substitution: two theories of recovery with application to neurobehavioral treatment, *J Clin Neuropsychol* 5:73-81, 1983.
37. Gianutsos R, Matheson P: The rehabilitation of visual perceptual disorders attributable to brain injury. In *Neuropsychological rehabilitation,* New York, 1987, Churchill Livingstone.
38. Marshall JF: Brain function: neural adaptations and recovery from injury, *Annu Rev Psychol* 35:277-308, 1984.
39. Bach-y-Rita P: Central nervous system lesions: sprouting and unmasking in rehabilitation, *Arch Phys Med Rehabil* 62:413-417, 1981.
40. Weinberg J, Diller L, Gordon WA: Visual scanning training effect on reading-related tasks in acquired brain damage, *Arch Phys Med Rehabil* 58:479-486, 1977.
41. Solan HA: A rationale for the optometric treatment and management of children with learning disabilities, *Optom Month* 12:10-15, 1981.
42. Matzke H, Foltz F: *Synopsis of neuroanatomy,* ed 4, New York, 1983, Oxford University Press.
43. Farber S: A multisensory approach to rehabilitation. In Farber S (ed): *Neurorehabilitation: a multisensory approach,* Philadelphia, 1982, WB Saunders, 115-123.
44. Padula W, Shapiro J: *Post-trauma vision syndrome caused by head injury: a behavioral vision approach for persons with physical disabilities,* Santa Ana, Calif, 1988, Optometric Extension Program Foundation, Inc., 1988.
45. Holtzman JD: Interactions between cortical and subcortical visual areas: Evidence from human commissurotomy patients, *Vision Res* 24:801-813, 1984.
46. Marx P: Supratentorial structures controlling oculomotor functions and their involvement in cases of stroke, *Eur Arch Psychiatry Neurol Sci* 239:3-8, 1989.
47. Warren M: Identification of visual scanning deficits in adults after cerebrovascular accident, *Am J Occup Ther* 44:391-399, 1990.

48. Trobe JR, Bauer RM: Seeing but not recognizing, *Surv Ophthalmol* 30:328-336, 1986.
49. Grüsser O-J, Landis T: Visual agnosias and other disturbances of visual perception and cognition. In Cronly-Dillon J (ed): *Vision and visual dysfunction*, Boca Raton, Fla, 1991 CRC Press, 12.
50. Walsh F, Hoyt W, Miller N: *Clinical neuro-ophthalmology*, ed 4, Baltimore, 1982, Williams & Wilkins.
51. Schneider GE: Two visual systems, *Am J Optom Physiol Opt* 163:895-902, 1969.
52. Trevarthen CB: Two mechanisms of vision in primates, *Psychol Forsch* 31:299-337, 1968.
53. Post R, Leibowitz HW: Two modes of processing visual information: implications for assessing visual impairment, *Am J Optom Physiol Opt* 63:94-96, 1986.
54. Cogan D: Ophthalmic manifestations of bilateral non-occipital cerebral lesions, *Br J Ophthalmol* 49:281-297, 1965.
55. Stein J: Representation of egocentric space in the posterior parietal cortex, *Q J Exp Physiol* 74:583-606, 1989.
56. Padula WV, Shapiro JB, Jasin P: Head injury causing post trauma vision syndrome, *N Engl J Optom* 12:16-21, 1988.
57. Trevarthen C, Sperry RW: Perceptual unity of the ambient visual field in human commissurotomy patients, *Brain* 96:547-570, 1973.
58. Leibowitz HW, Post RB: The two modes of processing concept and some implications. In Beck J (ed): *Organization and representation in perception*, Hillside, NJ, 1982, Lawrence Erlbaum Associates, 387.
59. Harrington DO, Drake MV: *The visual field: textbook and atlas of clinical perimetry*, ed 6, St Louis, 1990, Mosby.
60. Falke P, Abela BM Jr, Krakau CE, et al: High frequency of asymptomatic visual field defect, *J Intern Med* 229:521-525, 1991.
61. Krohel GB, Kristan RW, Simon JW, Barrows NA: Postraumatic convergence insufficiency, *Ann Ophthalmol* 18:101-104, 1986.
62. Stanworth A: Defects of ocular movement and fusion after head injury, *Br J Ophthalmol* 58:266-271, 1974.
63. Cohen M, Groswasser Z, Barchadski R, Appel A: Convergence insufficiency in brain-injured patients, *Brain Inj* 3:187-191, 1989.
64. Carroll RP, Seaber JH: Acute loss of fusional convergence following head trauma, *Am Orthop* 57-59, 1974.
65. Birnbaum MH: Noncomitant strabismus: evaluation and management, *J Am Optom Assoc* 55:758-764, 1984.
66. London R, Scott SH: Sensory fusion disruption syndrome, *J Am Optom Assoc* 58:544-546, 1987.
67. Pratt-Johnson JA, Tillson G: The loss of fusion in adults with intractable diplopia (central fusion disruption), *Aust NZ J Ophthalmol* 16:81-85, 1988.
68. Cohen AH, Soden R: An optometric approach to the rehabilitation of the stroke patient, *J Am Optom Assoc* 52:795-800, 1981.
69. Thompson NM, Ewing-Cobbs L, Fletcher JM, et al: Left unilateral neglect in a pre-school child, *Dev Med Child Neurol* 33:636-644, 1991.
70. Wilson B, Cockburn J, Halligan P: Development of a behavioral test of visuospatial neglect, *Arch Phys Med Rehabil* 68:98-102, 1987.
71. Perenin MT, Jeannerod M: Residual vision in cortically blind hemifields, *Neuropsychologia* 13:1-7, 1975.
72. Lynch J, McLaren J: Deficits of visual attention and saccadic eye movements after lesions of parietooccipital cortex in monkeys, *J Neurophysiol* 61:74-90, 1989.
73. Halligan P, Marshall J, Wade D: Visual field deficits after brain injury: Do visual field deficits exacerbate visuo-spatial neglect? *J Neurol Neurosurg Psychiatry* 53:487-491, 1990.

74. Gianutsos R: Computerized screening, *J Behav Optom* 2:143-150, 1991.
75. Cubelli R, Nichelli P, Bonito V, et al: Different patterns of dissociation in unilateral spatial neglect, *Brain Cogn* 15:139-159, 1991.
76. Albert ML: A simple test of visual neglect, *Neurology* 23:658-664, 1973.
77. Vallar G, Perani D: The anatomy of unilateral neglect after right hemisphere stroke lesions: a clinical/CT scan correlation study in man, *Neuropsychologia* 24:609-622, 1986.
78. Shelton P, Bowers D, Heilman K: Peripersonal and vertical neglect, *Brain* 113:191-205, 1990.
79. Halligan PW, Marshall JC: Left neglect for near but not far space in man, *Nature* 350:498-500, 1991.
80. Gordon WA, Ruckdeschel-Hibbard M, Egelko S, et al: Perceptual remediation in patients with right brain damage: a comprehensive program, *Arch Phys Med Rehabil* 66:353-359, 1985.
81. Kaizer F, Korner-Bitensky N, Mayo N, et al: Response time of stroke patients to a visual stimulus, *Stroke* 19:335-339, 1988.
82. Friedman PJ: Spatial neglect in acute stroke: the line bisection test, *Scand J Rehabil Med* 22:101-106, 1990.
83. Stone S, Wilson B, Clifford-Rose F: The development of a standard test battery to detect, measure and monitor visuo-spatial neglect in patients with acute stroke, *Int J Rehabil Res* 10:110, 1987.
84. Halligan PW, Wilson B, Cockburn J: A short screening test for visual neglect in stroke patients, *Int Disabil Stud* 12:95-99, 1990.
85. Halligan P, Marshall J, Wade D: Visuospatial neglect: underlying factors and test sensitivity, *Lancet* 2:908-911, 1989.
86. Bisiach E, Bulgarelli C, Sterzi R, Vallar G: Line bisection and cognitive plasticity of unilateral neglect of space, *Brain Cogn* 2:32-38, 1983.
87. Bender M, Teubr H: Spatial organization of visual perception following injury to the brain, *Arch Neurol Psychiatr* 58:721-739, 1947; 59:39-62, 1959.
88. Butter CM, Evans J, Kirsch N, Kewman D: Altitudinal neglect following traumatic brain injury: a case report, *Cortex* 25:135-146, 1989.
89. Rapcsak S, Cimino D, Heilman K: Altitudinal neglect, *Neurology* 38:277-281, 1988.
90. Halligan PW, Marshall JC: Figural modulation of visuo-spatial neglect: a case study, *Neuropsychologia* 29:619-628, 1991.
91. Ishiai S, Furukawa T, Tsukagoshi H: Visuospatial processes of line bisection and the mechanisms underlying unilateral spatial neglect, *Brain* 112:1485-1502, 1989.
92. Anton HA, Hershler C, Lloyd P, Murray D: Visual neglect and extinction: a new test, *Arch Phys Med Rehabil* 69:1013-1016, 1988.
93. Ishiai S, Sugishita M, Odajima N, et al: Improvement of unilateral spatial neglect with numbering, *Neurology* 40:1395-1398, 1990.
94. Riddoch MJ, Humphreys GW: The effect of cueing on unilateral neglect, *Neuropsychologia* 21:589-599, 1983.
95. Wouters B: "I don't see it so it must be to my left": Rehabilitation of visuospatially impaired adults, *J Vis Impair Blindness* 3:118-119, 1987.
96. Gianutsos R, Klitzner C: *Computer program for cognitive rehabilitation,* Bayport, NY, 1981, Life Science Associates.
97. Weintraub S, Mesulam MM: Visual hemispatial inattention: stimulus parameters and exploratory strategies, *J Neurol Neurosurg Psychiatry* 51:1481-1488, 1988.
98. Reitan RM, Wolfson D: The Halstead-Reitan neuropsychological test battery and REHABIT: a model for integrating evaluation and remediation of cognitive impairment, *Cogn Rehabil* 3:10-17, 1988.
99. Jurko MF, Smith RR: Recent developments in brain rehabilitation, *South Med J* 74:727-730, 1981.

100. Wallack EM: Diagnostic neurologic testing: a guide for patients and their families, *Cogn Rehabil* 5:26-29, 1987.
101. Friedberg ES, Ruskiewicz JP: When stroke threatens here's how and why to evaluate carotid bruit, *Rev Optom* 6:51-57, 1985.
102. Adamovich B, Henderson J, Auerbach S: *Cognitive rehabilitation of closed head injured patients: a dynamic approach*, San Diego, 1985, College-Hill Press.
103. Golden C: Using the Luria-Nebraska neuropsychological examination in cognitive rehabilitation, *Cogn Rehabil* 3:26-30, 1988.
104. Krasnow D: Fusional convergence loss following head trauma: a case report, *Optom Month* 1:18-19, 1982.
105. Berne SA: Visual therapy for the traumatic brain-injured, *J Optom Vis Dev* 21:13-16, 1990.
106. Nagafuchi M: Right unilateral spatial neglect of the left brain-damaged patients, *Tohoku J Exp Med* 161:131-138, 1990.
107. Kwartz J, Leatherbarrow B, Davis H: Diplopia following head injury, *Injury* 21:351-352, 1991.
108. Gianutsos R, Ramsey G: Enabling rehabilitative optometrists to help survivors of acquired brain injury, *J Vis Rehabil* 2(1):37-58, 1988.
109. Bracy O: Computer based cognitive rehabilitation, *Cogn Rehabil* 1:7-8, 18, 1983.
110. Craine JF, Gudeman HE: *The rehabilitation of brain functions: principles, procedures, and techniques of neurotraining*, Springfield, Ill, 1981, Charles C Thomas Publishing.
111. Stern JM, Stern B: Visual imagery as a cognitive means of compensation for brain injury, *Brain Inj* 3:413-419, 1989.
112. Bracy OL: Cognitive rehabilitation: a process approach, *Cogn Rehabil* 4(2):10-17, 1986.
113. Kreutzer J, Coulter S, Lent B, McNeny R: A glossary of cognitive rehabilitation terminology, *Cogn Rehabil* 3:10-13, 1986.
114. Soden R, Cohen AH: An optometric approach to the treatment of a noncomitant deviation, *J Am Optom Assoc* 54:451-454, 1983.
115. Hampton LD, Roth N, Meyer-Arendt JR, Schuman DO: Visual acuity degradation resulting from dispersion in polycarbonate, *J Am Optom Assoc* 62:760-765, 1991.
116. Lienert GA: Subject variables in perception and their controls. In Spillman L, Wooten BR (eds): *Sensory experience, adaptation, and perception*, Hillsdale, NJ, 1984, Lawrence Erlbaum Associates.
117. Forkiotis CJ: The prism: a choice optometric visual training therapy lens, *J Optom Vis Dev* 6(4):6-11, 1975.
118. Brunnett SM, Munson MT, Kirschen DG: Fresnel vs conventional prisms: their effects on the apparent fronto-parallel plane horopter, *Am J Optom Physiol Opt* 65:519-526, 1988.
119. Reading R: Prism-induced horopter distortions, *Ophthalmol Physiol Opt* 5:403-409, 1985.
120. Smith J: New pearls checklist. *J Clin Neuro Ophthalmol* 1981; 1:78.
121. Nooney T Jr: Partial visual rehabilitation of hemianopic patients, *Am J Optom Physiol Opt* 63:382-386, 1986.
122. Goodlaw E: Rehabilitating a patient with bitemporal hemianopia, *Am J Optom Physiol Opt* 59:617-619, 1982.
123. Greenwald I: *Effective strabismus therapy*, Santa Ana, Calif, 1979, Optometric Extension Program Foundation, 121-122.
124. Kaplan M: Vertical yoked prisms. In *Curriculum II, Continuing education courses: Vertical yoked prisms*, vol 51, Santa Ana Calif, 1978, Optometric Extension Program Foundation, 1-12.
125. London R: Monovision correction for diplopia, *J Am Optom Assoc* 58:568-570, 1987.
126. Griffin JR, editor: *Binocular anomalies: Procedures for vision therapy*, ed 2, Chicago, 1982, Professional Press, 277.

127. Cohen AH: Monocular fixation in a binocular field, *J Am Optom Assoc* 52:801-806, 1981.
128. Kreutzer J, Wehman P: *Cognitive rehabilitation for persons with traumatic brain injury: a functional approach,* Baltimore, 1991, Paul H Brookes Publishing.
129. Sohlberg M, Mateer C: *Introduction to cognitive rehabilitation: theory and practice,* New York, 1989, Guilford Press.
130. Jarvis P: The importance of patient friendliness in CACR software and tips for improving it, *Cogn Rehabil* 8:4:24-28, 1990.
131. Purdy M, Neri L: Computer-assisted cognitive rehabilitation in the home, *Cogn Rehabil* 7:34-38, 1989.

5

The Patient with Behavioral Disorders

Janice Emigh Scharre
Sandra Stein Block
Kelly A. Frantz

Key Terms

Behavioral disorders	Pervasive develop-	Pervasive develop-
Emotional disorders	mental disabilities	mental disorders
Attention deficit	Childhood	not otherwise
hyperactivity	schizophrenia	specified
disorder (ADHD)	Autism	(PDDNOS)

Children with behavioral disorders are a challenging and unique population for the optometrist. These behavioral disorders interfere with the primary eye care assessment and may contribute to the visual abnormalities detected. It is important for the eye care provider to understand them and to recognize the effect they can have on the visual system.

It is recognized that behavioral problems often coexist with mental retardation. In addition, the developmentally disabled child is at an increased risk for a wide range of psychiatric disorders.[1] Clinically, we frequently observe children with multiple handicaps, severe to profound mental retardation, and developmental delays who manifest behaviors that mimic the actions seen in children with "behavioral disorders." These may be self-stimulating and repetitive in nature (such as hand flicking, hand waving, light gazing, rocking, or spinning). Occasionally, the children will exhibit self-injurious tendencies (biting and head banging). Visual avoidance behaviors have also been observed. In these cases eye contact is limited or nonexistent or the child appears to actively avoid looking at the stimulus in question. It is important to recognize the behaviors manifested and their association or lack of association with other conditions; for example, not all children who manifest light gazing behavior are autistic. The behavioral disorders discussed in this chapter all have a number of characteristics or symptoms that aid in their differential diagnosis.

Understanding behavioral disorders is complicated by the terminology used to classify and describe the conditions. Since the publication of the third edition of the American Psychiatric Association's *Diagnostic and Statistical Manual of Mental Disorders (DSM-III-R)*, in 1980, psychiatric disturbances have been classified on the basis of descriptive data rather than presumed etiological mechanisms. In the current trend a psychiatric disorder is defined as a cluster of symptoms that occur within an individual and are associated with maladaptive behavior.[2] This chapter will identify and discuss the most frequently encountered behavioral disorders seen in children.

Attention Deficit Hyperactivity Disorder

The hyperactive child syndrome has received considerable focus in the literature during the past 10 to 15 years. It is one of the most common behavioral disorders seen in children. Historically it has been referred to as "hyperkinetic syndrome," "hyperactivity," "minimal brain dysfunction," and "maturational lag." Whereas its definition previously emphasized the hyperactive aspect of the condition, more recently the authors of the *DSM-III-R*[3] have seen fit to give primary status to its attentional problems.

Before the *DSM-III-R* revision,[3] attention deficit disorder had been described as a syndrome with two subtypes—that occurring with hyperactivity and that occurring without. It is currently referred to by the first of these designations or, in other words, as attention deficit hyperactivity disorder, (ADHD). This method of defining the condition was accepted by the American Psychiatric Association in 1987.

ADHD is characterized by three predominant features: impulsiveness, inattentiveness, and in some cases hyperactivity. Barkley[4] states that the prevalence of the condition is 3% to 5% (which would be equivalent to about one child in every classroom). Others[5] have suggested that it affects 10% to 20% of the school-age population. Boys outnumber girls 9:1.[2] ADHD is thought of as a childhood disorder, but recent research suggests the condition may persist into the adult years. Current estimates[4,6] are that about 50% to 65% of ADHD children will continue to manifest symptoms of the disorder into adolescence and adulthood.

A child is diagnosed with ADHD if he/she demonstrates at least 8 of the 14 behaviors listed in the box below. Furthermore, the behaviors must first have been observed before the age of 7 years and have been exhibited for at least 6 months. An affected child between the ages of 8 and 10 years (which are the primary ages for referral) will exhibit a number of signs and symptoms. It is generally assumed that a younger child will present with a greater number of more severe symptoms than an older child.

Diagnostic criteria for attention deficit hyperactivity disorder

A. At least eight of the following behaviors must have been present for at least 6 months

Often fidgets with hands or feet, or squirms in seat (in adolescents, may be limited to subjective feelings of restlessness)

Has difficulty remaining seated when required to do so

Is easily distracted by extraneous stimuli

Has difficulty following through on instructions from others, but not because of oppositional behavior or failure to comprehend directions (for example, fails to complete chores)

Has difficulty sustaining attention in tasks or play activities

Often shifts from one uncompleted activity to another

Has difficulty playing quietly

Often talks excessively

Often interrupts or intrudes on others (for example, butts into other children's games)

Often does not seem to listen to what is being said to him/her

Often loses things necessary for tasks or activities at school or at home (toys, pencils, books, assignments)

Often engages in physically dangerous activities without considering the possible consequences, but not for the purpose of thrill seeking (for example, runs into the street without looking)

B. These behaviors begin before the age of 7 years

Note: A criterion is met only if the behavior occurs more frequently in a child being assessed than in most children of the same mental age.

From American Psychiatric Association: *Diagnostic and statistical manual of mental disorders,* ed 3, Washington DC, 1987, American Psychiatric Association.

Even though the criteria for diagnosing ADHD have changed, the actual characteristics have not. Children with ADHD are usually described as being inattentive. They frequently have a short attention span, difficulty knowing where to attend, or if they know where to attend, no ability to sustain attention. Parents report that the children hear but do not appear to listen, and that they often exhibit problems in following multi-step directions.

Children with ADHD often act without realizing the outcome or consequences of their actions. They react impulsively, with uncontrolled outbursts, and are unable to wait for gratification. In the classroom they may ask frequent questions or shout out responses without waiting to be called upon. Aberrant behaviors (such as tantrums) cannot be adequately controlled.

Some children with ADHD display constant motor activity, whether it be running, jumping, or fidgeting; vocalizations; or the general inability to sit still. They may twirl their hair, click their tongue, or fall out of their chair. The amount of hyperactivity varies among children and may change over time in some children.[7]

The inattentiveness and impulsiveness seen in ADHD children often contribute to a sense of disorganization. They lose their place, cannot find their notebook, and do not know where to begin on an assignment. They are easily frustrated by what they perceive as complex tasks. They often show immature social skills and appear to be overly sensitive, inconsiderate, and unable to accept responsibility.[8]

ADHD has been statistically associated with perinatal complications, brain injury, twins, low birth weight, and a family history of learning problems.[9] Research has suggested that it is genetically transmitted. Zametkin et al.[10] identified a chemical imbalance in subjects with ADHD. Specifically, they found that glucose is used by the brain at a slower rate in subjects identified as ADHD. Recent magnetic resonance imaging studies have found subtle differences in their brain structure compared to nondisabled controls. Hynd et al.[11] noted that, ADHD children's scans were clinically normal with morphometric analysis showing the children to have a smaller corpus callosum. The authors suggested that these subtle deviations in normal corticogenesis might underlie the behavioral characteristics seen in the syndrome. It is now known that ADHD is a neurologically based medical problem, not the result of inadequate parenting or a poor diet.

Treatment for ADHD children has included dietary modifications, educational programming, and pharmacological intervention. The commercially available "cures" or special diets have limited scientific basis and have not been proven effective. Despite the research findings that show little or no effect of food coloring or additives on the behavior of these children, many parents and other adults are convinced of those effects and advocate dietary changes.[12]

The educational programming for a child with ADHD is critical. These children usually have difficulty completing assignments, doing two activities concurrently, attending to the task at hand, functioning at grade level, and working up to potential. It is important for the parent, educator, and other adults involved to be aware of the child's symptoms and how they affect the child in a learning environment. Situations should be structured to allow the child to act appropriately, become successful, and develop self-esteem. The child will need positive reinforcement. It is also important to develop consistent forms of behavior modification, which are carried over to the home setting. The child needs to know the consequences of his actions. The intent is to provide a well-structured environment with the rules, consequences, and expectations clearly explained. Programming is designed to increase appropriate behavior while decreasing negative behaviors.

A significant aspect of treating a child with ADHD is the use of medication. Studies[13] have reported on the success of stimulants in enhancing short-term learning in 25% to 80% of the children with ADHD. The drugs currently used are Ritalin (methylphenidate HCl), Dexedrine (dextroamphetamine sulfate), and Cylert (pemoline), with Ritalin the most widely used medication. Why these stimulant drugs calm and organize the child's behavior is unclear. The drugs are believed to stimulate the brain's neurotransmitters, allowing better regulation of the motor system, attention, and impulsive behavior. In contrast to the short-term improvements in learning and behavior, there is limited information that stimulant medications improve long-term academic achievement.[13] Varley[14] states, "No long-term study has demonstrated that medication alone improves the adaptation of ADHD children." The multimodal model studied by Satterfield et al.[15] of medication, individual educational programs, and appropriate psychotherapy appears to be the most successful documented approach to treating children with attention deficit disorders.

The optometrist should be aware of the possible ocular side effects of these medications. Although rare, Ritalin may cause blurred vision because of a cycloplegic effect.[16,17] It also can produce an allergic reaction of the lids and conjunctiva and, in toxic overdoses, pupillary mydriasis and hallucinations.[17] Dexedrine is known to produce mydriasis, and Cylert may result in nystagmus, oculogyric crises, and mydriasis.[16]

The optometric evaluation is most effective in a structured quiet examination environment; a minimum amount of auditory and visual stimulation is desired. The child should be informed of the next activity and given positive reinforcement of appropriate behavior during the examination. This reinforcement can be as simple as a compliment on "good sitting." The child's inability to attend for any extended period must be recognized, with the examination being completed in two sessions if attention appears to waver.

Children with developmental disabilities and clinical psychiatric syndromes (mental retardation, autism, pervasive developmental disorder, developmental speech and language disorders, anxiety disorders, affective disorders, childhood schizophrenia) can exhibit symptoms of ADHD. The differential diagnosis is based on an early history of motor activity and the fact that the symptoms are not episodic in nature. In some developmental disorders it has not been clearly defined whether there is co-occurrence of true ADHD or whether these behaviors are part of the primary developmental disorder.[18]

Pervasive Developmental Disabilities

Pervasive developmental disorders and childhood schizophrenia are a group of early-onset, severe, neuropsychiatric disorders that were once referred to as childhood psychosis. They are a broad spectrum of dysfunctions, the most severe being autism and the mildest a language-related disorder. Childhood schizophrenia is classified separately.[2] Schizophrenia occurring in childhood is very rare. The most recent edition of the *DSM-III-R* has a slightly different approach to the differentiation of these conditions. It presents "pervasive developmental disorders" which are subdivided into autism (infantile autism) and pervasive developmental disorder not otherwise specified (PDD-NOS). If the criteria for an autistic disorder are met, the additional diagnosis for schizophrenia should be made only when a child manifests delusions and hallucinations.[3] It is important to recognize that the child may have been diagnosed under a previously accepted terminology. The importance for optometry is not in the specific classification but rather in the characteristics and behaviors of each condition.

Autism

Frequently, early signs of autism (delays in social and language development) are unrecognized or mistaken for other conditions (such as deafness, hyperactivity, emotional disturbance, language disorder, or mental retardation).[19] Initially autism was regarded as a psychiatric condition; now it is being considered neurobiological. It is described,[20] however, as a behavioral syndrome characterized by abnormalities in social interaction, communication, and imaginative activity. The diagnosis is usually made by 30 months of age.

Autistic children exhibit atypical or delayed development and atypical responses to sensory stimuli, as well as disorders of communication and social interaction. They may be hypersensitive to touch or sound and have variable activity levels and sensitivities to pain. In all sensory areas, they can demonstrate hyporesponses or hyperresponses.[21,22] The behaviors identified are also observed in children with sensory integration disorders.[23] Autistic children often have unequal developmental profiles (splinter skills), in addition to significant deficits in speech and language development. When speech does develop, it tends to be peculiar with echolalia and unusual word usage (see box below).

Diagnostic Criteria for Autism

A. Impairment in reciprocal social interaction
   Substantial lack of awareness of the feelings or existence of others
   Abnormal or no seeking of comfort
   Impaired or no imitation
   Abnormal or no social play
   Impairment in ability to make peer friends
B. Impairment in verbal and nonverbal communication and in imaginative activity
   No method of communication
   Substantially abnormal nonverbal communication (lack of eye contact, staring, etc.)
   Absence of imaginative play
   Substantial abnormalities in the production of speech (such as pitch and volume)
   Peculiar speech patterns, such as immediate or delayed echolalia and idiosyncratic use of words or phrases ("Go on red riding?" to mean "I want to go on the swing")
   Impairment in initiating or sustaining a conversation with others, even when speech is present
C. Significantly restricted in types of activities and interests
   Stereotyped body movements (such as spinning, hand flapping, or head banging)
   Persistent preoccupation with parts of objects (spinning wheels, escalator railings)
   Extreme responses to small environmental changes (moving of a chair)
   Unreasonable insistence on following a routine, down to the smallest detail
   Restricted range of interests and preoccupation (arranging objects in a line, sorting of puzzle pieces)
D. Onset during infancy or childhood

At least eight of these items must be present—including two from A, one from B, one from C, and one from D.
From American Psychiatric Association: *Diagnostic and statistical manual of mental disorders: DSM-III-R* Washington DC, 1987, American Psychiatric Association.

Autism occurs in four to five individuals per 10,000. It is estimated that there are currently 90,000 to 110,000 autistic individuals in the United States. The disorder occurs four times more frequently in boys than girls.[24] Ritvo et al.[25] have reported an overall recurrence risk (having more than one child in a family with autism) of 8.6%.

The autistic syndrome is associated with viral infections during pregnancy, genetic disorders, neuroimmune system disorders, and disorders of neuronal development.[22,26,27] The symptoms suggest organic brain pathogenesis. However, the exact etiological factors of autism are unclear. It has been associated with the following conditions: fragile X syndrome,[28,29] rubella, herpes simplex, retinopathy of prematurity, phenylketonuria, Tourette's, congenital cytomegalovirus, Prader-Willi and Möbius syndromes,[30] Leber's congenital amaurosis,[31] and Joubert's syndrome.[32]

Current researchers in autism are investigating the presence of a central nervous system dysfunction. Courchesne et al.[33] found cerebellar hypoplasia in autistic individuals. A study by Gaffney et al.[34] compared magnetic resonance images of nonautistic and autistic individuals' brains, and found that autistic individuals had enlarged lateral ventricles and anterior horns, and a smaller right lenticular nucleus.

Autistic children are frequently suspected of having visual problems because of their "atypical" gaze or social "looking."[35] Clinically, this would appear as limited or no eye contact, visual avoidance behaviors, and observing a target from extreme lateral gaze. They also frequently manifest stereotypes (such as eye pressing, hand flicking, and light gazing).[21] These apparent sensory deficits often raise the suspicion of ocular abnormalities by parents[36] and educators.

There is limited information on the visual skills of autistic children, because the children are difficult to assess. Their poor language skills and cooperation present a challenge to the examiner. Their selective visual attention and hyperresponsiveness or hyporesponsiveness to stimuli may mimic or mask a visual deficit. Goodman and Ashby[37] reported on three boys who first presented with "slowness to see," described as delayed visual maturation (DVM), who subsequently manifested severe autistic behavior. In a broad sense, DVM refers to any apparently blind infant who subsequently sees, irrespective of coexistent neurodevelopmental or ocular abnormalities.[38]

Scharre and Creedon[39] evaluated 34 autistic children to determine whether their atypical visual behaviors were caused by significant visual abnormalities and to determine which clinical techniques might be applicable with them. The results showed that 44% of the children had a refractive error greater than 1 diopter (D) as measured by dynamic near retinoscopy. There were no trends for refractive error. Twenty-one percent of the children had an intermittent strabismus. Visual acuity was measurable in most of the children with the Teller Acuity cards. A significant number of children had difficulty with voluntary pursuit movements and gave atypical optokinetic nystagmus (OKN) responses, which may have been indicative of a cerebellar or attentional disorder.

Rosenhall et al.[40] studied oculomotor function in autistic children 9 to 16 years of age. Voluntary horizontal nonpredictable saccades were observed in 11 children with infantile autism or autism-like behaviors. These saccades were found to be abnormal in 55% of the population (hypometric and of reduced velocity). The investigators suggested that oculomotor dysfunction may be more common in the autistic population at large than their study found and stated that this supports the concept of cerebellar–brainstem dysfunction in autism.

Researchers have identified abnormal electroretinogram findings in some autistic individuals. Ritvo et al.[25] found that 48% of autistic individuals they studied had abnormally low b-wave amplitudes, which might indicate abnormal retinal function. These rod abnormalities resembled those seen in individuals with myotonic dystrophy, a hereditary muscle disorder. Realmuto et al.[41] also found abnormal electroretinograms but were unable to establish patterns of family transmission in their small sample.

No single treatment has been effective in the management of autism. Highly structured special education and behavior modification programs, including a 1:1 teacher/student ratio, have been utilized. Pharmacotherapy and nutritional interventions have had only limited success. Haloperidol, a low-dose, high potency neuroleptic, appears to reduce behavioral symptoms and improve discrimination ability in some children.[42-44] Megavitamin therapy, specifically vitamin B_6, has not been proven effective.[45]

Pervasive Developmental Disorders Not Otherwise Specified (PDDNOS)

Children with less severe forms of pervasive developmental disorders display a wide range of deficits in social and language skills yet are not as severely affected as autistic children. The onset of signs and symptoms is in early childhood, generally after 30 months of age. These children frequently have delays in speech and language development, particularly in understanding the nuances of communication. Although they have greater ability with appropriate social relationships than autistic children, they may still be viewed by their peers as eccentric. PDDNOS individuals outnumber autistic children by 3:1.[3,46]

Childhood Schizophrenia (Schizophrenia)

There are no diagnostic criteria in *DSM-III-R* for childhood schizophrenia. This may reflect the disagreements and confusion that surround this behavioral abnormality. To make the diagnosis of schizophrenia in a child, the signs and symptoms referable to the adult diagnosis must be present. Childhood schizophrenia appears to be genetically related to the adult type of schizophrenia. It is relatively rare, occurring in 1 or 2 children out of every 10,000 in the general population under 15 years of age. The onset is usually after 5 years.[2]

Childhood schizophrenia is characterized by rambling or illogical speech patterns, bizarre thought content, and difficulty with environmental reality. Affected children have an impaired ability to develop and maintain adequate social relationships, distortions in affective experiences, and intense and sometimes chronic anxiety. Many exhibit hallucinations or delusions, especially after the age of 8 years.[2] Some have stereotyped motor behaviors (such as twirling around) and inconsistent motor or cognitive behavior.[47]

Three common characteristics among schizophrenic children have been identified[47]: intense anxiety, perceptual difficulty in taking information from external stimulation, and defective self-awareness, especially of normal body feelings. Childhood schizophrenia has many symptoms of abnormal speech and unusual behavior, not unlike those observed in autism. A significant diagnostic distinction must be made between the child with autism and one with schizophrenia. A differentiating point between the conditions is the absence of delusions and hallucinations in autism.[3]

Considerable research[48,49] has been done on the oculomotor ability of schizophrenic adults. It has been noted that individuals with schizophrenia have impaired smooth pursuit movements but normal saccadic and vestibular movements. The studies reported did not include children with schizophrenia.

Emotionally Disturbed/Behavioral Disordered

Children with emotional disorders frequently have characteristics that mimic those in other behavioral disorders. Although these children have traditionally been described as showing behavioral or mental disorders, currently they are labeled as seriously emotionally disturbed. Public Law 94-142 (Education of the Handicapped Act) describes serious emotional disturbance as a condition exhibiting one or more of the following characteristics over a long period and to a marked degree that adversely affects educational performance:[50]

An inability to learn that cannot be explained by intellectual, sensory, or health factors

The inability to build or maintain satisfactory interpersonal relationships with peers and teachers

A general pervasive mood of unhappiness or depression or tendency to develop physical symptoms or fears associated with personal or school problems

This description includes children who have schizophrenia. Children with the most serious emotional disturbances exhibit abnormal mood swings, excessive anxiety, distorted thinking, and bizarre motor acts and are frequently identified as having a severe psychosis (a term no longer used) or schizophrenia.

Many children who do not have emotional disturbances display some of these behaviors throughout their development. However, in children with severe emotional disorders, such behaviors continue over a long period and signal an inability to cope with peers or the environment.[51] Children with emotional disturbances may manifest a number of characteristics and behaviors (listed in the box below).

Characteristics of Children with Emotional Disturbances

Hyperactivity, including short attention span and impulsiveness
Aggression/self-injurious behavior
Withdrawal (excessive anxiety or fear, failure to initiate interaction with others)
Immaturity (poor coping skills, temper tantrums)
Learning problems

From: National Information Center for Children with Disabilities: *Emotional disturbance*. Fact sheet H5(FS5), Washington DC, 1991. (This information is in the the public domain.)

The prevalence of emotional abnormalities is based on the number of children being served within the public school system. For the year 1988-89, 377,295 children and youths were identified with emotional and behavioral disturbances.[51] The causes of these disturbances have not been adequately determined. Research has identified various contributing factors, (such as heredity, diet, stress, brain disorder, and family functioning) but none has been shown to be the direct cause of the emotional disorder.

In a study of the frequency of visual problems in emotionally disturbed children, Lieberman[52] noted that 76% of the population (n=55) failed the vision screening. More than 50% of these individuals failed the tests of visual-motor development, visual-motor integration, form reproduction, saccaic fixations, and fusional ability. Thirty-seven percent exhibited a refractive error (spherical and astigmatic) of 1.00 D or more.

Conclusion

Children with behavioral disorders are a challenge to evaluate and require modifications of the examination procedures to elicit the maximum information. They may have significant visual dysfunctions that contribute to their overall behavioral problems. Early detection and intervention of visual abnormalities are a critical need for these children.

REFERENCES

1. Szymanski L: Psychiatric diagnosis of retarded persons. In Szymanski L, Tanguay P (eds): *Emotional disorders of mentally retarded persons*, Baltimore, 1980, University Park Press.
2. Clark R, Barkley R: Psychological aspects of pediatric and psychiatric disorders. In Hathaway W, et al (eds): *Current pediatric diagnosis and treatment*, Norwalk, Conn, 1991, Appleton & Lange, 727-769.
3. American Psychiatric Association: *Diagnostic and statistical manual of mental disorders: DSM-III-R*, Washington, DC, 1987, American Psychiatric Association.
4. Barkley R: *Attention deficit hyperactivity disorder: a handbook for diagnosis and treatment*, New York, 1990, Guilford Press.
5. Kavanagh JF, Truss JTJ (eds): *Learning disabilities: proceedings of the national conference*, Parkton, Md, 1988, York Press.
6. Klein RG, Mannuzza S: Long-term outcome of hyperactive children: a review, *J Am Acad Child Adolesc Psychiatry* 30:383-387, 1991.
7. Erickson R: *Child psych-pathology*, Englewood Cliffs, NJ, 1982, Prentice-Hall.
8. Fowler M: *Attention deficit disorder*, Washington, DC, 1991, National Information Center for Children and Youth with Disabilities.
9. Horowitz F (ed): *Review of child development research*, Chicago, 1975, University of Chicago Press.
10. Zametkin A, Mordahl T, Gross M, et al: Cerebral glucose metabolism in adults with hyperactivity of childhood onset, *N Engl J Med* 323:1361-1366, 1990.
11. Hynd GW, Semrud-Clikeman M, Lorys AR, et al: Corpus callosum morphology in attention deficit–hyperactivity disorder: morphometric analysis of MRI, *J Learn Disabil* 24:141-146, 1991.
12. Wender E: The food additive-free diet in the treatment of behavior disorders: a review, *J Dev Behav Pediatr* 7:35-42, 1986.
13. Swanson J, Cantwell D, Lerner M, et al: The effects of stimulant medication on learning in children with ADHD, *J Learn Disabil* 24:219-230, 1991.
14. Varley CK: Attention deficit disorder: a review of selected issues, *J Dev Behav Pediatr* 5:254-257, 1984.
15. Satterfield J, Hoppe C, Schell A: A prospective study of delinquency in 110 adolescent boys with attention deficit disorder and 88 normal adolescent boys, *Am J Psychiatry* 139:797-798, 1982.
16. Olin B (ed): *Drug facts and comparisons*, St Louis, 1992, Facts and Comparisons.
17. Lesher G: *A quick reference guide to the top prescription drugs*, Chicago, 1988, Illinois College of Optometry.
18. Cantwell DP, Baker L: Differential diagnosis of hyperactivity, *J Dev Behav Pediatr* 8:159-165, 1987.
19. Siegel B, Pliner C, Eschler J, Elliott G: How children with autism are diagnosed: difficulties in identification of children with multiple delays, *J Dev Behav Pediatr* 9:199-204, 1988.
20. Maurer R: Neuropsychology of autism, *Psychiatr Clin North Am* 9:367-380, 1986.
21. National Society for Autistic Children: Definition of the syndrome of autism: diagnosis and principles of management, *Pediatr Ann* 13:295, 1984.

22. Ornitz E: The functional neuroanatomy of infantile autism, *Int J Neurosci* 19:85-124, 1983.

23. Creedon M, Scharre J: Visual functional discrepancies in children with autism, *Occup Ther Pract* 3:69-76, 1991.

24. Ritvo E, Freeman B, Pingree K, et al: The UCLA–University of Utah epidemiologic survey of autism: prevalence, *Am J Psychiatry* 146:194-199, 1989.

25. Ritvo E, Jorde L, Mason-Brothers A, et al: The UCLA–University of Utah epidemiologic survey of autism: recurrence risk estimates and genetic counseling, *Am J Psychiatry* 146:1032-1036, 1989.

26. Ciaranello R, Vandenberg S, Anders T: Intrinsic and extrinsic determinants of neuronal development: relation to infantile autism, *J Autism Dev Disord* 12:115-145, 1982.

27. Hashimoto T, Tayama M, Mori K, et al: Magnetic resonance imaging in autism: preliminary report, *Neuropediatrics* 20:142-146, 1989.

28. Brown W, Jenkins E, Friedman E, et al: Autism is associated with the fragile-X syndrome, *Autism Dev Disord* 12:303-308, 1982.

29. Levitas A, Hagerman R, Braden M: Autism and the fragile X syndrome, *J Dev Behav Pediatr* 4:151-158, 1983.

30. Coleman M, Gillberg C: *The biology of the autistic syndromes*, New York, 1985, Praeger Scientific.

31. Roger S, Newhart-Larson S: Characteristics of infantile autism in five children with Leber's congenital amaurosis, *Dev Med Child Neurol* 31:598-608, 1989.

32. Holroyd S, Reiss A, Bryan R: Autistic features in Joubert syndrome: a genetic disorder with agenesis of the cerebellar vermis, *Biol Psychiatry* 29:287-294, 1991.

33. Courchesne E, Yeung-Courchesne R, Press G, et al: Hypoplasia of cerebellar vermal lobules VI and VII in autism, *N Engl J Med* 18:1349-1354, 1988.

34. Gaffney G, Kuperman S, Tsai L, Minchin S: Forebrain structure in infantile autism, *J Am Acad Child Adolesc Psychiatry* 28:534-537, 1989.

35. Hutt C, Ounsted C: The biological significance of gaze aversion with particular reference to the syndrome of infantile autism, *Behav Sci* 11:346-356, 1966.

36. Lovaas O, Newsom C: Behavior modification with psychotic children. In Leitenberg H (ed): *Handbook of behavior modification and behavior therapy*, Englewood Cliffs, NJ, 1976, Prentice-Hall, pp 303-360.

37. Goodman R, Ashby L: Delayed visual maturation and autism, *Dev Med Child Neurol* 32:808-819, 1990.

38. Fielder A, Russell-Eggitt I, Dodd K, Mellor D: Delayed visual maturation, *Trans Ophthalmol Soc UK* 104:653-661, 1985.

39. Scharre JE, Creedon MP: Assessment of visual function in autistic children, *Optom Vis Sci* 69:433-439, 1992.

40. Rosenhall U, Johansson E, Gillberg C: Oculomotor findings in autistic children, *J Laryngol Otol* 102:435-439, 1988.

41. Realmuto G, Purple R, Knobloch W, Ritvo E: Electroretinograms (ERGs) in four autistic probands and six first-degree relatives, *Can J Psychiatry* 34:435-439, 1989.

42. Campbell M, Anderson L, Cohen I, et al: Haloperidol in autistic children: effects on learning, behavior, and abnormal involuntary movements, *Psychopharmacol Bull* 18:110-113, 1982.

43. Campbell M, Anderson L, Small A, et al: The effects on haloperidol on learning and behavior in autistic children, *J Autism Dev Disord* 12:167-175, 1982.

44. Campbell M, Anderson L, Green W, Deutsch S: Psychopharmacology. In Cohen D, Donnellan A (eds): *Handbook of autism and pervasive developmental disorders*, New York, 1987, John Wiley & Sons, 545-565.

45. Raiten D, Massaro T: Nutrition and developmental disabilities: an examination of the orthomolecular hypothesis. In Cohen D, Donnellan A (eds):

Handbook of autism and pervasive developmental disorders, New York, 1987, John Wiley & Sons.

46. Rutter M: Infantile autism and other pervasive developmental disorders. In Rutter M, Hersov L (eds): *Child and adolescent psychiatry*, ed 2, London, 1985, Blackwell, 545-566.

47. Lavigne J, Burns W: *Pediatric psychology*, New York, 1981, Grune & Stratton.

48. Levin S: Frontal lobe dysfunctions in schizophrenia. I. Eye movement impairments, *J Psychiatr Res* 18:27-55, 1984.

49. Levin S: Frontal lobe dysfunctions in schizophrenia. II. Impairments of psychological and brain functions, *J Psychiatr Res* 18:57-72, 1984.

50. Public Law 94-142, *Fed Reg* 42:42478-42479, August, 1977.

51. National Information Center for Children and Youth with Disabilities: *Emotional disturbance*. Fact Sheet H5(FS5), Washington, DC, 1991.

52. Lieberman S: The prevalence of visual disorders in a school for emotionally disturbed children, *J Am Optom Assoc* 56:800-803, 1985.

APPENDIX 1

The following is a list of organizations that provide information on behavioral disorders.

Emotional Disorders

American Academy of Child and Adolescent Psychiatry
Public Information Office
3615 Wisconsin Ave., NW
Washington, DC 20016

Federation of Families for Children's Mental Health
1021 Prince St.
3rd Floor
Alexandria, VA 22314-2971

National Mental Health Association
1021 Prince St.
Alexandria, VA 22314-2971

Autism

Institute for Child Behavior Research
4182 Adams Ave.
San Diego, CA 92116

Autism Services Center
Douglas Education Building
Tenth Avenue and Bruce Street
Huntington, WV 25701

Autism Society of America
8601 Georgia Avenue
Suite 503
Silver Springs, MD 20910

Attention Disorder

Attention Deficit Disorder Association
80913 Ireland Way
Aurora, CO 80016

Children with Attention Deficit Disorders (CH.A.D.D.)
499 NW 70th Avenue, Suite 308
Plantation, FL 33317

6

Clinical Behavioral Objectives: Assessment Techniques for Special Populations

Darrell G. Schlange
Dominick M. Maino

Key Terms

Americans with Disabilities Act	PL 20/20 Vision Tester	Angle Kappa (Lambda)
Recognition Acuity	Teller Acuity Cards	Hirschberg Test
Broken Wheel Test	Detection Acuity	Krimsky Test
HOTV Visual Acuity Test	Candy Bead Visual Acuity Test	Cover Test
Tumbling E Test	STYCAR Miniature Toys Test	Lang Stereotest
Lea Symbols Test	Dot Visual Acuity Test	Random Dot E Test
Lighthouse Flash Card Test	Mohindra (Near Dynamic) Retinoscopy	Worth Four Dot Test
Allen Picture Cards	Brückner Test	MEM
Bailey-Hall Cereal Test		Tono-Pen XL
Resolution Acuity		

When first attempting any new diagnostic procedure, the student or practitioner may be confused about the specific steps required. A clinical behavioral objective breaks down each technique into short steps that allows the doctor to readily learn any unfamiliar procedure. This chapter will discuss diagnostic techniques used for special populations that assess visual acuity, binocularity, refractive status, and ocular health.

The diagnosis and management of the oculovisual abnormalities commonly found in special populations present many challenges to the optometrist. Approximately three million individuals in the United States have disabilities that interfere with their ability to work, play, and learn.[1]

CLINICAL PEARL

Approximately three million individuals in the United States have disabilities that interfere with their ability to work, play, and learn.

Early identification and intervention is important for appropriate cognitive, emotional, and psychosocial development. Furthermore, early intervention is cost-effective for society, prevents the development of secondary problems, and helps facilitate the benefits gained from other rehabilitation programs. Unfortunately many children and adults with disabilities face significant barriers to health and vision care. According to Kastner and Luckhardt,[2] these barriers include the following:

Health care system obstacles:
- Fragmentation of the delivery care system
- Poor planning
- Excessive governmental regulation
- Low financial rewards for the health care provider
- Excessive paperwork
- Increased provider/patient contact time

Consumer (patient) obstacles:
- Poor ability to communicate symptoms
- Little health care history information
- Complex medical/behavioral problems
- Questions concerning informed consent/guardianship

Health care provider barriers:
- Negative attitudes towards the handicapped[3]
- Architectural barriers
- Lack of transportation
- Lack of availability of health care providers
- Little or no training of the health care provider in the care of special populations

Direct care provider barriers:
- Poor training of direct care staff
- Excessive paperwork
- Crisis oriented health care

This chapter addresses the issue of the minimal clinical training (mentioned under *Health care provider barriers* above) the optometrist receives in diagnosing the numerous ocular health, binocular vision, and refractive anomalies present in the developmentally disabled population.[4,5,6,7] Specific clinical behavioral objectives have been designed by the faculty of the Illinois College of Optometry (and others)* to teach those clinical skills necessary to best meet the health and vision care needs of the handicapped.

A clinical behavioral objective is a step-by-step approach that breaks down the mechanics of each examination technique so that the student or clinician can easily adopt a diagnostic procedure into his/her examination sequence. The optometrist should seek out additional information relating to the efficacy, validity, specificity, and reliability of each diagnostic procedure described.[8,9,10]

Preparing For The Examination

One of the basic goals of the examination is to quickly obtain reliable clinical information in a relaxing and comfortable testing environment. This requires a strategy, developed early in the doctor-patient interaction, based on information that includes the case history, preexamination reports, other written/verbal communication, and the observation skills of the optometrist at the first patient visit.

CLINICAL PEARL

One of the basic goals of the examination is to quickly obtain reliable clinical information in a relaxing and comfortable testing environment.

Obtaining a complete case history is the first step in prioritizing the examination sequence so that you can conduct testing procedures that

---

*Harrington C, Magid L, Primm B: Policies and Procedures for Vision Screening of Difficult to Test Children in Georgia. Prepublication Draft (Publication date, 1993). Available from Lee T. Magid, Senior Speech and Hearing Specialist, Georgia Department of Human Resources, Children's Health Services Section, 260 Skyland Dr., Atlanta, GA 30109; 404-679-0526; fax, 404-679-4781.

will yield the most useful clinical information. A patient's complete history is often available if you work with children in a special education, rehabilitation, residential, or hospital setting. On the other hand, if you are examining these patients in your office or if you are working with an adult with disabilities, little medical, educational, or vocational information may accompany the patient.[8] Instruct the office staff to ask patients (or caregivers) at the time of appointment scheduling if there are any special concerns that the doctor should know prior to the appointment. These may include the patient's age,

---

Illinois College of Optometry
Illinois Eye Institute

CONSENT/RELEASE FORM

I, _____ , having presented myself at the Illinois Eye Institute of the Illinois College of Optometry for examination and/or treatment, do voluntary consent to the performance of examination, diagnostic procedures and/or treatment as deemed necessary or beneficial for my case.

I understand that any of the above measures may be performed by an optometrist, opthalmologist, other qualified specialist, intern, resident, student clinician, or technician under the supervision of either an optometrist, opthalmologist or qualified specialist.

I further acknowledge that no guarantees have been made to me as to the effect of such procedures on my condition.

I understand that as part of my vision examination, pharmaceutical agents will be utilized for the purpose of dilating my eyes. I further understand that the effects of these agents may include blurred vision and sensitivity to light, both of which could restrict my mobility making it unsafe to travel unassisted or operate a vehicle.

For research or scientific purposes I consent to the inspection/release of the records of my treatment by any person specifically authorized by the Administration of the Illinois Eye Institute.

_____   DATE:
PATIENT SIGNATURE

_____
GUARDIAN SIGNATURE

_____
WITNESS

Patient's Address/Phone:

FIGURE 6-1 Sample consent/release form.

medical conditions, medications taken, cognitive level, behavior disorders, present work or school activities, and specific disabilities. If needed, send consent/release (Fig. 6-1), case history, and report forms (Figs. 6-2, 6-3 and 6-4) to be completed before the patient is examined. These completed forms should be available at the time of evaluation.

Illinois Eye Institute of the Illinois College of Optometry
Pediatric Department
3239 South Michigan
Chicago, Illinois
(312) 225-6200

Teacher Report Form

Name _____ Date _____ Record # _____
School _____ Grade _____
Teacher_____

Information about academic achievement and progress in school is essential for the comprehensive vision care of the above named child. In order to complete our examination, we would like your assistance in providing the information requested below.

Please return this form to us addressed to the attention of the clinician caring for this child:

_____

1. Does this child have any major academic difficulties? Yes _____ No _____
   If so, please explain: _____
   _____

2. How does overall Academic Achievement compare with capability? _____
   _____

3. At what grade level does the child read? _____
   _____

4. How does reading achievement compare with reading capability? _____
   _____

5. Please check any special area of difficulty:

   _____ Vocabulary   _____ Word Recognition   _____ Oral Reading
   _____ Reading Rate   _____ Interpretation   _____ Silent Reading
   _____ Attention   _____ Comprehension   _____ Memory
   _____ Phonics   _____ Spelling   _____ Written Work

6. Has the child repeated a grade? Yes _____ No _____ If yes, which grade?
   _____

7. Is the child receiving any special educational help? Yes _____ No _____
   If yes, please explain: _____

Continued

FIGURE 6-2 Illinois College of Optometry teacher report form.

Please check only those responses which apply to the child while reading, writing, or doing other near work.

_____ Tilts head to one side	_____ Squints
_____ Covers or closes one eye	_____ Skips or rereads lines or words
_____ Rubs or blinks eye	_____ Holds reading too close or too far
_____ Complains of seeing double	_____ Uses finger or marker as a pointer
_____ Vocalize with lips or throat	_____ Complains of blur when looks up
_____ Daydreaming	_____ Puts head on arms while writing
_____ Confuses similar words	_____ Easily distracted
_____ Difficulty with recognition of words or letters	_____ Mirrors and/or reverses letters or numbers
_____ Has difficulty in completing assignments in allotted time	_____ Tends to become discouraged or frustrated easily
_____ Omits, substitutes, or reverses letters, numbers, or words while reading aloud	

8. Please include any additional information which you feel may be beneficial to us.

_____

Teacher   Date

I hereby give my consent to release the above information to the
ILLINOIS EYE INSTITUTE OF THE ILLINOIS COLLEGE OF OPTOMETRY.

_____

Parent or Guardian   Date

FIGURE 6-2, Cont'd.

The problem-oriented record is organized to promote an efficient, thorough, and comprehensive examination.[11] This includes a data base of the information obtained during the examination (e.g., test results, case history, report forms) that determines the patency of the visual system (e.g., visual acuity, refraction, binocular vision, ocular health). A problem list (Fig. 6-3) and assessment is then defined, followed by an appropriate treatment plan (including options and prognosis).

Scheduling patients with special needs will usually depend on the number of patients to be seen and the specific disabilities present. It is helpful to appoint exceptional individuals during the slow times of the day (e.g., early afternoon), so that there is sufficient time to conduct each evaluation free of distractions. You may wish to devote a morning a week to evaluate patients when you can schedule several individuals in sequence. The examination environment should be

ILLINOIS EYE INSTITUTE
Pediatric/Binocular Vision Service

Patient _____ DOB _____ File # _____

Clinician _____ Faculty _____

Pertinent Health Hx _____

Current Medications _____

Pertinent Educat. / Testing Hx _____

Current Grade / Classroom Type _____

Patient Progress Report/ Unit (date)

	Date	Specifics	1( )	2( )	3( )	4( )	5( )
Subjective	SP1						
	SP2						
	SP3						
	SP4						
	SP5						
Objective	OP1						
	OP2						
	OP3						
	OP4						
	OP5						
	OP6						
	OP7						
	OP8						
	OP9						
	OP10						

Codes: AB - Abated; B - Better; NC - No change; W - Worse

Assess. Diagnosis: 1._____ 3._____
2._____ 4._____

Plan
Treatment Recommended   VE   VP   S/A   Other _____
Prognosis _____   ETT(#Units) _____
Patching Program: Direct   Indirect   Binasal   Other _____
OD _____ hrs/day _____ days/week   OS _____ hrs/day _____ days/week
Fee for Therapy _____   Major Medical   Y / N   (*circle one*)

Rx Rec.
Date of Rx	OD	OS	Wearing Schedule
1			
2			

P/BV-MastProbList-5.91-1

FIGURE 6-3 Illinois College of Optometry, Department of Pediatrics and Binocular Vision master problem list.

ILLINOIS EYE INSTITUTE
Pediatric/Binocular Vision Service
3239 South Michigan Avenue
Chicago, IL 60616
Telephone: 312/225-6200 ext. 580

Visual Report

Name: _____   Date _____   File # _____

Address _____   DOB _____   Sex _____

City & State: _____   Zip _____   Phone _____

Listed below is a summary of the results of the visual assessment. Should you desire any further information, please do not hesitate to call the attending **staff Doctor** noted below. Only "checked" items apply to the above patient.

Eye Health:
A. External _____Normal_____Abnormal
B. Internal _____Normal_____Abnormal
C. Intraocular Pressure
_____Normal_____Abnormal
D. _____Unable to assess
Best Visual Acuity (With/Without Correction):
A. Distance:
Right Eye ____Left Eye ____Both eyes____
B. Near:
Right Eye ____Left Eye ____Both eyes____
C. Amblyopia of the _____eye is present. Best acuity is _____.
D. _____Unable to assess
Refractive Status:
A. Emmetropia--no significant amount
B. Myopia (nearsightedness) of a low/moderate /high degree
C. Hyperopia (farsightedness) of a low/moderate /high degree
D. Astigmatism of a low/moderate/high degree
E. _____Unable to assess
Binocularity:
A. Adequate/Inadequate
B. Strabismus (eye turn) is present/absent.
C. Direction of deviation _____Esotropia(inward)
_____Exotropia(outward)
_____Hypertropia(upward)
D. Stereopsis (depth perception) present/absent.
E. _____Unable to assess
Ocular Motilities or Eye Movement Skills:
A. Accurate/mildly/moderately/very deficient skills
B. Paresis/paralysis of an extraocular muscle is present/absent.
C. _____Unable to assess

Color Vision:
A. Adequate/Inadequate
B. _____Unable to assess
Peripheral (Side) Vision:
A. _____Normal _____Abnormal
B. _____Unable to assess
C. _____Not assessed at this time
Developmental Skills:
A. Adequate/Inadequate
B. _____Not assessed at this time
Disposition/Recommendations:
A.___Prescription lenses should not/should be worn.
B.___Glasses should be worn constantly/ distance only/near only.
C.___Optometric vision therapy is recommended.
D.___The patient was advised to return to the Illinois Eye Institute for _____
_____.
E.___The patient was referred to _____
_____for additional testing.
Comments:_____
_____
_____
_____
_____
_____
_____
_____

Attending Staff Signature:
_____
_____

P/BV-Visual Report-10.92-1

FIGURE 6-4   Illinois Eye Institute, Illinois College of Optometry, Summary Report Form.

pleasant, cheerful, brightly lit, colorful, and organized to help the patient relax and enjoy the evaluation.

CLINICAL PEARL

In January 1992 the Americans with Disabilities Act went into effect; it requires businesses to meet the special needs of handicapped persons. If your office is currently architecturally up to date (for example, it has wheelchair-accessible doorways and bathrooms), few physical changes will be required.

In January 1992 the Americans with Disabilities Act went into effect; it requires businesses to meet the special needs of handicapped persons.[12,13] If your office is currently architecturally up to date (for example, it has wheelchair-accessible doorways and bathrooms), few physical changes will be required.[14] You should contact the appropriate government offices for additional information.

All necessary instruments should be readily available so the examination routine flows with few interruptions. Be prepared with specially designed equipment for any posture needs or mobility problems the patient may have. Special positioning of the patient is important for maximizing comfort and performance during the examination. Avoid the distractions of a small, crowded, and messy examination room. Schedule one staff member to be available for assisting with the examination. The staff should be friendly and smile easily; be dressed neatly yet casually; project confidence; and present an appropriate demeanor with a caring and understanding attitude. This will help establish rapport with the patient and parent/guardian early in the examination. The entire staff should be cognizant of the unique problems these patients present and be flexible and adaptive to different developmental levels and behavioral responses. This may require flexible scheduling of more than one appointment for completion of all necessary procedures.

CLINICAL PEARL

The entire staff should be cognizant of the unique problems these patients present and be flexible and adaptive to different developmental levels and behavioral responses.

Patients may exhibit fear, anxiety, and apprehension about the examination. The following practices will help the examiner gain the patient's attention, cooperation, and trust.

- Greet the patient by his or her name (or nickname) and a hand shake if appropriate. Position yourself at the patient's eye level.

- Be on schedule so the patient doesn't have to wait.
- Consider the patient's wishes about family or friends being in the examination room.
- Direct your initial comments toward the patient, and then toward the accompanying family member as you briefly visit prior to the examination.
- Treat the patient as a person first; second, as a person with a disability (use terms like "person with a disability," not "disabled person"). Avoid showing pity and using negative terms (e.g., afflicted, wheelchair-bound, victim), for this attitude is offensive and patronizing.
- Seek to understand the patient's disability.
  1. Speak clearly.
  2. If there is a hearing impairment, speak in short simple sentences.
  3. If cognitive impairment is present, ask questions that can be answered in a few words.
  4. If there is speech impairment; listen carefully or ask the patient to write down what he or she is saying.
  5. If the patient is in a wheelchair, work at his or her eye level.
  6. If there is a visual impairment, identify and introduce yourself.
- Be honest with the patient. Explain in a gentle and nonthreatening voice what you will be doing and what he or she can expect to see or feel. Avoid negative facial expressions and intimidating body language.
- Understand the fears and concerns that the parent or guardian may also have about the examination. Encourage them to express these feelings openly. Avoid making the parent feel guilty, embarrassed, or negligent.

Case History

The case history is an essential part of the diagnostic process consisting of a brief summary of the patient's medical, developmental, and educational history. This will become a fundamental component of your minimum data base. This information will help you understand the chief reasons for the examination and give insights into other factors that may have influenced development, behavior, and learning. If possible attempt to obtain copies of any previous evaluations. Special-population patients have often received previous frustrating and disappointing examinations. The review of this history will help develop a caring and empathetic doctor-patient rapport. You should clearly identify the chief complaint and presenting symptoms. Describe these in the specific terms used by the patient, parent, guardian, or referring professional. Since many young patients are asymptomatic, this will frequently include observations made by the parent and others.

• Case History: Behavioral Objectives

Did you determine if:

1. The patient (or parent) was aware of any eye problems.
2. The patient (or parent) was aware of which eye(s) has the problem; when it happens; what the eye does (e.g., turn in, out, red appearance); associated conditions; and onset of problem.
3. There are any changes in the condition since it first appeared.
4. The patient can modify or compensate in any way for the problem.
5. There are any visually related symptoms that occur at home, school, or workplace (Teacher Report Form, etc.).
6. There is a family history of the same or similar conditions.
7. There has been previous treatment (glasses, surgery, VT, medications)?
8. There are related factors in the birth and development history, the medical history including medications, and the educational history.
9. There are specific goals that the patient (parent) may have.

Visual Acuity Assessment

The examination should provide early identification of visual and ocular anomalies so that prompt treatment can be initiated. The assessment of visual acuity is a critical element of this process because special-population patients have a higher incidence of ocular abnormalities that can affect visual acuity. These patients will have further complications with development and overall function when vision problems are left undiagnosed and untreated. Medical, legal, and our own professional standards mandate accurate visual acuity assessment as an essential component of our minimum database.[9] Patients with multiple handicaps have a wide range of abilities and behavioral responses secondary to dysfunctions of motor, sensory, cognitive, language, adaptive, and social/personal development. This may limit acuity assessment to doctor observation skills. However, in most cases, visual acuity optotypes ranging from basic detection to upper-level recognition acuity can be used. When assessing visual acuity, you should use the most efficient, accurate, and reliable procedures that are consistent with the individual's cognitive level and motoric abilities.[15]

CLINICAL PEARL

When assessing visual acuity, you should use the most efficient, accurate, and reliable procedures that are consistent with the individual's cognitive level and motoric abilities.

Recognition acuity threshold tests assess the patient's ability to discriminate or recognize a target (e.g., a letter or Landolt C pattern.) This includes the Snellen Acuity Chart, the Broken Wheel Visual Acuity Test (BWT),[16] the HOTV Visual Acuity Test, and the Tumbling E Test. Picture recognition targets include the Lea Symbols Test, the Lighthouse Flash Card Test, the Allen Picture Cards, and the Bailey-Hall Cereal Test. Letter recognition acuity is preferred over picture targets, and multiple targets with contour interaction are preferred over single targets. These latter optotypes are high contrast, can be used at various distances, and do not require cognitive, verbal, and directionality skills.

CLINICAL PEARL

Letter recognition acuity is preferred over picture targets, and multiple targets with contour interaction are preferred over single targets.

Resolution acuity threshold is assessed by requiring the patient to resolve a difference between two nonstandard optotypes, line gratings, or pictures. This includes the PL 20/20 vision tester and the Teller acuity cards. Patient responses are nonverbal and can be reinforced with operant conditioning (Fig. 6-5).[17,18]

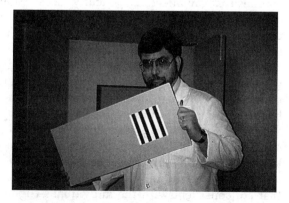

FIGURE 6-5 Teller acuity cards.

Detection acuity threshold is assessed by presenting targets that the child finds or detects. These tests include the Candy Bead Visual Acuity Test, the STYCAR Miniature Toys Test, and the Dot Visual Acuity Test.[19] These procedures tend to overestimate acuity, are conducted at near point, and may require extended test time. They can, however, provide insights into acuity deficiencies by comparing monocular differences between the two eyes. Optokinetic nystagmus (OKN) procedures provide a gross assessment of visual acuity. However, a positive response may be due to nonacuity functions (e.g., midbrain oculomotor responses, peripheral retinal detection).[20] Some patients may require a more objective procedure such as the VER (visually evoke response). This utilizes special electrodiagnostic techniques usually not available in private offices.[21] Patients with more severe disorders may require evaluation through observation of looking behavior, attention time, light awareness, localization, and fixation maintenance and preference.

Summary suggestions for visual acuity assessment

The following guidelines may help you conduct an effective and accurate assessment.[22]

- Use the highest-level assessment procedure that is consistent with the patient's developmental level. Be adaptable to different patient responses. If one test does not work, discontinue and try another procedure.
- Although many visual acuity tests are designed for specific age groups (i.e., BWT for children ages 2-5 years), they may be appropriate for special patients at any age. Compare test results with chronological norms but do not be limited by them.
- Some patients object to occlusion techniques (they resist occlusion or are tactually defensive); therefore, do binocular testing before monocular testing. Attempt both uncorrected and corrected acuity testing if possible.
- Use adaptive positioning for patients according to their unique postural or mobility needs (e.g., supine, in wheelchair, infant seat, bumper chair, etc.)
- Give your patients time to feel relaxed, comfortable, and unthreatened.
- Use friends or family members accompanying the patient as assistants for positioning, occluding an eye, instilling DPAs (diagnostic pharmaceutical agents), and facilitating attention.
- Maximize efficiency by having brief testing sessions with breaks to reduce fatigue and loss of interest.
- Randomize the presentation of optotype targets. Permit the patient to substitute any consistent response that indicates recognition of the target (e.g., always says "circle" for "apple").

- Help an easily distracted child maintain attention by using puppets, tokens, reinforcers (food), noise makers, flashing lights, singing, rocking, appropriate touching, giving praise for a "good job," and patient participation (e.g., blowing at the side with stripes, pointing to target using a finger/hand puppet the child holds, etc.)
- Present the test as a game (e.g., peek-a-boo and "Find the Zebra" for Teller cards).
- Always try both distance and near visual acuity tests.

• Visual Acuity Tests: Behavioral Objectives

Broken Wheel Visual Acuity Test

1. Present both demonstration cards at near and ask the patient to identify which car has the "broken wheel."
2. Determine the patient's reliability and level of comprehension of the task by presenting the demonstration cards more than once.
3. Administer the test at 3 meters (10 feet). Occlude an eye.
4. Present both cards at the same time (forced choice) at each acuity level.
5. Start with the larger targets and then progress to the smaller targets.
6. Randomly present the cards both horizontally (side by side) and vertically.
7. Check to make sure the patient is not squinting or peeking around the occluder.
8. Ask the patient to look carefully at both cards before making a choice.
9. Present targets that are close to the patient's threshold acuity level at least four times.
10. Discontinue testing when two or fewer responses were correct for a given acuity level.
11. Test right eye, left eye, and both eyes.
12. Record the results as that acuity level where more than 50% of the responses were correct (i.e., 3 out of 4 correct responses).
13. Record the visual acuity test used (Broken Wheel Acuity Test).

HOTV Visual Acuity Test

1. Present the demonstration cards (H, O, T, V) at near and ask the patient to identify each letter by pointing to or by matching the letter on the response card.
2. Determine the patient's reliability and level of comprehension of the task by presenting the demonstration cards more than once.
3. Administer the test at 3 meters (10 feet). Occlude an eye.
4. Start with the larger size targets and then progress to the smaller targets.
5. Check to make sure the patient is not squinting or peeking around the occluder.
6. Stop testing when only 4 out of 6 letters can be correctly identified on one test line.
7. Test right eye, left eye, both eyes.
8. Record the test results as a Snellen equivalent (10/10) for each eye.
9. Record the visual acuity test used (HOTV).

Lighthouse Flash Card Test

1. Present the large cards (House, Apple, Umbrella) at near and ask the patient to identify each object.
2. Determine the patient's reliability and level of comprehension of the task by presenting the large cards more than once.
3. Administer the test at 3 meters (10 feet). Occlude an eye.
4. Start with the larger targets and then progress to the smaller targets.
5. Give the patient 4 trials of each acuity level when approaching threshold acuity.
6. Randomly change the presentation order of the test targets.
7. Check to make sure the patient is not squinting or peeking around the occluder.
8. Discontinue testing when two or fewer correct responses were obtained at a given acuity level.
9. Test the right eye, left eye, both eyes.
10. Record the results as the test distance over the acuity level (10/20) where more than 50% of the responses were correct (3 out of 4).
11. Switch to the near acuity card.
12. Record the near visual acuity (right eye, left eye, both eyes).
13. Record the visual acuity test used (Lighthouse).

Lea Symbols Visual Acuity Test

1. Present the key card of demonstration symbols (house, apple, square, circle) at near and ask the patient to identify each object.
2. Determine the patient's reliability and level of comprehension of the task by presenting the demonstration symbols more than once.
3. Administer the test at 3 meters (10 feet).
4. Start with the top line of larger symbols and then progress to the smaller targets (15 lines of 5 symbols each, ranging in size from 10/100 to 10/5).
5. Encourage the patient to name, sign, or point (on the key card) to the symbols.
6. Avoid the patient's perception of failing the test by using a play format whereby the patient is encouraged to attempt answering correctly, even after exceeding the acuity threshold (when all symbols appear as circles or squares).
7. Use either the individual symbols or a mask over the large chart for those patients who cannot perform in a line test situation.
8. Check to make sure the patient is not squinting or peeking around the occluder.
9. Discontinue testing when only four out of the five symbols at a given acuity level are responded to correctly.
10. Test the right eye, left eye, both eyes.
11. Record the results as a Snellen equivalent (the test distance over the symbol acuity size, e.g., 10/20 −1) for each eye.
12. Switch to the near acuity card, using the cord attached to the chart to maintain a constant 40 cm viewing distance.
13. Record the near visual acuity in Snellen equivalent (right eye, left eye, both eyes).
14. Record the visual acuity test used (Lea Symbols).

Bailey-Hall Cereal Test

1. Present the largest of six pairs of 5-inch square cards (one with a picture of a round Cheerios cereal and the other a picture of a square box, same color and size) at near and ask the patient to identify the "cereal" or "Cheerio" using either verbal, pointing, or looking behavior.
2. Determine the patient's reliability and level of comprehension of the task by presenting the demonstration cards more than once.
3. Administer the test at a 1-foot distance. Occlude an eye. If three out of four correct responses are given, gradually move away from the child in 1-foot increments to the test distance designed for each card.
4. Start with the larger targets and progress to smaller ones, randomly presenting the two cards horizontally and vertically.
5. Check to make sure the patient is not squinting or peeking around the occluder.
6. Stop the test when there are inconsistent responses (less than 3 out of 4 correct responses).
7. Test and record for right eye, left eye, and both eyes.
8. Record the threshold acuity as the distance where the smallest card size is seen. (4/10 means correctly viewing the 10-foot card at a distance of 4 feet.)
9. Record the visual acuity test used (Bailey-Hall Cereal Test).

Teller Acuity Cards

1. Present the large grating cards before the patient and evaluate the looking behavior (fixation towards the side with the grating pattern, pointing to the side with the gratings, head movement in the direction of the side with the stripes, etc.).
2. Determine the patient's reliability and level of comprehension of the task by presenting the large cards more than once. Occlude an eye.
3. Administer the test at the appropriate distance (infants, 15 inches; 2 to 5 years, 22 inches; 4 years or older, 33 inches).
4. Start with the larger targets and then progress to the smaller stripes, randomly changing the presentation order.
5. Check to make sure the patient is not squinting or peeking around the occluder.
6. Request any assistant (parent or guardian) to refrain from cueing the child as to the location of the stripes.
7. Discontinue testing when the responses are random, inconsistent, or absent.
8. Test and record for right eye, left eye, and both eyes.
9. Record the visual acuity from the legend on each card, in cycles per centimeter (cycles/cm) or the Snellen equivalent.
10. Record visual acuity test used (Teller cards).

PL 20/20 Vision Tester

1. Position the patient 14 inches in front of the unit. Use dim room illumination.
2. Determine the patient's reliability and level of comprehension of the task by presenting the largest target size more than once.
3. Attract the patient's attention by activating the red LED light, the buzzer, or by tapping on the unit. Occlude an eye.
4. Start with the largest target at position 1 of the target wheel. Illuminate the target when the patient is attending appropriately.
5. Observe the looking behavior (fixation preference to the right or left) through viewing lens; record the response; and change to target position 2.
6. Continue with smaller targets until responses become random or inconsistent.
7. Check to make sure the patient is not squinting or peeking around the occluder.
8. Record the Snellen equivalent for the smallest target where more than 50% (3 out of 4 correct responses) of the responses were correct.
9. Test and record for right eye, left eye, and both eyes.
10. Record the visual acuity test used (PL 20/20 Vision Tester).

Candy Bead Visual Acuity Test (CBVAT)*

1. Present the candy beads at a distance of 6 inches and observe the patient's ability to look at or pick up and eat the candy bead.
2. Determine the patient's reliability and level of comprehension of the task by presenting the sample candy beads more than once.
3. Administer the test with candy targets on a plain contrasting background, initially at a viewing distance of 10 inches (25 cm), and positioned in front of the child on a table or feeding chair. Occlude an eye.
4. Place 1 or 2 candy beads on the table, using small nonpareils of approximately 1.1 mm size and encourage the child to pick up and eat the candy.
5. Check to make sure the patient is not squinting or peeking around the occluder.
6. Gradually increase the target distance (12 inches, 14 inches, and 16 inches) until the patient's response is absent or inconsistent.
7. Record the calculated Snellen equivalent for a threshold response (e.g., a 1.3 mm candy target viewed at 10 inches = 20/357)
8. Test and record for the right eye, left eye, and both eyes.
9. Record the visual acuity test used (Candy Bead Test).

---

*See Chapter 2 for CBVAT nomogram.

STYCAR Miniature Toys Test

1. Present the miniature toys at the near distance and ask the patient to identify them by name (toys: car, airplane, doll, chair, knives, fork, and spoon.
2. Determine the patient's reliability and level of comprehension of the task by requesting identification of the toys more than once.
3. Administer the test at 3 meters (10 feet). Occlude an eye.
4. Present the miniature toys in front of a high contrast background and request the child to identify them or point to a matching toy positioned near the child.
5. Start with the larger toys and then progress to the smaller ones.
6. Discontinue when the patient can not respond correctly with 75% accuracy (3 of 4 trials) or loses interest and attention.
7. Check to make sure the patient is not squinting or peeking around the occluder.
8. Test and record for right eye, left eye, and both eyes.
9. Record the results as 20/20 if correctly identifies the smaller toys or as 20/30 if correctly identified only the larger targets.
10. Record the visual acuity test used (STYCAR Miniature Toy Test).

Dot Visual Acuity Test (DVAT)

1. Present the DVAT unit before the patient and determine if they can see and touch the dot within the aperture (use largest dot).
2. Determine the patient's reliability and level of comprehension of the task by presenting the large dots more than once.
3. Administer the test at the appropriate distance of 10 inches. Occlude an eye.
4. Start with the larger dot targets (20/800 Snellen equivalent) and then progress to the smaller dots (20/20), presenting the targets in different locations within the test aperture.
5. Check to make sure the patient is not squinting or peeking around the occluder.
6. Use operant conditioning techniques (verbal or treat reinforcer) if necessary to sustain attention and performance.
7. Discontinue testing when the responses are random, inconsistent or absent.
8. Test and record for right eye, left eye, and both eyes.
9. Record the visual acuity according to the Snellen equivalent for the smallest dot seen.
10. Record visual acuity test used (Dot Visual Acuity Test).

Optokinetic (OKN) Drum Visual Stimulus Test

1. Present the OKN drum in front of the patient. Occlude an eye.
2. Initially position the drum at 1 foot from the patient. Rotate it slowly with the drum in the vertical position. Observe the eye movement response (OKN nystagmus).
3. Determine the patient's reliability and level of comprehension of the task by repeating this initial procedure more than once.
4. Attract attention to the drum by tapping, using noise, or a light.
5. Rotate the drum slowly (5 to 10 rotations/minute) in a clockwise and counterclockwise direction, in both vertical and horizontal positions.
6. Check to make sure the patient is not squinting or peeking around the occluder.
7. Record the presence of a persistent OKN eye movement response, for each direction of rotation, drum position, and distance from the patient (e.g., pediatric OKN +, CW & CCW, vertical & horizontal, 2 feet).
8. Discontinue testing when the response is inconsistent or absent.
9. Test and record for the right eye, left eye, and both eyes.
10. Record the visual acuity test used (OKN Drum).

Refractive Error Assessment

The assessment of refractive error in patients with multiple disorders often requires objective methods. Static, Mohindra (i.e., near retinoscopy method), and cycloplegic retinoscopy are commonly used techniques. Other techniques such as photorefraction and automated and electrodiagnostic refraction are helpful in specific cases.[23] The noncycloplegic static and Mohindra retinoscopy procedures are conducted first, utilizing techniques to control patient attention and fixation. Help the child enjoy this experience by proceeding in a cautious manner, and by giving the child time to become familiar with the test environment. Hand-held trial lenses, skiascopy lens bars, and trial frames should be used for neutralizing the refractive error. Corrected visual acuity (with the refraction in trial frame) is determined using the previously described acuity procedures.

The noncycloplegic and cycloplegic refractions should be compared when complex vision problems (e.g., strabismus, high refractive error, anisometropia and amblyopia) are present. Cyclopentolate 1% can be combined with phenylephrine 2.5% when a cycloplegic refraction and dilated fundus examination is required. Cases of patient drug sensitivity may contraindicate or limit the use of DPAs. In these situations drugs with reduced concentrations are often substituted. The use of atropine sulfate is advantageous when cyclopentolate is ineffective or when a more complete cycloplegia is necessary. The recommended dosage is a 1% solution administered at home three times each day (or 0.5% ointment at bedtime), three days prior to the examination. Many times it is best to leave DPA instillation till the end of the examination sequence.

Keratometry should be performed to determine the corneal component of refractive astigmatism. If patient cooperation or mobility limitations prevent the standard keratometer procedure; you can use the Placido's disc or Keeler Keratoscope. (Fig. 6-6) Subjective refraction is recommended if the cognitive and developmental level of the patient is appropriate. A trial frame refraction conducted in a relaxed position is preferred to using the chair stand, and phoropter. Variable or inconclusive retinoscopy results may require another appointment to repeat the procedure before prescribing treatment. Compare the refraction with the case history, the presenting signs and symptoms, and the visual acuity before determining an assessment and treatment plan.

CLINICAL PEARL

A trial frame refraction conducted in a relaxed position is preferred to using the chair, stand, and phoropter.

• Refractive Error Assessment: Behavioral Objectives

Mohindra (Near Dynamic) Retinoscopy

1. Arrange the lens bars or handheld lenses for easy access.
2. Explain to the patient that you will be turning off the lights. Have the patient look at your retinoscopy light while one eye is occluded.
3. Position the patient in a comfortable chair or on parent's lap.
4. Cover the eye not being evaluated.
5. Turn off all room lights.
6. Ask the patient to look at your light.
7. Perform retinoscopy at a 50 cm working distance.
8. Neutralize the primary meridians of each eye and record your gross findings on an optical cross.
9. Write your gross findings in spherocylindrical form.
10. Determine the net finding by adding a minus (–) 1.25 to the gross sphere power. (If gross finding = +2.00, adding –1.25 results in a net +0.75; if gross finding = –2.00, the net will equal –3.25.)

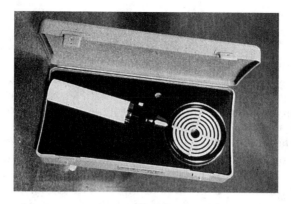

FIGURE 6-6   Keeler keratoscope.

Cycloplegic Refraction

1. Arrange the lens bars or handheld lenses for easy access.
2. Explain to the patient that you will place drops into their eyes and the drops may feel cold or sting for a few seconds. Tell them to hold onto something real tight and count to five, after which it will feel better.
3. Occlude the puncta before instilling any drops.
4. Instill one drop of topical anesthetic in each eye.
5. Record for each drop instilled into the eye, the time, name of drug, concentration, and number of drops used.
6. Wait a few minutes (1-3) before instilling the first drop of cyclopentolate 1% in each eye.
7. Instill a second drop of cyclopentolate after 5 minutes.
8. Instill a drop of phenylephrine 2.5% in each eye, if you are also going to conduct a dilated fundus examination.
9. Permit the patient to relax, play, or visit with family members while waiting 20 to 40 minutes for drug action.
10. Evaluate after 10 to 15 minutes to see if appropriate mydriasis and cycloplegia has occurred. If not instill additional drops as needed.
11. Perform retinoscopy with the patient attending to an appropriate target.
12. Neutralize each principal meridian and determine the spherocylindrical prescription. Determine your working distance and subtract this from the gross findings (e.g., gross +3.00, working distance 50 cm, subtract 2.00 D, Net = +1.00).

Binocular Vision Assessment

Patients with multiple problems have a higher than average incidence of binocular anomalies that interfere with normal development and function.[24] The assessment of binocular vision is an integral part of your examination and is important for the early detection and treatment of many disorders. You should initially determine if monocular oculomotor functions are appropriate by selecting threshold test targets that hold the patient's attention (letters, toys, pictures, puppets, etc.). The quality of monocular fixation should be determined according to centrality (central or eccentric), stability, and Angle Kappa (Lambda) alignment. The Physiological H test is used to determine the presence of "full range of motion" eye movements (FROM) or any paretic extraocular muscle disorder. The gross assessment of binocular alignment is made using examiner observation skills (looking at patient's eyes, head characteristics, etc.), the Hirschberg[25] and the Brückner tests.[26]

CLINICAL PEARL

The assessment of binocular vision is an integral part of your examination and is important for the early detection and treatment of many disorders.

Strabismus and other significant vergence disorders can be further evaluated using the Krimsky Test, unilateral cover test (UCT), and alternate cover test (ACT) sequence. If possible this should be performed in all diagnostic muscle action fields (DAFs). Any ocular deviation is described according to its laterality, direction, magnitude, frequency, distance, and concomitance. Nystagmus must be described according to wave form (jerk or pendular), velocity (fast or slow), amplitude (large or small eye movement), null point (where nystagmus is minimal), dampening conditions (convergence, bifocal to reduce accommodation, etc.), foveation characteristics (time on fovea), and other associated conditions (latent, periodic, etc.).

Patients with binocular anomalies have decreased sensory fusion that can be assessed with the Worth Four Dot Test and random dot stereograms (Random Dot E Test, Randot Stereotest, Lang Stereotest). Poor subjective responses by patients will limit the value of some of these tests, however.[27,28] Many subjective tests, including the Pola-Mirror[29] and Vis-à-Vis Polaroid techniques, require exceptional doctor observation skills and at times intuitive and inferential interpretation.

Motor fusion is determined by assessing the near point of convergence (NPC) and the relative vergence ranges. Use a prism bar or loose prisms for testing smooth and jump vergence ranges. Creative game playing may help the patient understand these subjective procedures (e.g., "It's magic . . . watch and tell me when this toy changes into two toys").

Accommodation is often deficient in patients with multiple disorders.[30] Therefore, tests of accommodation are a necessary component of the binocular vision evaluation. The monocular amplitude is assessed with either the minus lens or Donders push-up tests. The MEM (monocular estimation method) and amplitude tests are easier to perform on less responsive patients and are important for determining near point lens prescriptions.

• Binocular Vision Assessment: Behavioral Objectives

Brückner Test

1. Have patients wear their best optical correction.
2. Explain to the patient that you will turn off the lights for a few moments. Have him or her look at your light.
3. Turn off the examination room lights.
4. Stand at least 1 meter from the patient.
5. Shine your direct ophthalmoscope at the patient's nose bridge as he or she looks directly into your light.
6. Simultaneously illuminate both pupils so the retinal reflex can be seen in each eye.
7. Compare the brightness and whiteness of each retinal reflex.
8. Record if the reflexes were equal in whiteness/brightness or which eye had the whiter/brighter reflex.
9. Record the eye with the whiter/brighter reflex as the one suspected of having strabismus, uncorrected refractive error, or eye health abnormality.

Angle Kappa (Lambda)

1. Place yourself at eye level with the patient.
2. Position yourself at least 33 cm from the patient.
3. Occlude one eye.
4. Ask your patient to look directly at your penlight.
5. Monocularly sight over the barrel of your penlight.
6. Observe the corneal reflex position in the pupil center.
7. Estimate the amount of displacement from the center of the pupil in mm. (1 mm = 22 PD) and the direction of displacement (+ nasal, − temporal, up or down).
8. Repeat steps 3 through 7 for the other eye.
9. Record the displacement as eccentric fixation and indicate which eye, the magnitude, and direction.

The Hirschberg and Angle Kappa (Lambda) Test

1. Place yourself at eye level with the patient.
2. Position yourself at least 33 cm from the patient.
3. Have the patient wear their best optical correction.
4. Direct a light towards the bridge of the patient's nose and have the patient look at your light with both eyes unoccluded.
5. Monocularly sight over the penlight, looking at the corneal light reflexes.
6. Record the magnitude (1 mm = 22 PD) and direction (+ = nasal and − = temporal displacement) of the reflex of the Hirschberg test as the displacement from the center of each pupil.*
7. Conduct the Angle Kappa (Lambda) test on each eye.
8. Record if a strabismus was present, noting the magnitude, direction, which eye was affected, and the state of fixation.
9. Repeat the procedure in each of the nine diagnostic action fields (DAF) and identify any underacting/overacting muscles.

Krimsky Test

1. Have patients wear their best optical correction.
2. Evaluate both the Hirschberg and Angle Kappa tests before conducting the Krimsky test.
3. Place the appropriate correcting prism (based on the Hirschberg and Kappa results) before the fixating eye.
4. Shine your penlight at the bridge of the patient's nose and ask him or her to look at your light.
5. Monocularly sight over the penlight and note the corneal reflex position in the deviating eye.
6. Change the magnitude of the prism until the reflex of the deviating eye equals that of the fixating eye.
7. Record the magnitude and base of the neutralizing prism and the fixating eye.

---

*An optional method to approximate the magnitude of the deviation is to note a
- 30 PD magnitude if the reflex is at the border of the pupil
- 60 PD magnitude if the reflex is between the border of the pupil and the limbus, and a
- 90 PD magnitude if the reflex is at the limbus.

Always use caution with the Hirschberg/Kappa tests. Any pupil abnormality (e.g., anisocoria, displaced pupil) will affect the estimate of the deviation's magnitude.

Unilateral and Alternate Cover Test

1. Have patients wear their best optical correction.
2. Select an appropriate fixation target (e.g., Snellen letter, picture, toy, puppet, penlight).
3. Ask the patient to look at the distance target and keep it clear.
4. Unilaterally cover the right eye and watch the left eye for movement (bring occluder over the eye from a below or temporal position).
5. Unilaterally cover the left eye and watch the right eye for movement.
6. Give the patient *sufficient* time to fixate the target.
7. Record the direction of any movement of the noncovered eye (e.g., eye in, out, up, down).
8. Estimate the magnitude of movement (e.g.,~ 40 PD).
9. Alternately cover one eye, then the other (do not permit binocular viewing of the target).
10. Use a handheld prism (or prism bar) to neutralize any motion noted. Place the prism under the occluder before the covered eye; then alternate the occluder.
11. Record the eye with the prism in front and the prism power that neutralizes all movement.
12. Place the prism in front of the other eye and repeat steps 9 through 11.
13. Record the amount and base of the prism that neutralizes each fixating eye at distance (e.g., RE fixating, 30 PD Base-In; or LE fixating, 35 PD Base-In).
14. Repeat the procedure while fixating a near point target.
15. Record the frequency, laterality, distance and magnitude of the deviation (e.g., constant, alternating 30 PD exotropia at distance).

Lang Stereotest

1. Have patients wear their best near optical correction (*do not use Polaroid lenses*).
2. Place the test card at the patient's eye level (distance of 40 cm) using appropriate lighting.
3. Hold the card steady and instruct the patient to hold the head steady.
4. Have the patient identify any pictures seen and localize them by pointing.
5. Record the number of correctly identified pictures (e.g., 2 out of 3) and the stereo threshold (seconds of arc).

Random Dot E Test

1. Have patients wear their best optical correction and Polaroid filters.
2. Use adequate lighting and a test distance of 40 to 50 cm.
3. Determine if the patient can always point to the "Model E" card when also presented with the blank card.
4. Present the blank and the Random Dot E cards side by side if reliable responses were obtained in step 3.
5. Ask the patient to point to the Random Dot E card.
6. Randomize the two cards; present them to the patient; and ask the patient to again point to the Random Dot E card.
7. Present the cards at least four times and record if bifixation was seen (saw the "E" 4/4 or 5/6 times).
8. Record the stereopsis (seconds of arc) and test distance.

The Worth Four Dot Test

1. Have patients wear their best optical correction with anaglyph glasses.
2. Present the Worth Four Dot unit with the white dot at the bottom. Use normal room illumination.
3. Cover the patient's left eye and request they point to the green dots, or, if verbal, how many green dots are present. Continue if the responses are reliable.
4. Hold the light unit at 40 cm and ask the patient to tell you how many dots are seen (or point to the dots).
5. Repeat the procedure with the unit at 6 meters.
6. Record the patient responses (4 dots, normal; 5 dots, diplopia; 2 or 3 dots, suppression) and the test distance.
7. Repeat with neutralizing prism (if strabismic), perform the UCT, and record the responses (normal, anomalous retinal correspondence, etc.)

MEM Nearpoint Retinoscopy

1. Have patients wear their best optical correction.
2. Present an appropriate MEM target fastened to the front of the retinoscope at the patient's habitual near working distance.
3. Provide adequate illumination for reading the MEM target.
4. Pass the vertical streak of the retinoscope across the eye while estimating the amount of motion.
5. Quickly interpose an appropriate lens in the spectacle plane of the eye (quick dipping) while simultaneously passing the vertical streak of the retinoscope across the eye. Repeat for the vertical meridian of the eye.
6. Continue testing until the vertical and horizontal meridians of each eye have been neutralized.
7. Record the vertical and horizontal meridian findings for each eye as the Lag of Accommodation.

Near Point of Convergence Test

1. Begin testing with the patient's best optical correction.
2. Present a small threshold target (letter or toy) below eye level before the patient at a 40 cm distance.
3. Begin to move the target towards the bridge of the nose. Instruct the patient to inform you if the letters blur, double, or "look different."
4. Record the distance from the bridge of the nose when sustained blur or diplopia occurred.
5. Record when fusion recovered as the target was moved away.
6. Repeat the procedure five times. Note changes from trial 1.
7. Observe and record the distance where one eye appeared to turn out (even when patient did not report blur/diplopia).

Accommodative Facility Lens Flipper Test

1. Have patients wear their best optical correction.
2. Give instructions and demonstrate the technique.
3. Present an accommodative rock card with 20/30 print, single letters, at 16 inches.
4. Occlude one eye and quickly place the plus side of the lens flippers before the open eye. Instruct the patient to read the letter in the box when clear.
5. Quickly flip the lens so the minus side is before the same eye. Instruct the patient to read the letter in box 2 when clear.
6. Continue the alternation for one minute (calculate the cycles/minute rate).
7. Switch the occluder to the other eye and repeat.
8. Repeat with the patient binocular. Place suppression strips on the letters and Polaroids or anaglyphs on the patient.
9. Record the monocular and binocular cycles/minute; any suppressions; and which side (+/−) was more difficult.

Saccades and Pursuits

1. Use targets with 20/80-size letters.
2. Arrange two targets horizontally separated (25-30 cm) at 40 cm from the patient's eyes.
3. Give clear instructions. Demonstrate how to alternately fixate between the 2 targets.
4. Occlude one eye. Instruct patient to alternate 10 times between the 2 targets.
5. Occlude the other eye. Repeat procedure 4.
6. Perform the same procedure with the patient binocular.
7. Observe and record any uncontrolled head movement.
8. Observe, record and grade the saccades (4+ grading):
   - 4+   Smooth and accurate
   - 3+   Slight undershoot
   - 2+   Gross under/overshooting, increased latency
   - 1+   Inability to do the task.
9. Use a single target for pursuit testing (40 cm distance).
10. Occlude one eye. Observe pursuit ability while moving target horizontally, vertically, and diagonally.
11. Repeat steps 5 through 7, grading the pursuits (4+ grading)
    - 4+   Smooth and accurate
    - 3+   One fixation loss
    - 2+   Two fixation losses
    - 1+   More than 2 fixation losses, inability to do task.
12. Record any score of less than 3+ as poor performance.

Ocular Health Assessment

All special population patients require a thorough ocular health assessment. The basic purpose is to detect any abnormalities that may compromise ocular development, function, and health.[31] The anterior segment and ocular adnexia are examined using standard or handheld slit lamp techniques. Some patients will require the use of an illuminated hand magnifier (Burton lamp), transilluminator, or penlight. This should include an assessment of the lids/lashes anterior chamber, pupil function, iris, cornea, and conjunctiva. Your skill as an objective observer may be the primary source of information when more standard tests are not efficacious. Special attention must be given to the unique ocular health abnormalities typical of specific disorders.

Standard applanation tonometry (Goldmann) can be successfully completed for many patients with disabilities. Hand-held applanation instruments (such as the Tono-Pen XL) are an efficient and reliable alternative. Noncontact tonometers (Keeler Pulsair, AO-NCT) are also available in table and handheld units (Figs. 6-7 and 6-8). Tactile (digital) tensions may be used (record as soft, medium, or hard) if

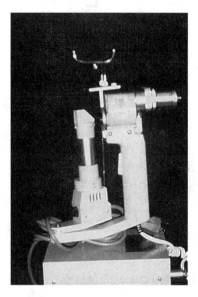

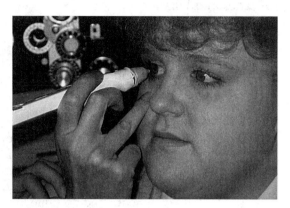

FIGURE 6-8 Tono-Pen XL.

FIGURE 6-7 Hand-held biomicroscope.

more conventional and quantifiable IOP procedures are unsuccessful. Patients who present with glaucoma-related signs and symptoms may require tonometry while under sedation. Various fixation devices with constant encouragement are often needed to control attention during tonometry.

The lens, vitreous, retina, and posterior pole must be evaluated through dilated pupils using both direct and indirect ophthalmoscopy. This may require special positioning (e.g., patient lying on floor, on parent's lap, or in a wheelchair, etc.) in order to examine the central and peripheral fundus. Record the optic disc characteristics (color, depth, rim, and cup/disc ratio); foveal area and macular reflex; retinal A/V vessel ratio; and health of the overall retinal field (note any vascular lesions, holes, tears, breaks, or pigment changes). Retinal photographs can be taken when appropriate.

Visual field disorders occur more frequently in patients with disabilities. Field screening can be accomplished using confrontation procedures with nonstandard targets (e.g., hand, toy, face, or other interesting item). Non-verbal responses are observed and recorded (e.g., fixation shift, pointing at the target, changes in head position) when charting field defects. The Ishihara Color Test (Children's version) is effective for detecting color vision deficiencies that may indicate the presence of ocular disease. The Wool (Yarn) Test is a color matching procedure that can be used if standard tests (Ishihara, D-15 Color Test, etc.) are inappropriate for your patient.

Electrodiagnostic evaluation is an objective procedure useful in the diagnosis of congenital or acquired ocular disease of unknown etiology.[32] The electroretinogram (ERG) records general retinal functions, while the visually evoked potential (VEP) records retinal and cortical macular functions.

• Ocular Health Assessment: Behavioral Objectives

Tono-Pen XL

1. Visually inspect the tonometer's probe for cracks, chips, or irregularities.
2. Cover the Tono-Pen probe tip with a new tip cover.
3. Complete a calibration check (not necessary prior to each use) by depressing first the reset button and then the activation switch. Observe if the previous calibration check was "good" as indicated by the LED display "---" and a beep. Perform the entire calibration procedure if the LED display shows "bAd" followed by a long beep.
4. Instill topical anesthetic into each eye.
5. Position the patient, seated or supine, and direct attention to a fixation target.
6. Tell the patient to look at the fixation target with eyes fully open. Hold the Tono-Pen XL as if a pencil, bracing your hand on the patient's cheek.
7. Depress and quickly release the activation switch prior to taking a measurement. A beep will sound indicating the instrument is ready. Touch the Tono-Pen to the cornea. Repeat several times.
8. Listen for a clicking sound and note the digital read out displayed for each valid IOP measurement. An average and statistical reliability is calculated after four valid readings.
9. Repeat the procedure for each eye and record the results.
10. Leave the tip cover on during storage and replace with new tip before each patient use.

Handheld (Kowa) Slit Lamp

1. Explain to the patient that you will be looking at their eyes with a special light held close to their face.
2. Remove the slit lamp from the hanging holder, turn the lamp on, and adjust for the appropriate illumination setting (direct view, vertical streak, cobalt blue filter, red-free filter, etc.).
3. Position the patient comfortably so you can slowly bring the instrument close to the eyes. Brace your hand on the patient's face or forehead to avoid hitting the eye.
4. Instruct the patient to look "straight ahead" while you begin with direct illumination. Inspect the lids, lid margin, lacrimal system, sclera, limbus, conjunctiva, cornea, iris, anterior chamber/angle, and lens.
5. Change to the small width vertical streak for more detailed inspection of the corneal layers, tear layers, anterior chamber depth, and lens.
6. Stain the cornea with fluorescene and further evaluate with blue light any corneal surface irregularities.
7. Evaluate the integrity of the pupil reflexes in both bright and dim lighting.
8. Evert the eyelid and inspect the palpebral conjunctiva.
9. Repeat for both eyes. Record your findings.

Assessment and Treatment Plan

After the examination database is compiled, you next complete the patient's assessment and treatment plan. Evaluate the findings in the various diagnostic areas and summarize specific problems on a master problem list (Fig. 6-3).[33] Determine an appropriate treatment plan for each problem area assessed. It is helpful to number the individual problems and give a corresponding number to the treatment plan for each problem. Specific treatment options may include prescription lenses (spectacles, contact lenses, low vision aids), vision therapy, environmental modifications, monitor with follow-up care, and referral to other professionals.[34] Identify for each of the treatment options the advantages and disadvantages, the treatment sequence, the prognosis/anticipated outcome, and the time/financial commitment. Also address the question "What if we do nothing now?" and the impact of delayed treatment.

CLINICAL PEARL

Identify for each of the treatment options the advantages and disadvantages, the treatment sequence, the prognosis/anticipated outcome, and the time/financial commitment.

A fundamental concern is whether treatment will enhance the patient's health and performance. Numerous studies[35] have documented positive treatment results even when the potential was unclear or discouraging at the onset. Explore all treatment possibilities. Maintain an open and positive attitude toward the potential benefits patients with disabilities may receive when treated appropriately. Follow the same management strategy for refractive errors[36] that you use with your nondisabled patients. There is evidence supporting the use of all types of lens prescriptions (spectacles and contact lenses) in both simple (single vision) and complex design (bifocals and low vision aids). The patient's special needs must be considered in the design of the lenses (e.g., bifocal height and power appropriate for the wheelchair table board). Observe the patient's environment (note any factors that may limit the wearing of glasses; the placement of bifocal seg heights, etc.) to determine the most appropriate lens treatment. Special frame design is needed in patients with head mobility limitations and unusual facial characteristics. When dispensing the spectacles review with the patient and/or guardian the care and handling; the recommended use; and the specific purpose. Many patients may become discouraged and discontinue wear if they do not understand why they have the glasses.

Vision therapy for the patient with disabilities is effective for the treatment of amblyopia, disorders of binocular vision, ocular motility, accommodation, eye-hand coordination, and visual perception. Therapy management should be consistent and involve 1 or 2 key therapists working in the most appropriate environment (office, home, school, or residence facility).[37] Modification of the home, school, work, and play environment should be considered for facilitating treatment and improving overall function. This may include modifying lighting, posture, working distance, room position, visual stimuli, support systems (e.g., computers, hand-eye coordination devices), and work or school activities (e.g., limit time, scope, and content). Patient education will help achieve a balance of compliance appropriate for their personal and social needs.

Your case presentation to the patient, parent, or guardian is critical for maximizing their understanding of the problems and your short- and long-term treatment goals. The verbal report offers an opportunity for questions, discussion, and the sharing of emotional and intellectual concerns about the normal course of the disability. A written report (Fig. 6-4) is essential for interprofessional communication and for providing documentation of your findings and treatment recommendations.[38]

Present a summary (Fig. 6-4) of each diagnostic area, possible etiologies, recommended treatment options, and prognosis. Relate this to the entering chief complaint, signs, and symptoms. Address patient questions such as "How clearly can I see?" (visual acuity); "Will glasses or contact lenses help me?" (refraction); "Are my eyes healthy?" (ocular health); "Do I have good visual efficiency for my schoolwork (job)?" (binocular vision); and "What can you do to help me see and perform better?" (treatment options). The underlying issue in many of these questions is the patient's need to feel better about themselves and their potential. All of this will assist your patients in identifying specific and realistic treatment goals.

Patients with disabilities require continuous care and management. Emphasize this need for follow-up as a part of your patient/parent education. The rapport established during the examination will continue to grow and support a discussion of disability-related issues. Never deny the patient an opportunity to pursue an appropriate treatment option even if it may seem to provide little or no potential benefit. If the patient pursues questionable treatment plans, you must schedule periodic assessment and progress reviews with the patient and family. These reviews should include updated written reports that always refer back to the original assessment and treatment goals. Permit the patient time to assimilate this information before deciding on treatment. You may also recommend that they obtain another medical opinion to assist in their decision-making process. The optometrist's participation on the "patient's team" can facilitate sharing of information and cooperation. You should assist the patient in the decision-making process, including the deciding of eligibility for legally mandated services. Always encourage communication with every member of the patient's health, education, and rehabilitation team. This will allow the patient to enjoy the full benefits of your professional services.[35]

Summary

1. You will learn to enjoy your patients more if you treat them as a person having similar cares and needs as the non-disabled.
2. People with disabilities are frequently mistreated by the health care system. They are cautious and tentative about examinations, but do respond to a friendly and honest approach.
3. Become comfortable with the assessment procedures described. Practice them on your able-bodied patients and become efficient in their use.
4. Be flexible and adaptable with the examination routine. Work within the patient's developmental and behavioral characteristics.
5. Consider all treatment alternatives. Realize that your treatment's potential for success is only possible when attempted, monitored, and modified.
6. Plan ongoing training for you and your staff. Have appropriate references available for consultation when needed.[39] Include informal staff meetings and formal educational programs.

7. Maintain open communications between your office and the patient, the patient's family or guardian, and other professionals providing social, medical and educational services.
8. Children and adults with developmental disabilities need your special services and expertise. Many agencies serving the handicapped value the services you give. Do not hesitate to contact those agencies and provide optometric vision care for individuals diagnosed as special.[40]

REFERENCES

1. Elkind J: The incidence of disabilities in the United States, *Hum Factors* 32:397-405, 1990.
2. Kastner K, Luckhardt J: Medical services for the developmentally disabled, *NJ Med* 87:819-22, 1990.
3. Ettinger ER: Affirmative action issues within optometry, *J Am Optom Assoc* 63:611-13, 1992.
4. Maino D, Maino J, Maino S: Mental retardation syndromes with associated ocular defects, *J Am Optom Assoc* 61:634-40, 1990.
5. Geering J, Maino D: The patient with mental handicaps: a primary care perspective, *South J Optom* 10:23-7, 1992.
6. Maino D, Wesson M, Schlange D, et al: Optometric findings in the fragile X syndrome, *Optom Vis Sci* 68:634-40, 1991.
7. Maino D, Scharre J: Poland-Mobius syndrome: a case report, *Optom Vis Sci* 66:621-25, 1989.
8. Ettinger E: Optometric evaluation of the patient with cerebral palsy, *J Behav Optom* 2:115-22, 1991.
9. Frantz K, Caden B: Diagnosis and management of common eye diseases in infants, toddlers, and preschool children. In Schieman M (ed): *Pediatric Optometry Problems in Optometry Series* 2:420-37, 1990.
10. Schieman M: Assessment and management of the exceptional child. In Rosenbloom A, Morgan M (eds): *Principles and practice of pediatric optometry,* Philadelphia, 1990, JB Lippincott Co, 388-419.
11. Maino J: The problem oriented record, *J Am Optom Assoc* 50:915-18, 1979.
12. Randle W: Opening opportunities for disabled: Confusion, debate still trail new law, *Chicago Tribune Business Section* 7;12/1/91:1,4.
13. Dorning M: Opening opportunities for disabled: Firms trying to meet access rules, deadlines, *Chicago Tribune Business Section* 7;12/1/91:1,4.
14. Anonymous: Disabilities act to impact optometric practices, *AOA News* 1:1, 1991.
15. Richman J: Assessment of visual acuity in preschool children. In Scheiman M (ed): *Pediatric Optometry Problems in Optometry Series* 2:319-32, 1990.
16. Richman J, Petito G, Cron M: Broken wheel acuity test: a new and valid test for preschool and exceptional children, *J Am Optom Assoc* 55:561-5, 1984.
17. Mayer D, Dobson V: Visual acuity development in infants and young children as assessed by operant perferential looking, *Vis Res* 22:1141-51, 1982.
18. Birch E, Halek L, Stager D, et al: Operant acuity and developmentally delayed children with low vision, *J Pediatr Ophthalmol Strabismus* 24:64-9, 1987.
19. Kirschen D, Rosenblaum A, Ballard E: The dot visual acuity test: a new acuity test for children, *J Am Optom Assoc* 54:1055-9, 1983.
20. London R: Optokinetic nystagmus: a review of pathways, techniques, and selected diagnostic applications, *J Am Optom Assoc* 53:791-8, 1982.

21. Lovasik J, Woodruff M: Increasing diagnostic potential in pediatric optometry by electrophysiological methods, *Can J Optom* 45:69-83, 1983.

22. Rouse M, Ryan J: The optometric examination and management of children. In Rosenbloom A, Morgan M (eds): *Principles and practice of pediatric optometry*, Philadelphia, 1990, JB Lippincott Co, 155-92.

23. Bobier W, Schmitz P, Strong G, et al: Comparison of three photorefractive methods in a study of a developmentally handicaped population, *Clin Vis Sci* 7:225–35, 1992.

24. Maino D: An eye care delivery service model for children and adults with developmental disabilities: a program of the Easter Seal Society of Metropolitan Chicago and the Illinois College of Optometry. Presented during the Access to Health Care Symposium American Association on Mental Retardation 116th Annual Meeting, New Orleans, LA; May 29, 1992.

25. Wick B, London R: The Hirschberg test: analysis from birth to age 5, *J Am Optom Assoc* 51:1009-10, 1980.

26. Griffin J, Cotter S: The Brückner test: evaluation of clinical usefulness, *Am J Optom Physiol Opt* 63:957-61, 1986.

27. Ciner J, Scheiman M, Schanel-Klitsch E, Weil L: Stereopsis testing in 10 to 35 month old children using operant preferential looking, *Optom Vis Sci* 66:782-7, 1989.

28. Lang T, Lang J: Eye screening with the Lang stereotest, *Am Orthop J* 38:48-50, 1988.

29. Griffin J: Screening for anomalies of binocular vision by means of the polaroid mirror method, *Am J Optom Arch Academ Optom* 48-689-92, 1971.

30. Duckman R: Accommodation in cerebral palsy: function and remediation, *J Am Optom Assoc* 4:281-3, 1984.

31. Blackman J: Mental retardation. In Blackman J (ed): *Medical aspects of developmental disabilities in children, birth through three*, Rockville, Md, 1983, Aspen Pub, 47-55.

32. Kuroda J, Adachi-Usami E: Evaluation of pattern visual evoked cortical potentials for prescribing spectacles in mentally retarded infants and children, *Doc Ophthalmol* 66:253-9, 1987.

33. Amos J: The problem-solving approach to patient care. In Amos J (ed): *Diagnosis and management in vision care*, Boston, 1987, Butterworths, 1-7.

34. Hoffman L, Rouse M: Referral recommendations for binocular function and/or developmantal perceptual deficiencies, *J Am Optom Assoc* 51:119-25, 1980.

35. Bader D, Woodruff M: The effects of corrective lenses on various behaviors of mentally retarded persons, *Am J Optom Physiol Opt* 57:447-59, 1980.

36. Ciner E: Management of refractive errors in infants, toddlers, and preschool children. In Schieman M (ed): *Pediatric Optometry Problems in Optometry Series*, 2:394-420, 1990.

37. Clunies-Ross G: The development of children with Down's syndrome: lessons from the past and implications for the future, *Aust Pediatr J* 22:167-, 1986.

38. Zambone A: Optometrists on the team: holistic care and the patient-parent-educator interface. In Rosenbloom A, Morgan M (eds) *Principles and procedures of pediatric optometry*. Philadelphia, 1990, JB Lippincott Co, 560-76.

39. Fatt H, Griffin J, Lyle W: *Genetics for primary eye care practitioners*. 2nd ed Boston, 1992, Butterworth-Heinemann.

40. Gnadt G, Wesson M: A survey of the vision assessment of the developmentally disabled and multi-handicapped in University Affiliated Programs (UAPS), *J Am Optom Assoc* 63:619-25, 1992.

• Appendix: Equipment Resources

Bailey-Hall Cereal Test
Bailey-Hall Preferential Looking Test
Multimedia Center
School of Optometry
University of California, Berkeley
Berkeley, CA 94720

Broken Wheel Test of Visual Acuity
Optokinetic Drum Visual Stimulus
 Test
Worth Four Dot
Skiascopy lens bars, other items
Bernell Corporation
750 Lincoln Way East
PO Box 4637
South Bend, IN 46634
800-348-2225

Candy Bead Vision Screening
Nonpareils (1.1 mm width)
Any grocery store

Handheld Slit Lamp
Haag-Streit Services, Inc.
7 Industrial Park
Waldwick, NJ 07463

HOTV Vision Test
Dot Visual Acuity Test
Good-Lite Company
1540 Hannah Ave.
Forest Park, IL 60130
708-366-3860
708-366-7295 (fax)

Keeler Instruments
456 Parkway Ave.
Broomall, PA 19008

Lea Symbols
Precision Vision
721 North Addison Road
Villa Park, IL 60181
708-833-1454
708-833-1520 (fax)

Lighthouse Flashcard Vision Test
Lighthouse Low Vision Products
2602 Northern Blvd.
Long Island, NY 11101

Compuserve
Online Resources and References
Disabilities Forum (GO
 DISABILITIES)
Handicapped Users' Database (GO
 HUD)
IBM Special Needs Forum (GO IBM-
 SPECIAL)
Computer Database Plus (GO
 COMPDB)

PL 20/20 Vision Tester
Optical Technology Corporation
515 E. 22nd Terrace
Lawrence, KS 66046

Random Dot Butterfly
Other Random Dot targets
Synthetic Optics Corporation
903 Mohawk Road
Franklin Lakes, NJ 07417

STYCAR Vision Screening Test
STYCAR Graded Balls Test
STYCAR Miniature Toys Test
NFER-Nelson Publishing Company
Danville House
2 Oxford Road East
Windsor, Berkshire
England SL41DF

Teller Acuity Cards
Random Dot E
Lang Stereo Test
Stereo Optical Company, Inc.
3539 N. Kenton
Chicago, IL 60641
800-344-9500

Teller Acuity Cards
VisTech Consultants Inc
1372 North Fairfield Road
Dayton OH 45432

Tono-Pen XL
Mentor O & O Inc.
3000 Longwater Dr.
Norwell, MA 02051
800-628-5227

7

Ocular Health Anomalies in Patients with Developmental Disabilities

Dominick M. Maino
Joseph H. Maino
Gerhard W. Cibis
Frederick Hecht

Key Terms

Congenital glaucoma	Fragile X syndrome	Laurence-Moon-Biedl syndrome
Lowe syndrome	Neurofibromatosis	Brain-retina neuroembryodys-genesis
Apert syndrome	Tuberous sclerosis	
Crouzon syndrome	Sturge-Weber syndrome	Microcephaly
Down syndrome	Congenital amaurosis of Leber	
Fetal alcohol syndrome		

It has been estimated[1] that up to 3% of the population may exhibit a developmental disability that seriously affects the individual's ability to learn, work, or contribute to society in a meaningful way. This chapter describes several mental retardation syndromes that have significant ocular and systemic health abnormalities that will require advanced diagnostic and treatment tools. The primary care optometrist should be prepared to appropriately manage these quality of life–threatening defects and assist the rehabilitation team and their patients in the decision making process.

CLINICAL PEARL

The primary care optometrist should be prepared to appropriately manage these quality of life–threatening defects and assist the rehabilitation team and their patients in the decision making process.

Syndromes Associated with Congenital Glaucoma

Glaucoma is frequently associated with syndromes involving developmental delay (i.e., Stuge-Weber, Reiger, and Lowe syndromes), various postsurgical complications, and trauma. It may also be associated with retrolental fibroplasia, retinoblastoma, and juvenile xanthogranuloma. Up to 45% of these secondary glaucomas demonstrate anterior segment dysgenesis and other anatomical/developmental defects. It is imperative that routine monitoring of intraocular pressue (IOP) occur.[2]

Although applanation pressures can be performed on an awake infant, it is easier to determine the IOP while the child is being examined under anesthesia. An infant's IOP (about 10 mm Hg) tends to be lower than an adult's. Depending on the stage and the length of time of anesthesia, the infant IOP will measure somewhat lower than you would normally expect in the unanesthetized state. For consistent results it should be measured as soon as the child is intubated.[2] If examination under anesthesia is not feasible because of medical contraindications or parental concerns, the optometrist should be aware that IOP readings may be extremely variable.[3]

The typical neonatal cornea measures approximately 10 to 10.5 mm and grows by 0.5 to 1 mm the first year. Since increased corneal diameter (buphthalmos) can be the first indication of congenital glaucoma, assessing the size of the cornea in both vertical and horizontal dimensions is vital. Haab striae and epiphora may also indicate increased IOP in a young child.

Corneal dystrophies may be associated with congenital glaucoma and can have epithelial edema as a result of abnormal corneal endothelium. IOPs in this instance will vary. Individuals with corneal dystrophies usually do not exhibit developmental delay. Glaucoma-induced epithelial edema has bullae and clears with the application of pressure or glycerin, scraping the epithelium, or using medication to decrease the IOP. Anatomical angle structures in developmental glaucoma include high iris insertion on the trabecular meshwork, a thickened meshwork (Barkan's membrane), and iris strands.[4-6]

Medical therapy alone is not an effective mode of treatment for congenital glaucoma but often is used as adjunct therapy after surgical intervention. Therapeutic pharmaceuticals (such as beta blockers) may be used until surgery can be performed or to increase the successful management of the glaucoma after surgery. The surgical procedures of choice include both goniotomy and trabeculotomy. Changes in the IOP and the axial length of the eye, along with optic nerve cupping, must be monitored at all follow-up visits. If any abnormalities of the anterior chamber are noted, follow-up evaluations under anesthesia should be conducted at approximately 3 month intervals for the next year. Yearly in-office evaluations of intraocular pressures are then recommended.[2,5,6]

CLINICAL PEARL

Medical therapy alone is not an effective mode of treatment for congenital glaucoma but often is used as adjunct therapy after surgical intervention.

Lowe Syndrome (oculocerebrorenal syndrome)

Lowe syndrome is a sex-linked recessive metabolic disorder with its onset in early infancy. Clinical features include mental, psychomotor, and growth retardation. Muscular hypotony, reduced reflexes, and hyperactivity (including strange choreoathetoid movements with screaming) are frequently noted. The ocular anomalies include nystagmus, congenital glaucoma, miotic pupils, and ectropion uveae. Poor or absent pupillary reactions, malformations of the iris and anterior chamber angle, and blue sclera, cloudy corneas, and buphthalmos may all be present. Characteristic flat disciform cataracts, microphakia, and strabismus are also seen.[7a]

Treatment for patients with Lowe syndrome includes cataract surgery (after the first week of birth) and the application of aphakic glasses or contact lenses. The development of corneal keloids, however, is often a contraindication to contact lenses.[8,9] If no deprivation amblyopia or glaucoma-induced damage has occurred, many patients will achieve normal visual acuities.

Cranial Deformity Syndromes

Apert and Crouzon syndromes are two of the more frequently encountered cranial abnormalities. Mental retardation is often the result of chronic hydrocephalus secondary to premature closure of the sutures. Apert syndrome (acrocephalosyndactyly) is an inherited disorder with oxycephaly (towerskull), syndactyly, and agenesis of the spinal bones and limbs. Ocular findings include shallow orbits, exophthalmos, hypertelorism, and ptosis. Strabismus, nystagmus, moderate to high refractive error (hyperopia), and exposure keratitis are noted as well. Other patients with Apert syndrome may have ophthalmoplegia, cataracts, ectopia lentis, retinal detachments, and/or papilledema with optic atrophy.[1,7b]

Crouzon syndrome (dysostosis cranio-facialis oxycephaly) is an autosomal dominant disorder with manifestations apparent at birth. The numerous clinical characteristics include prognathism, synostosis of the coronal and lambdoid sutures, parrot-beaked nose, and a widening of the temporal fossae. Exophthalmos, hypertelorism, nystagmus, cataracts, and strabismus are common ocular anomalies. Other eye findings include blue sclera, exposure keratitis, papilledema, optic atrophy, and corneal dystrophy.[1,7c]

Surgical correction of the strabismus for individuals with cranial deformities should occur after the midface reconstructive surgery has deepened the orbits. This will reduce the typical V pattern exotropia. Any amblyopia present should be managed with appropriate refractive correction and patching.

Down Syndrome

Down syndrome (trisomy 21) is the most frequent cause of mental retardation due to a genetic etiology.* Common physical/clincial/systemic features are moderate mental retardation, low-set ears, hypertelorism, epicanthal folds, leukemia, and skeletal abnormalities. There may also be short fifth fingers, a fissured tongue, transverse palmar creases, and various heart abnormalities. The more numerous ophthalmic problems seen include blepharoconjunctivitis, nystagmus, strabismus, moderate to high refractive error, lens opacities, and keratoconus.[7d]

CLINICAL PEARL

Down syndrome (trisomy 21) is the most frequent cause of mental retardation due to genetic etiology.

Surgical management of the strabismus and downward-slanting palpebral fissures may be beneficial for Down patients who function at

*See Chapter 2.

a higher cognitive level. Treatment of the blepharitits with appropriate lid hygiene (lid scrubs and warm compresses) reduces the likelihood of other opportunistic infections. Uncorrected refractive error, amblyopia, keratoconus, esotropia of an accommodative nature, and other learning-related vision disorders can be managed with the application of contact lenses, glasses, and orthoptics/vision therapy as required.[1,7d,10]

Fetal Alcohol Syndrome (FAS)

When taking the history of a child with dysmorphic features, you should not only include questions concerning the eye but also inquire into the family history to ascertain whether either parent abused drugs.[11] The prevalence of FAS is as high as 1 per 750 live births with 30% to 40% of the children born to alcoholic mothers having the syndrome. FAS is one of the most preventable causes of mental retardation (Figure 7-1).

 CLINICAL PEARL
FAS is one of the most preventable causes of mental retardation.

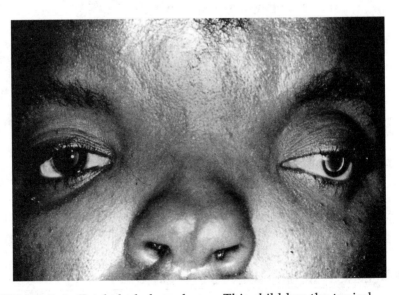

FIGURE 7-1 Fetal alcohol syndrome. This child has the typical facial characteristics of FAS. Note the flat philtrum, slightly upturned nose, telecanthus and ptosis. This child also exhibited exotropia, amblyopia, Peters anomaly and high myopia.

The clinical findings most frequently associated with high alcohol intake during pregnancy are[12-15]

- Growth retardation in both height and weight that persists in the postnatal period
- Central nervous system dysfunction (intellectual defects, micro cephaly, and hyperactivity)
- Characteristic craniofacial anomalies (telecanthus with shortened palpebral fissures, flat philtrum, short upturned nose, thin upper vermillion border, epicanthal folds, and ptosis)
- Other systemic, cardiovascular, and urogenitial system disorders

FAS cannot be diagnosed by a laboratory test but must be determined by supportive physical findings and a maternal history of heavy alcohol consumption during pregnancy. Most children with FAS are the end result of mothers who consumed 6 to 7 drinks a day early in the pregnancy. Unless the physical signs and history both confirm it, FAS can only be presumed to be present.

Some children may not meet the full criteria for diagnosis of FAS and are referred to as having FAE, or fetal alcohol effect. It has been suggested that binge drinking results in a number of children with FAE depending on the time of insult, amount of alcohol consumed, and other genetic and environmental factors. Even though the diagnosis of FAS or FAE may be strongly supported by both the physical factors and the case history, a full genetic workup should be conducted when appropriate to rule out other etiologies that could cause the developmental delay noted.

The ocular findings of FAS include antimongoloid slant of the lid fissures, lateral displacement of the inner canthi, and ptosis. Amblyopia, moderate to high amounts of refractive error, and anisometropia are frequently seen as well. Up to 50% of the children will exhibit strabismus, with most demonstrating an esotropia. The most serious ocular anomalies are malformations (hypoplasia) of the optic nerve with a resultant reduction in visual acuity. Nystagmus may be present, with tortuosity of the retinal vessels a common finding.

Anterior segment anomalies have been seen in up to 10% of children with FAS—ranging from posterior embryotoxon to severe corneal opacification with perforation in the neonatal period. The most typical developmental malformation is Peters anomaly. As with all individuals demonstrating an anterior segment abnormality, it is important to monitor the IOP for the development of glaucoma.[7e,13-15]

Fragile X Syndrome (Unstable DNA)

The fragile X syndrome has emerged as the most common heritable cause of mental retardation, one of the first genetic etiologies of learning disabilities, and the first genetic disease noted to be caused by a DNA nucleotide-repeated sequence.[16,17a,18] It affects approximately 1 per 1000 males and 1 per 2000 females with a gene frequency estimated to be 1 per 625 in the general population. The clinical picture includes nonspecific development delay in infancy and moderate to severe retardation later in childhood, with boys being more adversely affected than girls.

CLINICAL PEARL

The fragile X syndrome has emerged as the most common heritable cause of mental retardation, one of the first genetic etiologies of learning disabilities, and the first genetic disease caused by a DNA nucleotide-repeated sequence.

Numerous physical characteristics are present—and may include a large body size, long narrow head, reduced intercanthal distance (<3.5 cm), protruding or low-set ears, and large hands and feet. The young child may also exhibit hypotonia, seizures, and recurrent otitis media. A connective tissue dysplasia is commonly seen, with mitral valve prolapse, long digits, hyperflexible joints, flat feet, and macroorchidism (in 80% of affected men) being noted.[19-21]

Fragile X females demonstrate similar physical characteristics—but usually to a lesser degree—and may show a reduced IQ, learning disabilities, math and language delays, sensory integration abnormalities, attentional dysfunctions, and various psychiatric illnesses. They will have a tendency to be very shy, and many exhibit the typical gaze avoidance associated with fragile X.[17b]

If any suspicion of the fragile X syndrome arises based on your clinical assessment or family history, appropriate laboratory testing is required. There are several ways to proceed with these laboratory tests:[22-25]

- Cytogenetics only
- Cytogenetics and linkage
- Cytogenetics and DNA probes (currently recommended)
- Cytogenetics and linkage and DNA probes
- DNA probes only (in the near future)

Cytogenetics is still a prerequisite for diagnosis at this time. The fragile site is on the X chromosome in band q27.3, where it manifests most often by showing gaps in the continuity of the chromosome. Frank chromosomal breaks or polyradial formations may also indicate the presence of this syndrome. These manifestations are visible through the light microscope in lymphocytes (and other cells) grown in a laboratory culture medium deficient in folic acid and thymidine or to which methotrexate or 5-fluorodeoxyuridine (FUDR) has been added.

Molecular genetic studies are the wave of the future, however. Direct DNA analysis of the fragile X gene has given us startling information. For instance, it has been found that

- The fragile X gene is made up of DNA that is unstable.
- This unstable DNA has a repeating nucleotide sequence.
- The repeat is cytidine phosphate–guanosine (CpG).
- This repeating nucleotide sequence gets longer with each succeeding generation.
- The length of the repeating sequence can vary between siblings and even within different cell populations in an individual.
- The longer the CpG repeating sequence, the more severe are the clinical phenotypes.

The elongation of this repeating sequence provides a biological basis for anticipation. Anticipation is the progressively earlier appearance and greater severity of a genetic disease in successive generations.

Oculovisual and visual/perceptual motor abnormalities associated with fragile X are numerous. Maino et al.,[26,27] Maino and King,[28] Amin and Maino,[29] and Storm et al.[30] have all noted moderate to high amounts of refractive error (59% hyperopia, 17% myopia, 22% astigmatism [$>/= +1.00$ D]) with a third to half of the population exhibiting strabismus (esotropia more frequently than exotropia). Nystagmus is seen in approximately 13% of the fragile X population.

Other learning-related oculovisual anomalies include amblyopia, anisometropia, accommodative insufficiency, and convergence excess and insufficiency as well as mild to severe dysfunctions in visual motor integration, ocular motilities, laterality/directionality, visual figure ground, visual closure, visual form constancy, visual memory, and visual sequential memory.[28,29]

The optometrist should be aware that many patients currently under their care may have undiagnosed fragile X. Dibler and Maino[31] have noted that a thorough and complete differential diagnosis should be conducted for each individual suspected of having this important syndrome. It has also been suggested[28] that any child with mental retardation of nonspecific etiology who presents with a strabismus should routinely be screened for fragile X.

CLINICAL PEARL

The optometrist should be aware that many patients currently under their care may have undiagnosed fragile X.

Phakomatoses

The phakomatoses include neurofibromatosis I and neurofibromatosis II, tuberous sclerosis, Sturge-Weber syndrome, ataxia-telangiectasia, von Hippel–Lindau and Wyburn-Mason syndromes. The last three are relatively rare and will not be discussed in this review.

Neurofibromatoses

The neurofibromatoses include at least two distinct clinical entities: NF1 (von Recklinghausen disease), caused by a mutation of chromosome 17, and NF2 (bilateral acoustic neurofibromatosis), caused by a mutated chromosome 22. The differential diagnosis becomes challenging when a patient presents with multiple cutaneous or CNS tumors. In the patient with NF1, neurofibromas and gliomas are frequently noted; but in NF2 schwannomas, meningiomas, and ependymomas typically occur.

If two or more of the following are noted, the differential diagnosis for NF1 can be made:

- Six or more café-au-lait spots larger than 5 mm in diameter in prepubertal individuals
- Six or more café-au-lait spots over 15 mm in diameter in postpubertal individuals
- Two or more neurofibromas of any type or one plexiform neurofibroma
- Axillary or inguinal freckling
- Optic glioma
- Two or more Lisch nodules (iris hamartomas)
- A distinctive osseous lesion (sphenoid dysplasia of the long bone with or without pseudarthrosis)
- A first-degree relative with diagnosed NF1

Individuals with NF1 will also exhibit an autosomal dominant genetic etiology with 100% penetrance in adulthood. Because of this etiology, all immediate relatives should be informed and appropriately evaluated. Other systemic manifestations include growth anomalies, spontaneous fractures, and facial hemihypertrophy. Glaucoma, proptosis, cataracts, optic atrophy, and ptosis are frequently seen as well.

The diagnostic criteria of NF2 are

- Bilateral eighth nerve (vestibulocochlear) masses
- A first-degree relative with NF2 and/or
  Unilateral eighth nerve mass
  Two of the following:
  Neurofibromas of any type
  Meningiomas
  Gliomas
  Schwannomas
  Juvenile posterior subcapsular cataracts (40%)

Prenatal and presymptomatic DNA diagnosis is possible in familial cases; therefore, genetic counseling and regular follow-up visits are important for patients with NF1 and NF2. The presence of amblyopia as a consequence of lid neurofibromas is common. Surgical intervention in this instance is palliative, not curative, in nature. Appropriate amblyopia therapy should be initiated. The differential diagnosis for recalcitrant amblyopia includes determining whether optic gliomas, afferent pupillary defects, and café-au-lait spots are present.[32,33,34,35]

Tuberous sclerosis

Tuberous sclerosis (Bourneville disease) is the classical phakomatosis associated with mental retardation. Retinal astrocytic harmatomas are found in 87% of these patients, with the incidence age dependent. The harmatomas may be present at birth and increase during the first decade of life. Other fundus findings include punched-out depigmented areas of the retinas, atypical colobomas, and optic nerve atrophy (Fig. 7-2). Papilledema, angiofibromas of the eyelids, a sixth nerve (abducent) palsy, and strabismus occur frequently[36] (Fig. 7-3).

Sturge-Weber syndrome

Sturge-Weber syndrome is a phakomatosis characterized by port-wine stain (nevus flammeus), facial hypertrophy, jacksonian epilepsy, and cognitive impairment. It is a congenital vascular disorder with leptomeningeal angiomas (arachnoid and pia mater) of the cerebral cortex. The port-wine stain covers roughly the area of the first and second divisions of the trigeminal nerve (Fig. 7-4).

Seizures occur in up to 55% of this population, their onset indicating the beginning of neurological and other cognitive involvement. As the patient ages, the seizures become more frequent and severe. Mental retardation is present in about 60% of this population and is usually mild to moderate in nature.

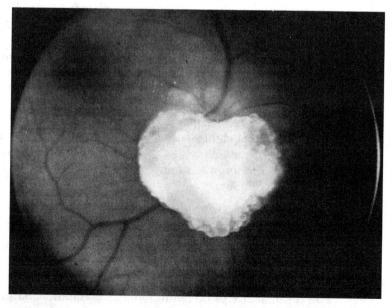

FIGURE 7-2 Retinal astrocytoma in tuberous sclerosis.

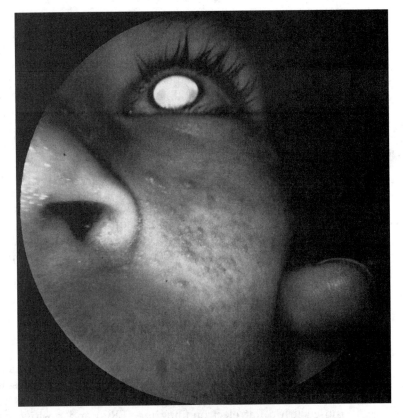

FIGURE 7-3 Facial angiofibromatoma in tuberous sclerosis

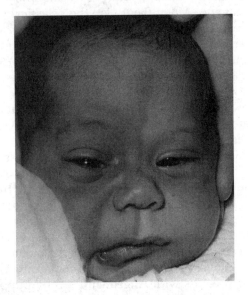

FIGURE 7-4 An infant demonstrating nevus flammeus
(Sturge-Weber syndrome).

The most frequently encountered ocular findings are glaucoma, buphthalmos, diffuse chorodial hemangiomas (40%), and angiomas of the episclera, conjunctiva, and iris. Tortuous and dilated retinal vessels and retinal detachments may also occur. Approximately 30% of the individuals with Sturge-Weber develop glaucoma, and 60% of these have glaucoma and buphthalmos before 2 years of age. This glaucoma is typically unilateral (on the side of the port-wine stain) and is diagnosed more often when the upper eyelid is involved.[37-39]

Cerebral Palsy

Cerebral palsy is a diverse nonprogressive syndrome usually resulting from insult to the motor centers of the brain. Oculovisual and visual/perceptual/motor abnormalities are numerous. The most common ocular findings include strabismus, optic atrophy, extraocular muscle dysfunction, nystagmus, and accommodative abnormalities. Mental retardation may be present in up to 60% of the population.[40-42] (See Chapter 2 for additional information.)

Tapetoretinal Degenerations

Individuals with congenital amaurosis of Leber exhibit both neurological defects and mental retardation. However, modern imaging, biochemical and molecular biological techniques are placing that classification in doubt. At this time congenital amaurosis is accepted as a diagnosis only when normal intelligence is present without neurological defect. A more appropriate diagnostic classification for those with a flat electroretinogram (ERG) and positive neurological involvement is retina-brain neuroembryodysgensis.[43]

Laurence-Moon-Biedl is the classical example of a retinal pigmentary/mental retardation syndrome. Ocular findings include ptosis, nystagmus, strabismus, night blindness, progressive ERG deterioration, and retinitis pigmentosa (Fig. 7-5). Obesity, hypogenitalism, and short stature are also commonly observed.[7f] Prader-Willi (PW) syndrome patients[44] have a similar obesity and hypogonadism with retardation as do Laurence-Moon-Biedl patients but do not demonstrate tapetoretinal degeneration. Prader-Willi involves chromosome 15, as does Angelman syndrome.[45]

Different clinical outcomes between these two syndromes may be due to differential imprinting (variations in the expression of the genetic material is dependent on whether the transmitting parent is the father or mother). If the deleted chromosome 15 is from the father, the patient will have PW (with almond-shaped upward-slanting palpebral fissures and obesity, caused by binge eating); even before the obesity is evident, the baby is hypotonic and has small hands and feet. Conversely, if the deleted chromosome 15 is from the mother, the child presents with Angelman ("happy puppet") syndrome which is characterized by severe developmental delay, a puppetlike gait, par-

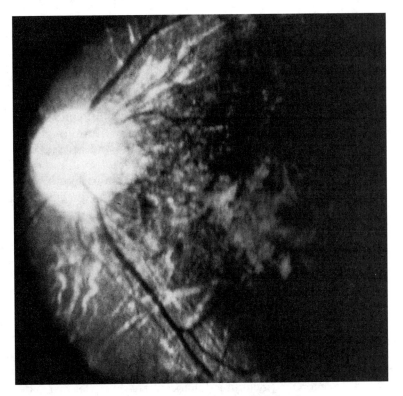

FIGURE 7-5 Laurence-Moon-Biedl tapetoretinal fundus.

oxysmal bouts of laughter, and hypopigmentation of the iris and choroid.

Brain-Retina Neuroembryodysgensis (BRN)

There is a spectrum of developmental brain anomalies associated with varying patterns of abnormal ERGs. Shared mechanisms of BRN can explain these findings. The ERG is helpful in providing further clinical markers to describe conditions and differentiate etiologies when visual impairment is associated with developmental brain anomalies. Until these etiologies are determined, the descriptive term BRN should be used.

The embryonic retina is an extension of the brain, so very early genetic, chromosomal, and teratogenic influences can affect its development. Colobomas of the optic disc[46] or retina, abnormal disc size,[47] and retinal pigmentary changes often predict brain defects.[48,49] New imaging techniques (computed tomography [CT] and magnetic resonance imaging [MRI]) allow detailed assessment of any brain abnormalities. Anomalies associated with ERGs are often allied with brain malformations and dysfunctions. Because of this, both dark and light as well as oscillatory potentials can be affected. Characteristically, the

ERGs may show increased implicit times with decreased amplitudes or may be extinguished, attenuated, or negative in nature. (An ERG whose b-wave is of less amplitude than its a-wave for the same response is referred to as being negative.) It is often associated with congenital stationary night blindness and is described as a Schubert-Bornschein type of ERG.[50]

The negative ERG associated with BRN is not a classical Schubert-Bornschein, however. It is more like those seen in quinine toxicity, which exhibit delayed implicit times and decreased amplitudes. These negative ERGs indicate a possible defect in neural transmission that may not be seen on histological examination.[51,52]

Abnormal ERGs in conjunction with optic nerve hypoplasia signify early retina-brain maldevelopment, not a tapetoretinal degeneration, with intrauterine onset. Individuals with fetal alcohol syndrome and microcephaly as well as those with Peter, Rieger, and Axenfeld anomalies fall into this category of patients.[53] BRN is a descriptive term, not a diagnosis. It indicates a disruption of early embryonic events in the formation of neural brain and retina. This group includes patients with various genetic, metabolic, and other yet unknown etiologies. (Syndromes with mental retardation, strabismus, blindness, or decreased vision and an abnormal ERG include Walker-Warburg, Fukuyama's dystrophy, Joubert, Zellweger, Dandy-Walker, and Aicardi: also included are agenesis of the cerebellar vermis, lissencephaly [including microcephaly, hypertelorism, dysmorphic facies, mental retardation, and other organ malformations], and holoprosencephaly). A full workup that includes an ERG evaluation to determine the underlying pathogenesis is required.

Microcephaly

When assessing microcephaly, the optometrist must obtain a thorough pre- and postnatal history. Although microcephaly can be readily apparent at birth, it may not be noticeable until the growth of the body and head has become substantially disproportional. Postnatal causes include meningitis, intraventricular hemorrhage, and trauma. Prenatal etiologies include viral infection, radiation, and various teratogens (such as alcohol and cocaine). Familial microcephaly occurs with both autosomal recessive and autosomal dominant inheritance. The presence of a chorioretinitis could indicate TORCH syndrome (*t*oxoplasmosis, *r*ubella, *c*ytomegalovirus, *h*erpes simplex).

The use of brain imaging (MRI and CT) differentiates between the many etiologies of microcephaly. MRI is appropriate when you need to assess myelination patterns, differentiate between gray and white matter, and evaluate atrophied gray matter islands. And whereas CT only hints at an agenesis of the corpus callosum, the MRI will show the corpus in detail. MRI will also allow you to appreciate microgyria, polygyria, and macrogyria more readily.

Agenesis of the corpus callosum, optic nerve hypoplasia, and polygyria, along with holoprosencephaly and lissencephaly, are often caused by intrauterine viral and other infections early in embryogenesis. It is important to differentiate genetic from teratogenic etiologies that may result in similar brain structural abnormalities. The use of CT, MRI, and ERG can assist the primary care optometrist in their differential diagnosis.[54-56]

Summary

For a more complete review you are referred to the many excellent articles and texts on the subject.[58-61] Optometrists can and should play an important role in the care of individuals with developmental, cognitive, and physical disabilities. Armed with a basic understanding of the underlying disorder, we can assist our patients to maximize their potential and to live more meaningful and enriching lives.[57]

REFERENCES

1. Maino D, Maino JH, Maino SA: Mental retardation syndromes with associated ocular defects, *J Am Optom Assoc* 61:707-716, 1990.
2. Hoyt, Lambert S: Childhood glaucoma. In Taylor D (ed): *Pediatric ophthalmology*, Boston, 1990, Blackwell Scientific, 319-332.
3. Frantz K, Peters R, Maino D, Gunderson G: Effect of resisting the tonometry procedure upon intraocular pressure. Accepted for publication, *J Am Optom Assoc*, 1994.
4. Cibis GW, Tripathi RC: The differential diagnosis of Descemet's tears (Habb's striae) and posterior polymorphous dystrophy bands, *Ophthalmology* 89:613-620, 1982.
5. Cibis GW: Congenital glaucoma, *J Am Optom Assoc* 58:728-733, 1987.
6. Waring GO, Rodriquez NM, Laibson PR: Anterior chamber cleavage syndrome: a stepladder classification, *Surv Ophthalmol* 20:3-14, 1975.
7. Roy FH: *Ocular syndromes and systemic disease*, ed 2, Philadelphia, 1989, WB Saunders, a, 262; b, 29; c, 114; d, 134-135; e, 157; f, 173.
8. Cibis GW, Waeltermann JM, Whitcraft CT, et al: Lenticular opacities in carriers of Lowe's syndrome, *Opthalmology* 93:1041-1045, 1986.
9. Tripathi RC, Cibis GW, Tripathi BJ: Pathogenesis of cataracts in patients with Lowe's syndrome, *Ophthalmology* 93:1046-1051, 1986.
10. Catalano RA: Down syndrome, *Surv Ophthalmol* 34:385-398, 1990.
11. Miler M: Fetal alcohol syndrome. In Cibis GW, Tongue AC, Stass-Isern ML: (eds): *Decision making in pediatric opthalmology*, St Louis, 1993, Mosby (Decker imprint).
12. Hanson JW, Jones KL, Smith DW: Fetal alcohol syndrome: experience with patients, *JAMA* 235:1485-1460, 1976.
13. Stromland K: Ocular involvement in the fetal alcohol syndrome, *Surv Ophthalmol* 31:277-284, 1987.
14. Stromland K: Ocular anomalies in the fetal alcohol syndrome, *Acta Ophthalmol Suppl* 63:1-50, 1985.
15. McCarus CL: Ocular manifestations of fetal alcohol syndrome, *Am Orthop J* 41:132-136, 1991.

16. Fatt H, Griffin J, Lyle W: *Genetics for the primary eye care practitioner,* ed 2, Boston, 1992, Butterworth-Heinemann, 54.

17. Schopmeyer B, Lowe F: *The fragile X child,* San Diego, 1992, Singular Publishing, a, 1-5, 10-17; b, 19.

18. Sutherland G, Richards R: Fragile x syndrome: the most common cause of familial mental retardation, *Acta Paediatr Scand* 35:94-101, 1994.

19. Patel BD: The fragile x syndrome, *Br J Clin Pract* 48:42-44, 1994.

20. Martinez S, Maino DM: A comprehensive review of the fragile x syndrome: oculo-visual, developmental, and physical characteristics, *J Behav Optom* 4:59-64, 1993.

21. DeVries LBA, Halley DJJ, Oostra BA, Niermeijer MF: The fragile x syndrome: a growing gene causing familial intellectual disability, *J Intellect Disabil Res* 38:1-8, 1994.

22. Hecht B, Hecht F: Fragile x syndrome: unstable DNA. In Cibis GW, Tongue AC, Stass-Isern ML (eds): *Decision making in pediatric ophthalmology,* St Louis, 1993, Mosby (Decker imprint), 130.

23. Sutherland GR, Gedeon A, Kornman L, et al: Prenatal diagnosis of fragile x syndrome by direct detection of the unstable DNA sequence, *N Engl J Med* 69:634-640, 1991.

24. Sabaratnam M, Laver S, Butler, Pembrey M: Fragile x syndrome in North East Essex: towards systematic screening: clinical selection, *J Intellect Disabil Res* 38:27-35, 1994.

25. Rousseau F: The fragile x syndrome: implications of molecular genetics for the clinical syndrome, *Eur J Clin Invest* 24:1-10, 1994.

26. Maino DM, Wesson M, Schlange D, et al: Optometric findings in the fragile x syndrome, *Optom Vis Sci* 68:634-640, 1991.

27. Maino D, Schlange D, Maino J, Caden B: Ocular anomalies in fragile x syndrome, *J Am Optom Assoc* 61:316-323, 1990.

28. Maino DM, King R: Oculo-visual dysfunction in the fragile x syndrome. In Hagerman R, McKenzie P (eds): 1992 International Fragile X Conference Proceedings, Dillon, Colo, 1992, Spectra Publishing, 71-78.

29. Amin V, Maino DM: The fragile x female: visual, visual perceptual, and ocular health anomalies, Accepted for publication, *J Am Optom Assoc,* 1994.

30. Strom RL, Pebenito R, Ferretti C: Ophthalmologic findings in the fragile x syndrome, *Arch Ophthalmol* 105:1099-1102, 1987.

31. Dibler LB, Maino DM: Martin-Bell phenotype, fragile x syndrome, and very low birth weight children: the differential diagnosis. Accepted for publication, *J Optom Vis Dev* 1994-95.

32. Pulst S: Neurofibromatoses. In Cibis GW, Tongue AC, Stass-Isern ML (eds): *Decision making in pediatric ophthalmology,* St Louis, 1993, Mosby (Decker imprint), 134-135.

33. National Institutes of Health Consensus Development Conference statement on neurofibromatosis, *Arch Neurol* 45:575-577, 1988.

34. Lubs MLE, Bauer M, Formas ME, Djokic B: Iris hamartomas in the diagnosis of neurofibromatosis. I, *Int Pediatr* 5:261-265, 1990.

35. Kaiser-Kupfer MI, Kupfer C, Pulst SM: The association of posterior capsular lens opacities with bilateral acoustic neurofibromas in patients with neurofibromatosis type 2, *Arch Ophthalmol* 107:541-542, 1989.

36. Lee KY, Cibis GW: Abnormalities of the retina without diagnostic electroretinography. In Cibis GW, Tongue AC, Stass-Isern ML (eds): *Decision making in pediatric ophthalmology,* St Louis, 1993, Mosby (Decker imprint), 174.

37. McCartan MJ, Maino DM: Sturge-Weber syndrome: a case report. Accepted for publication, *J Optom Vis Dev* 1994-95.

38. Tripathi BJ, Tripathi RC, Cibis GW: Sturge-Weber syndrome, encephalo-trigeminal angiomatosis. In Gold DH, Weingeist TA (eds): *The eye in systemic disease,* Philadelphia, 1990, JB Lippincott, 443-447.

39. Cibis GW, Tripathi RC, Tripathi BJ: Glaucoma in Sturge-Weber syndrome, *Opthalmology* 91:1061-1069, 1984.

40. Maino JH: Ocular defects associated with cerebral palsy: a review, *Rev Optom* 69:70-72, 1979.

41. Scheiman M: Optometric findings in children with cerebral palsy, *Am J Optom Physiol Opt* 61:321-323, 1984.

42. Duckman R: The incidence of visual anomalies in a population of cerebral palsied children, *J Am Optom Assoc* 9:1013-1016, 1979.

43. Cibis GW: Brain-retina neuroembryodysgenesis. In Cibis GW, Tongue AC, Stass-Isern ML (eds): *Decision making in pediatric ophthalmology,* St Louis, 1993, Mosby (Decker imprint), 62-63.

44. Libov A, Maino DM: Prader-Willi syndrome, *J Am Optom Assoc* 65:355-359, 1994.

45. Schneider B, Maino DM: Angelman syndrome, *J Am Optom Assoc* 64:502-506, 1993.

46. Cook CS, Sulik KK: Keratolenticular dysgenesis (Peters' anomaly) as a result of acute embryonic insult during gastrulation, *J Pediatr Opthalmol Strabismus* 25:60-66, 1988.

47. Cook CS, Nowotny AZ, Sulik KK: Fetal alcohol syndrome, *Arch Ophthalmol* 105:1576-1581, 1987.

48. Weleber RG, Lovrien WE, Isom JB: Aicardi's syndrome: case report, clinical features, and electrophysiologic studies, *Arch Ophthalmol* 96:285-290, 1978.

49. Warburg M: Ocular malformations and lissencephaly, *Eur J Pediatr* 146:450-452, 1987.

50. Schubert G, Bornschein H: Beitrag zur analyse des menschilchen elektroretinogramms, *Ophthalmologica* 123:396-413, 1952.

51. Cibis GW, Burian HM, Blodi CF: ERG changes in acute quinine poisoning, *Arch Ophthalmol* 90:307, 1973.

52. Ripps H: Night blindness revisited: from man to molecules. Proctor lecture, *Invest Ophthalmol Vis Sci* 23:588-609, 1982.

53. Katz LM, Fox DA: Prenatal ethanol exposure alters scotopic and photopic components of adult rat electroretinograms, *Invest Ophthalmol Vis Sci* 32:2861-2872, 1991.

54. Harbord MG, Lambert SR, Kriss A, et al: Autosomal recessive microcephaly, mental retardation with nonpigmentary retinopathy, and distinctive electroretinograms, *Neuropaediatrie* 20:139-141, 1989.

55. Manning FJ, Bruce AM, Berson EL: Electroretinograms in microcephaly with chorioretinal degeneration, *Am J Ophthalmol* 109:457-463, 1990.

56. McKusick VA, Stauffer M, Knox DL, Clark DS: Chorioretinopathy with hereditary microcephaly, *Arch Ophthalmol* 75:597-600, 1966.

57. Geering J, Maino DM: The patient with mental handicaps: a primary care perspective, *South J Optom* 10:23-27, 1992.

58. Press L, Moore B: *Clinical pediatric optometry,* Boston, 1993, Butterworth-Heinemann.

59. Grisham D: Management of nystagmus in young children. In Scheiman M (ed): *Pediatric optometry problems in optometry,* Philadelphia, 1990, JB Lippincott, 496-527.

60. Abplanalp P (ed): *Modern diagnostic technology problems in optometry,* Philadelphia, 1991, JB Lippincott.

61. Rosenbloom A, Morgan M (eds): *Principles and practice of pediatric optometry,* Philadelphia, 1990, JB Lippincott.

8

Clinical Decision Making in Special Populations: Dealing with Incomplete Data

Ellen Richter Ettinger

Key Terms

Clinical decision making	Strategies for optimum patient management	Closed-loop systems
Ambiguous clinical data	Open-loop systems	Problem solving

Clinical decision making is a challenging process for any patient population. A full set of data is helpful in providing a framework for the doctor to determine appropriate diagnoses and patient management plans. When the information available to the doctor is limited, the task of decision making becomes even more demanding and difficult.

Uncertainty and an incomplete data base are common features of clinical decision making in special populations. The uncertainty comes mainly from two factors:

1. **Quantity of data.** Patients from special populations have a wide range of cognitive abilities and skills, with many unresponsive to traditional optometric tests (visual acuities, subjective examinations). This decreases the quantity of data that is usually available for diagnosis.

2. Quality of data. The quality of the data collected may be limited as well, since the patient's responses may be questionable. Patients may respond to subjective tests, to some degree, but the level of their responsiveness and sensitivity will limit the quality of these responses. In the non-affected population, optometrists usually work to fine-tune a subjective refraction to the nearest 0.25 diopter (D). Patients from special populations may function with larger just noticeable differences. Those who can respond to the subjective refraction examination may not notice differences of 1.00 or more diopters. Ambiguous or vague responses contribute to a clincian's uncertainity.

CLINICAL PEARL

In order to improve the clinical decision making in special populations, try to improve the quality and quantity of data collected.

Optometrists have recently gained a much greater understanding of the ocular problems commonly associated with special populations. Ocular anomalies of patients with cerebral palsy,[1-3] Down syndrome,[4-6] mental retardation,[7-11] fragile X syndrome,[12-13] and other disabilities[14-17] have been described. Being familiar with the associated ocular dysfunctions of these patients helps optometrists provide quality vision care for them. The objective of this chapter is to discuss strategies that will strengthen and improve the decision-making process used in the diagnosis and management of special populations.

Dealing with Limited and Ambiguous Data

Clinical decision making in special populations is like trying to solve a puzzle when pieces are missing. If a clinician is accustomed to working with a normal, highly responsive, patient population, working with clinically fuzzy (ambiguous) data can be intimidating. The strategy used when dealing with limited data is to try to maximize the quality and quantity of information gathered. This allows the clinician to be as well prepared as possible for the decision-making process.

Optimizing the Quality and Quantity of Data

Obtaining sufficient information is a fundamental component of good clinical decision making. The doctor who is working with special populations can use several strategies that help provide valuable information. Many of the recommendations that are useful in expanding the quantity of clinical information also help to enhance the quality of the information. To optimize the quality and quantity of data obtained, the clinician should:

1. Use alternative clinical tests (such as the Broken Wheel Test[18] and Allen Picture Cards[19]) when traditional tests (Snellen Acuity) cannot be performed.

2. Consider doing traditional tests in more creative, nontraditional, ways. For example, patients who are nonverbal can point to letters on a communication board as they view them on a Snellen chart instead of reading them out loud. Patients who are hearing impaired may respond better to written instructions. They may prefer to write letters that they see on a Snellen chart rather than to say them aloud. When motor skills do not allow a patient to sit in front of traditional optometric equipment (slit lamp and tonometer), handheld models should be used.

3. Be flexible in your testing sequence. If a patient seems to be tiring during the examination, move on to another area. Changing tests is similar to giving the patient a short break. You can always return to complete the unfinished test when the patient is more attentive. The two key words to remember in carrying out the testing sequence are *priority* and *variety*. If you anticipate that limited information will be accessible from a patient, try to get the most important information first. If the patient has a decreased attention span, performing retinoscopy and making a determination about the refractive error at an initial visit may be more important than obtaining data on visual perceptual skills. Additional information can be gathered later during the examination, or at another visit. You should work quickly and use a variety of diagnostic procedures to maintain the patient's attention. Some patients will need additional time to formulate and communicate their responses. By providing this extra time, you can improve the quality and quantity of the data obtained.

4. Make the patient as comfortable as possible in the clinical setting. Patients who are at ease both physically and emotionally will often be more cooperative and motivated. Patients from special populations are usually under the care of more than one health-care professional. Multiple visits to a variety of professionals are seldom a rewarding experience. Making sure your patients feel safe, secure, and welcome should not be underestimated in your approach to patient care.

5. Enlist the assistance of the patient's care-givers (parents, teachers, social workers, and other health-care professionals) to obtain more information about an individual's health and visual function. When a patient's responses are limited, care-givers may be

able to provide information concerning his or her visual function. If possible, have the primary care-giver bring the child's medical and eye care records. If these are not available, have this person send them to your office.

6. Consider an incremental approach when an examination yields limited data. With an incremental approach, the doctor gathers information over several visits rather than obtaining all the information in a single visit. This approach may enable you to acquire data that would otherwise be inaccessible.

7. Learn as much about the patient as possible. To be able to design optimum testing strategies and management plans the optometrist must be familiar with the patient. What types of activities and hobbies does the patient enjoy? How does the patient use vision? What is the severity of the disability (mild, moderate, or severe)? Are there any associated problems (mental retardation, allergies, seizure disorders)? Is the patient under medical care for other health problems?

"An entry sheet for the cerebral palsy patient"[3] has been designed to help optometrists become familiar with cerebral palsied patients (Fig. 8-1). Similar information can be collected to gain comprehensive insight into all your patients with special needs. On this sheet motor status is of major importance, because cerebral palsy is a motor problem. For other disabilities you should note the syndrome and the severity of any deficits. You should also be aware of any associated medical, sensory, and perceptual problems. Understanding the patient's disability will help you formulate management plans that are relevant to the patient's visual needs and personal goals.

Becoming More Confident in Objective Test Results

Optometrists who are experienced in working with disabled individuals are used to relying on their objective test results. Clinicians who are new to these populations often will feel astounded at the need to depend so heavily on objective findings.

Why does this apprehension in relying on objective test results occur? In nonhandicapped patients, we are able to confirm our objective test results with the use of subjective findings. Since we have a mechanism to validate objective findings in the general population, we often think of an objective finding as more an *estimate*, with a built-in tolerance for error. The ambiguity does not bother us as much when we know that we can verify or fine-tune our findings with a subjective procedure.

With special populations objective test results become more important. How can we gain confidence in these results? One way is to remember that there are other methods that will assist us in confirm-

Entry Sheet for the Cerebral Palsy Patient

Name _____ DOB _____ Date of Exam _____

Patient profile (age, race, gender)

Is person accompanying patient assisting with history?
  If yes
            Name of person
            Relationship to patient

Patient's visual needs
    Primary activities
            If child: Grade in school/any type of special program
            If adult: Occupation/primary activity
    Other activities, hobbies, visual needs

Motor status
    Neuromuscular classification (spasticity, dyskinesia, ataxia, mixed types)
    Portion of body affected (hemiplegia, paraplegia)
    Time of onset of CP and cause, if known (prenatal, mother had rubella,
            postnatal head injury)

Associated problems (mental retardation, seizure disorders, hearing loss,
            perceptual problems)

Current medical problems/medications taken/other health professionals
            involved in caring for patient

Visual problems known from previous exams

Chief complaint

FIGURE 8-1. Entry sheet for the cerebral palsy patient. (From
Ettinger ER: *J Behav Optom* 2:115-122, 1991.)

ing the findings. For example, a clinician can trial frame a prescription
from retinoscopy and see how the patient responds. Frequent
follow-up evaluations and progress visits will help confirm data
previously collected.

Many clinicians place greater importance on the precision of
objective test results than is actually needed. As mentioned, the
patient may exhibit a large just-noticeable difference that allows for a
minimum level of error without interfering in comfort or function.
The clinician should attempt to be as precise as possible; however,
small magnitudes of error may not affect a patient's comfort or ability
to function efficiently. Trial-framing, follow-up testing, and feedback
from care-givers can all assist you in identifying proper clinical
endpoints. As you work more with special populations and begin to
rely on your objective test results, you will become confident in your
findings.

Optimizing the Steps in Decision Making

We usually think of clinical decision making as an outcome or a final product. This can be intimidating. If decision making is considered to be a *process* rather than an outcome, it becomes manageable. There are three steps in this model (Fig. 8-2).

Evaluate the Patient's Status

The strategy for patient evaluation is to maximize the data available. Using nontraditional and objective assessment techniques will maximize the quantity and quality of your data.

Consider the Available Management Alternatives

You must consider all options when addressing a problem. Do not ignore available possibilities. We often decide on a treatment plan because it is the first option that comes to mind. "Snap-reacting" is a common phenomenon in which we pick the most familiar solution or the one with the stamp of tradition and the force of habit.[20] By taking the time to consider all alternatives and weighing the predicted outcomes of each, we can choose the most appropriate treatment program. By "snap-reacting," we eliminate many opportunities for managing a problem. For example, if a patient has a complaint about his/her glasses, we may consider the following options:
1. Change the prescription
2. Change the form of the correction (as from a bifocal to single vision)
3. Adjust the current frame to fit more comfortably
4. Provide environmental recommendations (such as improving the lighting in the room)

If we consider only a change in the prescription, we ignore other alternatives that could improve the patient's function. Every problem has several possible solutions. We must consider the full range of options when searching for an optimum treatment alternative.

Make Decisions

When you maximize the quality and quantity of your data and consider all treatment options, your ability to make decisions is

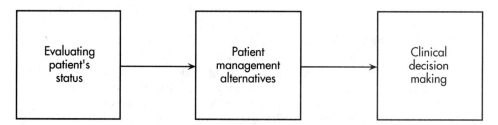

FIGURE 8-2. The three steps involved in clinical decision making.

strengthened. Optometric management plans often include the use of lenses, prisms, vision therapy, surgery, low vision devices, environmental recommendations, and consultation/referrals (Table 8-1). In addition to traditional optometric intervention, educational recommendations and interdisciplinary communications can be particularly helpful for these patients. For example, the optometrist can use information on the patient's visual status and perceptual motor development to provide valuable input regarding educational placement. Similarly, you can provide helpful insights to other health-care professionals (such as occupational therapists) who are treating these patients.[21,22]

Common decisions made by optometrists for patients with disabilities include:

When to prescribe glasses

When to make a change in the prescription

When to recommend vision therapy

How to design an effective vision therapy program

How to advise the patient about other health care options (for example, ocular surgery)

TABLE 8-1

Strategies for Optimum Patient Management

Optometric Intervention	Comments
Lenses	The decision to prescribe glasses can be complicated when caring for special populations (A decision tree to assist in strategies on prescribing glasses is provided in Figs. 8-3 and 8-4)
Prisms	Prisms can be helpful in special populations; consider the patient's response and adaptation to them and also follow-up to assess their acceptance
Vision therapy	Vision therapy can be a viable option for patients with special needs
Ocular surgical procedures	In considering surgical procedures for patients from special populations, always evaluate the risks versus benefits; invasive procedures should be considered with caution
Low vision devices	When a disabled patient has a visual condition that suggests the need for a low vision aid, consider whether his/her cognitive and motor abilities are consistent with those required to use the device
Environmental and educational recommendations	Make recommendations on classroom seating and educational placement; recommendations on lighting and other environmental conditions may also be helpful
Consultation/referral	Remember: Optometric intervention is best when it is part of interdisciplinary patient care; consult with pediatricians, special education teachers, occupational or physical therapists, speech therapists, and other health-care professionals as needed

Decision Making

Prescribing Glasses

A commonly encountered dilemma when working with special patients is deciding when to prescribe glasses. With lower-functioning patients, we often wonder whether an individual will really benefit from glasses. Is this patient able to appreciate an improvement from a correction? Is the visual benefit attained worth the effort of getting the patient to wear the glasses?

Two clinical questions are particularly important in this decision-making process (1) Does the patient have any vision related symptoms? and (2) Is a significant refractive error present? Refractive errors within special populations are considered significant at a magnitude of 1.50 D or more (myopia, hyperopia, or astigmatism).[3] However, presbyopic patients may warrant correction for even lower magnitudes of hyperopia.

The first step is to consider whether the patient has any symptoms of blurred vision. Scenarios 1 and 6 (Fig. 8-3), the two extremes of the decision tree, are the easiest to evaluate.

Scenario 1

If the patient has symptoms of blurred vision and a significant refractive error is found, then the patient should benefit from wearing a correction. Glasses should be prescribed in this situation.

Scenario 6

If the patient has no symptoms and no significant prescription is found, glasses are not required.

The more complex cases (scenarios 2 to 5, Figure 8-3) are those between the extremes. In these situations trial-framing the prescription is helpful in determining whether the patient can benefit from a correction.

Scenario 2

This is an example in which the patient presents with symptoms of blur. The prescription found is not substantial, but the patient responds well to trial-framing. Since there is a positive response and the patient has symptoms without correction, glasses are indicated.

Scenario 3

If the patient complains of blurred vision but has no significant refractive error, consider other areas (such as visual skills, perceptual anomalies, or ocular health problems) that might affect vision.

Scenario 4

If the patient has no visual symptoms but a significant refractive error is found, the correction should be trial-framed. If vision appears to be

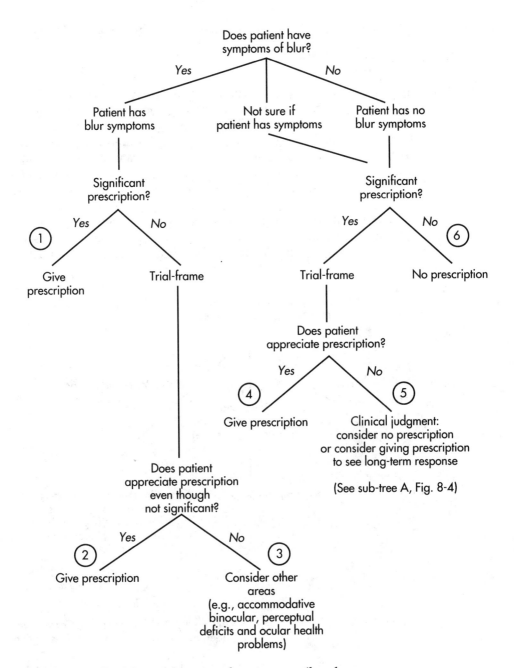

FIGURE 8-3. Decision making in when to prescribe glasses.

better or the patient's visual behavior improves glasses should be prescribed.

Scenario 5

This is one of the most difficult scenarios presented. The patient has no symptoms, has a significant prescription, but responds poorly when trial-framed. Will the patient really accept a prescription? Will there be a real benefit from wearing glasses? Your clinical judgment, on a case-by-case basis, must be used. An important clue is to consider whether the patient has had any previous experience with a similar prescription. The following three possibilities should be considered (Fig. 8-4):

1. If the patient has unsuccessfully tried a similar prescription (subtrees C and D), you need to ask whether giving the same prescription will offer any benefit. If the patient's current situa-

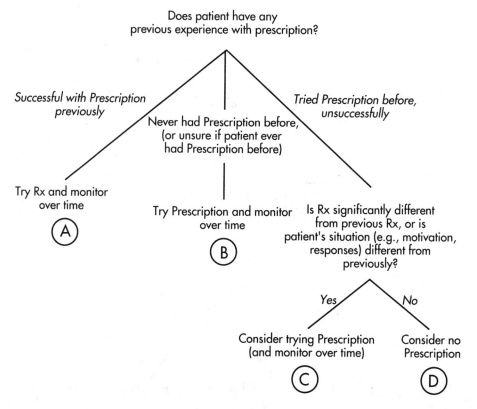

FIGURE 8-4. Subtree A: decision making for scenario 5 of Figure 8-3. The patient has no blur symptoms. A significant prescription is found, but the patient does not respond well to trial-framing. The clinical dilemma is whether the patient will benefit from a prescription.

tion is different from previous conditions (improved motivation or improved responses to visual stimuli), then trial-framing should be tried or glasses prescribed and the patient reevaluated at a later date (C). If the prescription is the same as the one that was tried unsuccessfully and the patient's situation is unchanged, then there is no indication for giving this prescription (D).

2. If the patient was successful in wearing a similar prescription previously, this is a positive indicator. A common example would be the individual who has lost a pair of glasses. If this person was successful with a similar prescription before, there is reason to believe he will benefit from the correction. The prescription should be given (subtree A). If desired, the clinician has the option of trial-framing or having the patient return for a subsequent reevaluation.

3. If the patient has not worn glasses or the doctor is unsure whether glasses have been worn, it is appropriate to give them a try (subtree B). Allow the patient sufficient time to adapt to them.

The last scenario to discuss is at the center of the top branch in figure 8-3 (not sure if the patient has symptoms). This sometimes occurs if the patient is not communicative or when responses are questionable. You should determine if a significant refractive error is present by using appropriate objective examination techniques and prescribe when necessary.

CLINICAL PEARL

Trial-framing the proposed prescription and having the patient back for frequent reevaluations will aid you in determining the most appropriate prescription for your patient.

When Prescription Changes Are Indicated

Decisions on whether a patient needs a change in prescription can be analyzed (similarly to the process noted in the preceding section). Does the patient have any symptoms with the prescription? Is the change in prescription significant? (A change of 1 D, or even less, may be considered significant depending on the patient's sensitivity and visual demands.) If the change is consistent with a patient's symptoms, then a change in prescription should be given.

When the change is not significant or the patient does not have symptoms, the decision can be more complex. Trial-framing may then help you determine the benefits of a change.

CLINICAL PEARL

Vision therapy for patients with developmental disabilities is most appropriate when your patient and care-giver are highly motivated.

Vision Therapy Recommendations

When should the optometrist recommend a program of vision therapy? The most obvious answer is "When you think it can help." The decision as to whether or not to recommend vision therapy will depend greatly on (1) whether the patient's problem is considered amenable to vision therapy (2) whether he/she is assessed to be a good candidate for vision therapy and (3) whether there is a support system that will enable him to maintain the commitment to such a program.

Does the patient have a condition that is receptive to treatment by vision therapy?

Recent reports in the literature have identified which types of ocular problems in special patients are amenable to vision therapy. Cerebral palsied patients, for example, have a high prevalence of strabismus,[1-3] but this may be neurological in nature.[2,23] Vision therapy for strabismus is generally not effective for patients within this population.[2,3,24] Unless an eye turn is believed to be functional (as with an intermittent exotropia), strabismus therapy is usually not initiated. On the other hand, certain ocular disorders have been found to be more responsive. Vision therapy for accommodative problems, oculomotor dysfunction, and perceptual deficits can be effective for this population.[25]

Is the patient cooperative and motivated?

Vision therapy works best when the patient is highly motivated. If the patient participates and cooperates, he/she has a better chance of succeeding. If motivation is absent, the usefulness of a vision-therapy program is questionable.

Does the patient have a support system available to help maintain commitment to a vision-therapy program?

Will a parent bring the child to the doctor for the vision therapy sessions, or will a teacher, social worker, or other care-giver be able to bring the child? Will these individuals see that the patient works on any techniques that are prescribed for home or school? Knowing that a patient will attend vision therapy sessions regularly and will follow through on techniques prescribed is a positive factor for recommending vision therapy.

Designing Successful Vision-Therapy Programs

Designing effective vision therapy can affect the outcome of clinical care for your special patients. The following questions should be asked when designing vision therapy programs:

1. What symptoms and signs does the patient have? Evaluate the optometric problems and identify which can be treated by vision therapy. These can be your goals for vision therapy remediation.
2. What are the patient's visual needs and goals? To design a relevant program you should be familiar with a patient's visual tasks and activities. In addition, to help patients develop additional skills, you should attempt to gain insights into their personal goals and aspirations. It is appropriate to ask a patient, "In what activities would you like to be involved?"

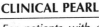

CLINICAL PEARL

For patients with short attention spans, consider brief sessions that occur several times a week rather than a long session once a week.

3. Does the patient's disability affect vision therapy? In some cases a disability does not affect a vision-therapy program. When it does, however, it is important to take this into account. For example, if you are planning to work on eye-hand coordination and the patient has motor problems, activities must be planned at an appropriate level. It is not enough just to know the patient's visual status. You must also understand the patient's disability and how it affects function.
4. What individuals in the patient's life can be involved in reinforcing the gains achieved through a vision therapy program? Parents, special educators, social workers, occupational and physical therapists, and other health care professionals can all be part of the team that will help the child develop and maintain improvements attained through vision therapy.

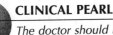

CLINICAL PEARL

The doctor should be conscious of the patient's sense of accomplishment or frustration. Work at a level that challenges the patient but does not create frustration.

Hints for Planning a Successful Vision-Therapy Program

The following are three steps that can help you set up a program of visual therapy for special patients:

1. Choose activities that the patient will enjoy. This will maintain his/her interest, cooperation, and motivation.
2. For patients with short attention spans, adjust the duration of the sessions. Consider brief sessions that occur several times a week rather than a long session once a week. For some children, two 15-minute sessions in your office per week and two at home may be more effective than a 1-hour in-office session. The more training techniques completed at home or school, the better. Working in the patient's habitual environment is usually advantageous.
3. Be conscious of the patient's sense of accomplishment or frustration. Work at a level that challenges the patient but does not create frustration. Remember: A goal of vision therapy is to build the patient's confidence in visual skills and abilities, not to develop frustration and anger at limitations.

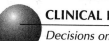

CLINICAL PEARL

Decisions on recommendations for surgery should consider both the benefits and risks of the procedure.

Ocular Surgery

Optometrists are often asked for their advice on whether ocular surgery is advisable for special patients. In many cases the decision is entirely based on the patient's ocular status and general medical condition, independent of any disability. Surgery is then recommended on the same basis as it would be for any individual from the general population. In some cases the patient's disability will affect your decision. For example, strabismus is a common finding in patients with cerebral palsy; however, strabismus surgery is not considered an effective therapeutic measure for treatment in this population. Other types of surgery may be beneficial. For example, in a child with a congenital cataract, surgical removal of the lens is recommended as long as there are no medical contraindications.

The following are some questions that the optometrist considering ocular surgery may want to address:

1. What benefits can the patient derive from the procedure, and what will happen if the patient does not have the procedure?
2. What is the full range of possible outcomes of the surgery, and the probabilities of success for each?
3. What are the possible risks of this surgical procedure in general, and for this patient?
4. What are the possible post-surgical complications, and what effect would they have on this patient?

Uncertainty and the Benefits of "Closed-Loop" Thinking

Consider the following two models of decision making (Fig. 8-5): In model A you evaluate the patient's status, consider available alternatives, and make a decision. The evaluation of the patient's status and a consideration of management options are the inputs to clinical decision making. For example, model A is a simple refractive decision in which the doctor evaluates the patient's refractive status, considers the possibilities (changing the prescription, changing the bifocal type, making no changes) and then decides which of the alternatives is most appropriate. In model B, the clinician performs all of the steps in model A, but also gets feed back on the decision that was made. This feedback allows the doctor to reevaluate the situation and make any corrective changes as needed.

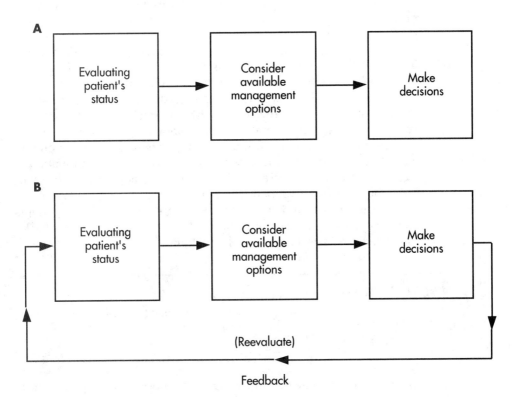

FIGURE 8-5. The two models of decision making. **A,** An open-loop system. Evaluation of the patient's status and a consideration of the clinical management options are the inputs to this model. The third step (decision making) is the end of the process. **B,** A closed-loop system. The same three steps as in model *A* are shown, but reevaluation provides a mechanism for feedback after the clinical decision is made.

In model A, problem solving occurs with an open-loop system: a decision is made and is itself essentially the end point; there is no feedback. In model B, a closed-loop system, you evaluate the consequences of any decisions made and thus have the opportunity to make corrections as needed to optimize the outcome.

CLINICAL PEARL

When the doctor is highly confident of the decision, an open-loop system may suffice (that is, the action taken is expected to solve the problem easily) and a closed-loop system would not provide any additional information.

Open- and closed-loop systems are major issues within the area of problem solving.[20] When you are highly confident of your decision, an open-loop system may suffice; that is, the action taken can be expected to solve the problem easily and a closed-loop system would not provide any additional information. When making simple changes in refractive corrections, you generally do not ask the patient to return for reassessment of the new glasses. If a presbyope needs a small increase in the add and it is consistent with the patient's age and previous prescription, you are usually confident that it will be accepted. Similarly, if a low myope has mild distance vision symptoms, the prescription is usually given without much concern. Based on your experience with patients and your knowledge of optics, you feel confident that the patient will do well with these changes. Often you just tell the patient to return whenever the next full examination is recommended. We usually do not receive feedback in these types of cases, but our past experiences assure us that the actions taken will benefit the patient. In many instances we also assume that if patients have a problem, they'll come back (i.e., no feedback is good feedback). This is not necessarily true in all situations.

CLINICAL PEARL

The advantage of closed-loop problem solving is that the doctor can evaluate the consequences of any actions and do what is necessary to maximize the outcomes.

Sometimes, however, you lack enough information to predict how the patient will respond to a given action. You may be uncertain as to whether the patient will (1) do better with a new prescription, (2) have trouble with the prescription, or (3) show no significant response, good or bad. This uncertainty can be immobilizing and may make the clinician uncomfortable about these decisions. The advantage of closed-loop problem solving is that it lets you evaluate the consequences of your actions and do what is necessary to maximize the outcomes. For example, you may decide to change the prescription and have the patient back in 2 weeks for a progress evaluation. Reevaluating a patient over time and getting input from others (parents, teachers, social workers, health-care providers) can help in assessing the effects of your interventions.

Strategies for Clinical Decision Making in Special Populations

A set of strategies for each of the components involved in clinical decision making is presented in Table 8-2. It is helpful to remember several rules for optimizing decisions in special populations:

1. Maximize your inputs. Obtain a detailed case history and comprehensive database. These are the first steps toward good clinical decision making.
2. Consider all the patient-management options available. By looking at *all* of your options, you can select the best alternative.

TABLE 8-2.
Strategies for Improving Decision Making in Caring for Special Populations

Case history	1. Get to know the patient well
	2. Obtain a comprehensive case history
	3. Demonstrate a warm and caring attitude
	4. Put the patient at ease to gain cooperation and participation
Clinical testing	1. Optimize the quantity of clinical information
	a. Use appropriate testing procedures for each patient:
	(1) Consider standard tests done in creative ways, (2) Consider alternative testing procedures (Broken Wheel Test)
	b. Make the patient comfortable and at ease during testing
	c. Remain flexible in your clinical testing sequence
	2. Optimize the quality of clinical care
	a. Allow the patient extra time to respond to the questions
	b. Use appropriate testing procedures based on a patient's abilities and function; see (1) and (2) above
Decision-making strategies for patient management	1. Obtain enough clinical information to support the decision-making process
	2. Optimize your knowledge base on the special populations you encounter
	3. Consider all of the patient management options; see Table 8-1
	4. Do not be intimidated by complex cases; set priorities when dealing with multiple problems
	5. Choose final management plans that are relevant to the special needs and goals of each patient
	6. Consider family-focused management plans that involve the support of family and care-givers
	7. Use feedback and reevaluate over time

3. Make educated and informed decisions based on a thorough knowledge of the patient and his clinical profile.

4. Use feedback. You can (a) monitor the patient over time, (b) solicit information from people who interact with the patient (parents, care-givers, teachers, social workers, other health-care professionals), and (c) make corrective changes as necessary.

5. When cues to decision making are limited, consider an incremental approach to patient care. With an incremental approach the doctor can continue testing over several sessions. You may choose to make several small changes over time, rather than one large change all at once. In this way, you can monitor the patient's progress and fine-tune the clinical data obtained. The incremental method allows you to approach the decision-making process in discrete stages, when it may be difficult to meet all of your patient's needs at one time.

6. Do not be overwhelmed by the complexities of a case. Patients from special populations often have associated medical problems. Multiple ocular anomalies may also be present. It is best to prioritize these and use an incremental approach to solving them.

7. When a patient's responses are limited, rely more on objective testing. Experience in using objective test results in clinical decision making will improve your confidence level in patient management.

8. Be familiar with information concerning eye-care problems in special populations. More articles on these patients have become available in recent years. By expanding your knowledge base you can make more appropriate clinical observations and decisions. Articles on the vision problems of individuals with cerebral palsy,[1-3] Down syndrome,[4-6] mental retardation,[7-11] fragile X syndrome,[12,13] and other disabilities[14-18,26] can be found.

9. Consider family-focused management plans that involve the care-givers. Adhering to clinical recommendations often relies on the actions of parents and other care-givers. Linder[27] and Bailey et al.[28] have discussed the concept of family-focused (as opposed to child-focused) programs. By stimulating the involvement, participation, and support of parents and care-givers, you inspire a higher level of adherence to clinical recommendations. Focusing only on the child can result in plans that are unrealistic for the situation or environment. By involving the care-givers, you will put into action management plans that are more applicable to a patient's life and family situation.

10. Remember that each patient is an individual and that, when working with these patients individual management plans are essential. A patient's visual demands, the severity of his condition, and any disabilities that are present all play a role in determining optimum treatment. By considering the unique set

of needs and goals for these individuals, you will be able to select more effective optometric interventions.

11. Become part of the team. Interdisciplinary interactions are paramount in caring for a disabled individual. By interacting and communicating with parents and family members, special educators, pediatricians, social workers, physical therapists, occupational therapists, and others involved in the care of the patient, you can obtain input that is important in the decision-making process. In addition, you can provide information that will be helpful in the patient's overall management.

Conclusion

Clinical decision making for patients from special populations can be complex and challenging. Appropriate strategies are needed to make incomplete or ambiguous data more useful. By utilizing effective strategies for clinical testing and decision making, optometrists can significantly enhance a patient's ability to function at his/her highest level.

Advances in technology have led to the creation of mobility and assistive communication devices that allow disabled individuals to function at higher levels than was previously possible. Efficient visual skills can help these patients to take full advantage of all technological advances available. To use a communication board, the individual must be able to see the pictures. To use a closed-captioned television system, a hearing-impaired patient must be able to read the captions. To use mobility devices optimally, the person must be able to see where he is going.

The optometrists' abilities to make improvements in the visual status of a patient extend far beyond the patient's visual function; they can involve giving the patient improved mobility, independence, opportunities for education, and options for employment. The patient may also develop a greater sense of self-confidence and self-esteem. All patients who are cognitively, physically, or emotionally challenged should have single, clear, comfortable, binocular, and pathology-free vision. Through appropriate clinical decision making, the optometrist will be able to ensure high quality and accessible eye care for all special population patients.

REFERENCES

1. Duckman RH: The incidence of visual anomalies in a population of cerebral palsied children, *J Am Optom Assoc* 50:1013-1016, 1979.
2. Duckman RH: Visual problems. In McDonald ET (ed): *Treating cerebral palsy,* Austin, Tex, 1987, Pro-Ed, 105-131.
3. Ettinger ER: Optometric evaluation of the patient with cerebral palsy, *J Behav Optom* 5:115-121, 1991.
4. Fanning G: Vision in children with Down's syndrome, *Aust J Optom* 54:74-82, 1971.

5. Long F: Systemic and ocular manifestations of Down's syndrome, *Am J Optom Med* 6:1-4, 1989.
6. Warshowsky J: A vision screening of a Down's syndrome population, *J Am Optom Assoc* 52:605-607, 1981.
7. Pesch R, Nagy D, Caden B: A survey of the visual and developmental-perceptual abilities of the Down's syndrome child, *J Am Optom Assoc* 9:1031-1037, 1978.
8. Maino DM, Maino JB, Maino SA: Mental retardation syndromes with associated ocular defects, *J Am Optom Assoc* 61:706-716, 1990.
9. Levy B: Incidence of oculo-visual anomalies in an adult population of mentally retarded persons, *Am J Optom Physiol Opt* 61:324-326, 1984.
10. Bradley B: Differential responses in perceptual ability among mentally retarded brain-injured children, *Optom Weekly* 55:31-33, 1964.
11. Mackay D, Bankhead I: Fine motor performance in subjects of subnormal, normal, and superior intelligence, *Aust NZ J Dev Dis* 11:143-150, 1985.
12. Maino DM, Schlange D, Maino JH, et al: Ocular anomalies in fragile X syndrome, *J Am Optom Assoc* 61:316-323, 1990.
13. Maino D, Wesson M, Schlange D, et al: Optometric findings in the fragile X syndrome, *Optom Vis Sci* 68:634-640, 1991.
14. Mankinen-Heikkinen A, Justonen E: Ophthalmic changes in hydrocephalus: a follow-up examination of 50 patients treated with shunts, *Acta Ophthalmol* 65:81-86, 1987.
15. Alexander J: Ocular abnormalities among congenitally deaf children, *Can J Ophthalmol* 8:428-433, 1973.
16. Johnson D, Caccamise F: Rationale for performing visual assessments with hearing-impaired persons prior to conducting speech reading research and training, *J Acad Rehabil Audiol* 16:128-142, 1983.
17. Ronis M: Optometric care for the handicapped, *Optom Vis Sci* 66:12-16, 1989.
18. Richman JE, Petitio GT, Cron MT: Broken wheel acuity test: a new and valid test for preschool and exceptional children, *J Am Optom Assoc* 55:561-656, 1984.
19. Allen HF: A new picture series for preschool vision testing, *Am J Ophthalmol* 44:38-41, 1957.
20. Albrecht K: *Brain power: Learn to improve your thinking skills,* New York, 1980, Prentice Hall.
21. Kalb L, Warshowsky JH: Occupational therapy and optometry: principles of diagnosis and collaborative treatment of learning disabilities in children, *Occup Ther Pract* 3:77-87, 1991.
22. Hellerstein LF, Fishman G: Vision therapy and occupation therapy: an integrated approach, *J Behav Optom* 1:122-126, 1990.
23. Duckman RH: Vision therapy for the child with cerebral palsy, *J Am Optom Assoc* 58:28-35, 1987.
24. LoCascio GP: Treatment for strabismus in cerebral palsy, *Am J Optom Physiol Opt* 64:861-865, 1987.
25. Duckman RH: Effectiveness of visual training on a population of cerebral palsied children, *J Am Optom Assoc* 51:607-614, 1980.
26. Thorn F, Thorn S, Ziemian DM: TV captions are difficult to read with small amounts of blur, *NEWENCO Res Ser,* 1-4, 1991.
27. Linder TW: *Transdisciplinary play-based assessment: a functional approach to working with young children,* Baltimore, 1990, Paul H Brooks Publishing.
28. Bailey DB, Simeonsson RJ, Winston PJ, et al: Family-focused intervention: a functional model for planning, intervening, and evaluating individualized family service, *J Division Early Child* 10(2):156-171, 1986.

9

Management of Functional and Perceptual Disorders in Patients with Developmental Disabilities

Robert H. Duckman

Key Terms

Functional and perceptual disorders	Record player pursuits	Monocular minus lens rock
Cerebral palsy	"Lazy Susan" rotations	Near-far monocular accommodative rock
Mental retardation	Spelling flashlight	
Visually impaired	Object localization	Movement through space
Developmentally delayed	Chalkboard saccadics	Directional concepts
Positioning	Grid activities	Rote memory of right/left
Tube rotations	Tic-tac-toe grids	Directional arrows
Mirror rotations	Cops-and-robbers	Directional maps
Object tracking	Picture fixations	Moving around in space
Swinging ball	Monocular accommodative pushout	Form perception
Magnet motilities		
Racetrack motility		
Groffman tracking		

Providing appropriate eye and vision care for individuals with developmental disabilities can be very challenging. Providing treatment for the numerous functional and perceptual disorders present in these special populations has either been ignored or done without proper optometric input. This chapter has been written because:

1. The medical/optometric literature is replete with citations supporting the fact that there is significantly greater prevalence of ocular/visual anomalies in handicapped populations. That, however, is generally where the literature stops. Very little (although it is increasing) has been written about therapy for these patients.

2. Special populations are made up of individuals with real needs. Their visual needs have been ignored and not given the importance they deserve. In addition, clinicians have received little, if any, training in working with these patients. Early intervention to resolve visual problems of patients with developmental disabilities has the potential for increasing each individual's overall functional ability and quality of life. Optometrists are uniquely equipped to manage the visual needs of these special populations since they are the only eye care professionals trained in both the medical and functional areas. Every patient must be assessed in relation to his or her functional capabilities. The most effective programs will be those that acknowledge these patients as emotional beings who are not handicapped in their ability to express an appreciation for your help and their own achievement.

3. By outlining specific visual therapy activities, practitioners with little prior experience in this area will be able to provide therapy for patients who were previously believed to be nontreatable.

4. As our medical technology improves and more high-risk infants survive, you will examine a greater number of special population patients in private practice. Since legislation mandates thorough care for these children (such as PL 94-142, the Education for All Handicapped Children Act) you will need to develop the skills for the diagnosis and treatment of individuals with developmental disabilities.

Several case reports will illustrate how to manage visual programs for children and adults with disabilities. The therapy approaches discussed here can be generalized to any special population. People with disabilties may look different, have difficulties giving subjective responses, and may respond more slowly than their non-affected peers. This may often give the misperception that they are "slow." In fact, they may have a superior intellect and poor expressive skills. This slowness misleads many practitioners to grossly underestimate the abilities of their patients.

It has been noted[1] that the most significant finding was not the extraordinary prevalence of visual anomalies within this group but the total disregard for the treatment of these visual deficits within the health care–delivery system. Ten years after publication of this research, Ronis[2] wrote of similar issues. "The need for vision care in this population is substantial, yet many get none or less than they need. These patients often need more than treatment of eye disease or an accurate spectacle correction."

It is not, however, always a simple matter of needing vision care. As I will discuss later, many of these patients have multiple handicaps, and each requires treatment. It is necessary for the rehabilitation team to prioritize the treatment needs. Since many of these children may be medically fragile, visual problems are often placed on the bottom of the medical priorities list. The occupational, physical, and speech/language therapists can, when possible, combine therapy activities. As an example, many children with developmental disabilities need communication devices for which accurate eye movement and/or fixational skills are required. Thus, improving a patient's eye movement skills can have enormous importance in achieving the goals of the therapist.

Background

Little exists in the literature that reviews treatment of visual problems within special populations. The following provides a discussion of the limited research in this area. Correa and Poulson[3] worked with a small sample of young blind and mentally handicapped children to improve reaching and grasping exploratory behaviors. Children 2 to 4 years of age were administered a graduated prompting teaching program to train motor skills utilizing positive reinforcement schedules. Over the training period the clinicians were able to increase the reaching/grasping responses of these children. Responses that were 100% appropriate to midline, right, and left stimulus placements occurred. They suggested that these children would have a better chance of learning about their environment because of the improved exploratory skills.

A case report by Bader[4] described improved gross and fine motor skills in a 5½-year-old child with cerebral palsy. Attentional, behavioral, and academic enhancement was noted as a result of spectacle correction of a moderate myopic refractive error in both eyes. One of the more impressive studies was conducted by Bader and Woodruff,[5] who showed the positive effect of corrective lenses on various behaviors of individuals with mental retardation. The authors posited that sensory deprivation caused by defects of the ocular refractive system tends to deprive the individual of visual input and such deprivation may inhibit further sensory, perceptual, and cognitive development. They developed a questionnaire to probe the following areas:

1. Social and emotional skills

2. Gross and fine motor skills
3. Reading and writing skills

Bader and Woodruff[5] divided their groups into three age categories, as well as an experimental group, and three control groups. Each subject was evaluated before the application of refractive correction or placement into one of the control groups and again at 2- , 4- , and 8-week post-treatment intervals. Their results suggested a strong relationship between improved visual inputs and development. Positive behavioral changes occurred to a greater extent in the "new glasses" group (those who had need of a refractive correction or a significant change in refraction) than in the various control groups. The new-glasses group showed significant improvements in their ability to identify objects and people, their sociability, their eye contact and classroom behavior, their posture while eating and walking, and their gross motor skills (catching, kicking, and throwing a ball) and fine motor skills (reaching and grasping, stacking blocks, stringing beads, cutting paper, and tracing), along with a greater neatness and speed of working. In addition, there were fewer teacher complaints regarding these children. The changes were greatest in the youngest (0 to 6 years) experimental group. The study concluded that many social/emotional behaviors, gross and fine motor skills, and academic performance levels can be improved with the correction of refractive errors in the mentally retarded population and, furthermore, the earlier the intervention takes place, the more enhanced the performance can be.

In another study on the effectiveness of visual therapy in a population of children with cerebral palsy,[6] it was noted that adapted therapy techniques administered by occupational, physical, and speech therapists showed significant improvements in ocular motility (100%) and accommodative function (66.66%). Because accommodative function was poor or absent in all the children in this sample, it was postulated that cerebral palsy might affect the brain centers controlling accommodation. This study suggests, however, that accommodative dysfunction can be successfully treated with appropriately applied vision therapy.

Harrison[7] has recognized the importance of a stable central body and eye position in terms of sensory input. She states that "once body and eye position are not easily maintained centrally, reception and use of sensory input can be distorted." The thrust of her therapy program is to "help these children achieve a stable central body position (the physiotherapist's task) and as normal eye position and muscle movement as possible." She emphasizes ocular motility and hand/eye coordination in home-based programs, having found that, although visual function in some children does not improve, most patients demonstrate visual improvements in a matter of weeks or months. Another interesting finding from her study is that many fathers have found the daily treatment enables them to begin to relate to and form relationships with their handicapped children.

Vision in the Multiply Handicapped Child

Factors that cause visual problems in the general population also produce visual problems in the multiply handicapped child. Neuromuscular dysfunction may disturb visual development in other ways. For example, some children cannot stabilize their head position, which means that their eyes never have a stable position from which to search their environment and learn clues for orientation. Other ocular/motor problems occur when neuromotor dysfunction affects eye muscles. Development of visual/motor skills is adversely influenced by the difficulty of coordinating direction of gaze and hand movement, and early visual development is also affected. Any young child with a visual dysfunction will encounter roadblocks to their early learning experiences. When this occurs in multiply handicapped children, it is an added and confounding problem.

Early intervention and visual stimulation in individuals with disabilities can significantly affect overall function.[8] In Down syndrome and other developmental disabilities this stimulation increases the repertoire of cognitive responses the child has at his or her disposal. The positive outcomes of visual stimulation/therapy on children with disabilities have been impressive.

CLINICAL PEARL

Early intervention and visual stimulation in individuals with disabilities can significantly affect overall function.

All factors (cognitive level, physical health, motor/sensory function) must be realistically assessed before deciding which goals are attainable for each individual. As an example, many multiply handicapped children cannot communicate verbally and must depend on language boards. Frequently these necessitate appropriate fixation, pursuit, or saccadic abilities, but the child's ocular/motor skills are poor.[1] Teaching the patient to improve fixation on a language board display (even if there is no carry over into other types of fixational activities) may be enough to allow that individual to effectively communicate with others.

Much of this chapter concentrates on vision therapy approaches and techniques as applied to the multiply handicapped population. It should not be forgotten, however, that vision therapy involves other aspects of visual care. We will discuss some of these non–"visual training" therapies and then attempt to construct a rationale for, and a means of administering vision therapy within a population of multiply handicapped children. Factors that cause visual problems in the general population also operate to produce visual problems in multiply handicapped populations. Because of frequent neuromuscular dysfunction in these patients, visual development may be disturbed in other ways.[9] For example, some children cannot stabilize their head position; hence, their eyes never have a consistent position from which to search their environment and learn clues for orientation. When neuromotor dysfunction affects eye muscles, ocular/motor problems ensue. Development of visual skills is adversely influenced by difficulty of coordinating gaze direction and hand movement. Early visual development is also disturbed. When this occurs in the multiply handicapped child, it is an added and confounding problem. Early detection and remediation are important, especially for multiply handicapped children.

CLINICAL PEARL

Some children cannot stabilize their head position; hence, their eyes never have a consistent position from which to search their environment and learn clues for orientation.

Ocular Motor Disorders

Studies of visual function in the multiply handicapped child show a significantly higher incidence of visual anomalies. There is a large variance in prevalence data because of differences in the nature of the groups studied. In the general population of children age 6 to 17 years, the incidence of strabismus ranges between 5.5% and 6.7%.[10,11] In an approximately equivalent age range of cerebral palsied children, the percentages range from a low of 15%[12] to a high of 60%.[13,14] In a review of the ocular anomalies commonly found with mental retardation syndromes, Maino et al.[15] noted that all have significant refractive errors, strabismus, and nystagmus. Pigassou-Albuoy and Flemming[16] suggest that the high incidence of strabismus in the cerebral palsy population is due to lesions in the motor centers of the brain, which could affect the elaboration of higher cortical processes (such as binocular vision). They further hypothesize that the difficulty in curing strabismus in this population is because a significant component of the strabismus is neurological in nature and not uniquely functional as in non-affected children. The frequent occurrence of strabismus in multiply handicapped children has focused attention on this anomaly, often to the exclusion of others. The treatment of strabismus in these special populations, however, is very difficult.

Optometric Therapy for the Multiply Handicapped Patient

The primary goal of any optometric therapy program is to allow the patient to interact with his or her environment in a manner that best meets his or her needs. "Needs" is the key word. The individual's intellectual and physical capabilities must be considered when planning a therapy program. In the treatment of visual problems of multiply handicapped children, it is important to define carefully the full scope of visual deficits and evaluate how these affect performance. After determining which deficits can be treated, goals and objectives should be outlined and an appropriate treatment plan designed. Vision therapy must be integrated with other therapies to produce the best results and aid in fulfilling the patient's objectives. Multiply handicapped children are usually involved in many different therapies. Even if the vision therapy is top priority, it is yet *another* therapy program that the parent and child have to fit into their schedules. If it can be incorporated into the other therapies, it becomes less onerous and more feasible.

CLINICAL PEARL

The primary goal of any optometric therapy program is to allow the patient to interact with his or her environment in a manner that best meets his or her needs.

The first objective is to diagnose all ocular diseases and refer or treat as needed. Once the organic anomalies have been determined, you have a better idea of what can or cannot be accomplished. Defined goals of therapy should always reflect consideration of these anomalies. The next step is to correct any refractive error. Glasses should be prescribed when there is a significant refractive problem that interferes with function. However, the level of intellectual function should also be taken into account when prescribing, because behavioral characteristics (such as tactile defensiveness, self-stimulation, head banging, eye pressing, poor head/neck support, or self-abusive actions) can affect the outcome of any therapy prescribed. When intellectual function is impaired, it is suggested that you follow the guidelines below:

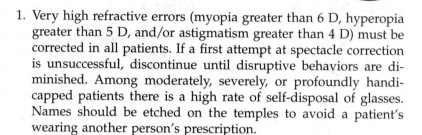

CLINICAL PEARL

To properly use a bifocal segment, the patient must have appropriate head, neck, and trunk control, along with adequate visual/motor skills. If these are not present bifocals may be contraindicated.

1. Very high refractive errors (myopia greater than 6 D, hyperopia greater than 5 D, and/or astigmatism greater than 4 D) must be corrected in all patients. If a first attempt at spectacle correction is unsuccessful, discontinue until disruptive behaviors are diminished. Among moderately, severely, or profoundly handicapped patients there is a high rate of self-disposal of glasses. Names should be etched on the temples to avoid a patient's wearing another person's prescription.
2. Moderate refractive errors (2 to 6 D myopia, 2 to 5 D hyperopia, 2 to 4 D astigmatism) are a gray zone. Clinical judgment should be used when prescribing.
3. Low refractive errors (less than 2 D myopia, hyperopia, or astigmatism) need not be prescribed unless the patient has intellectual functioning that allows symptoms to be communicated.

When intellectual function is mildly or not impaired, the criteria for prescribing for distance are no different from what they are for the non-disabled. The application of a near vision prescription requires careful consideration. As noted above, accommodative function is depressed in this population. It is necessary to prescribe plus lenses for near tasks. Motor abilities must be taken into account, which may preclude the use of an add for near point. To properly use a bifocal segment, the patient must have appropriate head, neck, and trunk control and visual/motor skills. If these are not present, bifocals may be contraindicated. It is often possible to give plus lens prescriptions in single-vision lenses for classroom and/or near use. Multiply handicapped children are usually in small classrooms with most material presented at near distances. Chalkboards, if used at all, are typically not more than 6 to 8 feet away. In addition, teachers can be asked to present material on the chalkboard larger than usual, or at the child's desk, which will decrease the effect of distance blur experienced in the classroom.

Low vision devices can be considered when required. However, their use may be difficult because of the cognitive or motor disabilities present. The most successful devices include high plus lenses for near and handheld telescopes for distance. The telescopes are worn on a neck chain or strap. Parents should be informed of the costs involved and the possibility that the devices may become lost or need replacement.

Case Reports

Too often a practitioner will discredit the value of conventional therapies because of a patient's disability. Unconventional therapies may be totally discounted. What follows are four case reports that illustrate how optometric management significantly increased visual function for a patient and improved the quality of life.

Patient F.R.

This 14-year-old mentally retarded, visually impaired boy lived in an institution. His right eye was phthisic and had no light perception. His left eye had peripheral retinal detachments, a subluxated lens, and visual acuity of about 20/400. He would not tolerate spectacles even though they corrected the left eye to 20/200. His behavior in school was disruptive, and his mobility was severely limited. Three other visual examinations had produced similar results, i.e., spectacles prescribed and quickly discarded by the patient. A 6× handheld telescope was given, which he wore around his neck. With it the acuity in his left eye improved to 20/40. He became extraordinarily dependent on it, to the point where he would not let anyone touch it. He even wore it to bed (at night). His attention, mobility, and academic performance in class improved. The telescope gave him sufficient visual function to feel more secure with regard to moving around in space.

Patient C.S.

This aniridic, visually impaired, developmentally delayed 4-year-old boy came in for an initial evaluation as a result of referral from a social-service agency. He had significant pendular nystagmus that nulled in superior gaze. His grandmother reported that he spent much of the time with his head bent down. His physical therapist was concerned about long-term postural effects. He had no communication skills except for a consistent "yes/no" response. Visual acuity was 20/200 as measured with the Mentor BVAT Picture Acuity Optotypes. By experimentation, the correct amount of base-down prism that would remedy the postural defect was determined (16 Δ BD, OU). The child's grandmother, teacher, and physical therapist all reported improvement in his function directly related to the application of the prism. (This is an excellent example of optometric therapy aiding the goals of other therapists.)

Patient E.K.

This 7-year-old girl with cerebral palsy was evaluated for ocular/ motor dysfunction. She was emmetropic, had a full range of ocular motility, and exhibited good visual acuity (measured with American Optical pictures and a pointing/matching paradigm); but she demonstrated only momentary contact with her visual environment. During acuity testing, she would make a rapid glance at a projected picture and then at the near-point card. Pointing was always done while her head was positioned *away* from the card. At times it seemed as if she was "actively" avoiding vision as a sensory modality. Her motor involvement was significant (athetoid quadriplegia), and she used a wheelchair. She had the cognitive skills to drive a power wheelchair, but not the visual/motor skills. It became apparent that she had appropriate visual memory skills and was able to function by using short-term memory. She had difficulty driving the power wheelchair and using visual input at the same time. Ocular/motor training and hand-eye activities were prescribed to increase fixation time and pursuit/saccadic eye movements. Within 7 months she had sufficiently improved visual/motor skills to begin using a power wheelchair. Her use of this device motivated her to continue improving fixational, pursuit, and saccadic skills. As these skills improved, she was allowed more time in the chair. (This is another example of where the goals of optometric therapy aided the goals of other therapists on the rehabilitation team.)

Patient B.G.

A 21-month-old boy with developmental delay and juvenile glaucoma presented as an agency referral. He had had 15 glaucoma surgeries and was so photophobic that his parents could not take him out in the daytime without a blanket wrapped around his face. He was enrolled in an early intervention program for visually impaired children. Little progress had been made, however, because of his inability to tolerate normal illumination. With the minimal information that could be acquired during the examination because of this intolerance, he was prescribed NoIR ½%[21] filters mounted into swimming goggles. The goggles were made of clear plastic, with the outside painted black. He was given this appliance and was soon able to tolerate room lights. He also responded appropriately when taken into normal daylight. After 2 weeks his parents and teachers noted significant improvement in his classroom activities. (This case demonstrates how innovatively applying filters for severe photophobia can result in significant functional improvement.)

Vision Therapy and the Patient with Multiple Disabilities

Therapy must begin at an appropriate level. It is important to start at a level where the child is challenged, but also where with conscious effort, he/she can succeed. You should keep in mind that progress with these children is often slow. Your therapy goals must be precisely defined, realistic, and short term. Whenever possible, use positive reinforcement schedules to strengthen the child's motivation for working at tasks. In the section below, various visual activities are described. When selecting tasks for training, be sure to consider the child's intellectual function, the physical and visual limitations that exist, and the child's personal preferences.

CLINICAL PEARLS

In the supine position, with the face toward the ceiling the oculomotor effort is the same in all directions.

CLINICAL PEARL

For oculomotor therapy, find the position where the child is most relaxed, most likely to be able to concentrate, and least likely to hyperextend or spasm.

Ocular/Motor Activities

Ocular/motor activities are indicated when children have poor fixational, pursuit, and saccadic ability. These skills are essential for many educational activities and for using language boards. Therefore educational and communication goals may be easier to achieve once the goals of vision therapy are attained.

Positioning

Start your ocular motility therapy with the patient supine. The rationale for this is that in a seated position the child has to exert different amounts of effort as the eyes move down and up (toward and against the pull of gravity) but in a supine position, with the face toward the ceiling, the ocular/motor effort is the same in all directions. However, there are many children who cannot comfortably lie supine without going into hyperextension patterns or muscle spasms. Always keep in mind that positioning may be altered as needed. The primary consideration is to find the position where the child is *most relaxed*, most likely to be able to concentrate, and least likely to hyperextend or spasm. If you work with a child in the sitting position, it is important that the head and shoulders be kept in alignment while hip posture is maintained. Hypotonic children can be assisted by using posture-supporting devices (slant boards, pillows, even a parent's or therapist's arms). Hypertonic children can be relaxed by posturing them in appropriate ways. Consult the child's occupational therapist for additional information.

Environment

It is essential to start your ocular/motor therapy in a protected and visually quiet environment. A large well-illuminated room with multiple stimuli is significantly more distracting than a small, darkened, empty room. Once the child is comfortable working within this protected environment, normally occurring sensory "noise" can be gradually reintroduced.

Head movements

Ultimately you want the child to follow a moving target using eye movements only. This may be unrealistic at first. Start your therapy by allowing head movement. This will help establish foundations for a fovea to target match. As the skills improve, an attempt can be made to separate the eye, head, and neck systems. The head may be stabilized by your hands or by sandbags.

Presentation of targets

Select targets that will maintain the patient's attention. The greater the number of high-interest targets identified, the better your chance of maintaining the patient's attention throughout a training session. These targets should be constantly alternated during a session.

Practice is required to learn at what speed targets should be moved. The eye can track a maximum velocity of 30°/second,[17] but children with poor pursuit skills require a slower speed. It is better to move the target too slowly than too quickly. To maintain the child's interest, therapy procedures should be changed frequently and tedious activities should be intermingled with enjoyable ones. Even with a child whose attention span is short, attempts at tracking are worth the effort. The objectives should always be to increase fixation time and extend the range of successful tracking.

Monocular versus binocular presentation

Initially, training should be done monocularly. Once equality of monocular performance is obtained, you can start binocular therapy.

Therapy Activities to Improve Fixation and Pursuit Skills
Tube rotations

When no other task can be successfully handled, put the child in the position of maximum relaxation in a *totally* darkened room. Hold a cardboard cylinder (an empty paper towel tube) up to one eye while the other eye is occluded. At the far end of the tube (the end away from the eye), present an illuminated target. The target may be a transilluminator or pen light, a transilluminator inside a translucent finger puppet, or a transilluminator covered by colored cellophane. (For reasons that I have been unable to explain, multiply handicapped children will often be captivated by certain colors. Children who will not follow a transilluminator by itself or one with a red or blue filter will suddenly visually track one when a yellow filter is placed over the light. The color a particular child will attend to must be identified by trial and error.) While keeping one end of the tube about an inch from the eye, slowly move the target at the other end of the tube. Move your light in horizontal, vertical, or circular patterns. If the tube is held close to the eye and the only stimulus available is the illuminated target at the other end, it is likely that as the light is moved the child will track the target. As the ocular/motor skills start to improve (that is, as the child starts to follow the target more accurately and for a longer period), gradually start moving the tube further from the eye. Initially you will hold the tube about an inch from the eye (which will allow more than enough room to observe motility skills). As ocular motor skills improve this distance may be increased gradually. Eventually, remove the tube and present the illuminated target in a totally darkened room.

The initial purpose of the tube is to isolate visual stimulation and define the environment for the purpose of setting up a fovea-fixation target match. Once this match is developed, it must be generalized to a normal environment. You should gradually increase room illumination so the child can follow the target in the therapy room with peripheral stimulation present. As the tube is eliminated, you can move the target randomly. With improvement in the child's skill, change the target from a flashlight to a finger puppet, a racing car moving on a track, a computer-generated object on a video-display terminal, or any target that will enhance fixation and pursuit movements. Tactile reinforcement (having the child touch the target as it is being moved) will often increase the accuracy of eye movements and the duration of fixation.

Mirror rotations

This activity can be done in any position. The target for fixation and pursuit movements is the child's own eye. A small plane mirror is held in front of one eye (about 6 to 8 inches) while the other eye is patched. The child is instructed to look at and follow his or her eye as you *slowly* move the mirror horizontally, then vertically, and finally in circular, oblique, and random patterns. Watch the performance at all times and give verbal feedback whenever the child loses fixation. Remember: The feedback should always be positive. For example: "You are doing so nicely, keep watching your eye" or "Try looking at that beautiful eye of yours." There are many variations on the mirror theme that can be incorporated into any therapy program. A child can be placed in front of a larger mirror while objects or people move slowly within the field. The child is instructed to keep watching the rabbit or the bird, or the teacher, as they move around or are moved around in the room behind the child.

Object tracking

The more internal movement an object has, the more likely it will draw the visual attention of the individual. Take a plastic tube of about 18 inches, fill it with oil, and drop a marble into it. The marble should have some internal component, such as glitter. The tube should be carefully sealed at both ends. The child is asked to fixate the marble as the tube is turned from end to end. The allure of the glitter in the marble will be enhanced if there is a light source nearby. Marbles can be changed if the child loses interest. Another form of this object-tracking activity is to get a child to track a wind-up or friction toy, or an object placed on an electric train set in front of the child. Additional attention-getting fixation targets can include wind-up toys that move through water.

Swinging ball

Suspend a sponge ball, a yarn ball, or a Nerf ball at eye level, 2 to 3 feet in front of the child. Slowly swing the ball in a plane parallel to the child's frontal plane. Instruct the child to follow the ball as it moves from side to side. Yarn balls are texturally more interesting and seem to quickly capture the child's attention. Other types of light-weight balls can be used as well. If the child has enough hand control, you can stand opposite him while the ball swings between you. Tell the child to try to strike the ball with his or her hand so it hits the therapist (have the child "aim" for you). If the child successfully "hits" you, act as if he/she has hurt you by yelling "ouch." This seems to motivate most children to try harder. They realize it is being faked and think it is funny.

Magnet motilities

Using a magnetic wand and forms, place a form on one side of a sheet of poster board facing the child. Hold the wand on the other side and slowly move it around asking the child to watch the "floating circle." If the child has reasonable hand control, you can ask the child to move the wand to make the circle move either in random or in predeter-mined patterns.

Racetrack motility

Racetrack motility may be done as a pursuit activity alone or with hand-eye coordination depending on the motor and cognitive skills of the child. On a chalkboard or large piece of paper, draw a racetrack at eye level. Place this 3 feet away on a wall opposite the child. The track is drawn with a specific degree of difficulty, ranging from a simple wide oval (Fig. 9-1) to a complex, convoluted, variable-width track (Fig. 9-2). Either you or the child can hold a flashlight. If you hold it, the child's task is to pretend that the light is a car and to follow it as it goes around the track. If the flashlight goes outside the path of the track (and you should frequently do so on purpose), the child must indicate, by some predetermined response code, that this has happened. A child who can manipulate the flashlight should be encouraged to "drive" the light around the track *slowly*, keeping it in the track. This is a very motivating activity for most children, but some enjoy crashing the car or jumping the path. They may do this on purpose, and for these individuals, little in the way of ocular/motor training will be accomplished. (This procedure is contraindicated for these children.) Patients with optical head pointers and sufficient head/neck control may also do their own driving.

Follow the leader

This can be done only with children who are able to manipulate a flashlight or optical head pointer. You and the child each hold a flashlight and sit about 5 to 6 feet opposite a blank wall in a totally darkened room. Slowly move the light around on the wall while the child tries to keep his or her light directly on yours so it appears as if there is always a single light. You may have color filter paper on top of at least one of the lights so the child has feedback as to which of the two is his or hers.

Groffman tracking

This is a more enjoyable activity for children than most, but technically it does not train ocular pursuit ability. Rather, it trains accuracy of small saccadic eye movements and fixation skills. It is grouped here

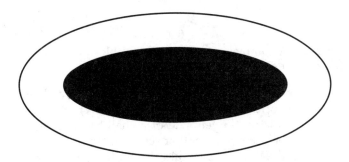

FIGURE 9-1. A simple wide oval for use in racetrack motility exercises.

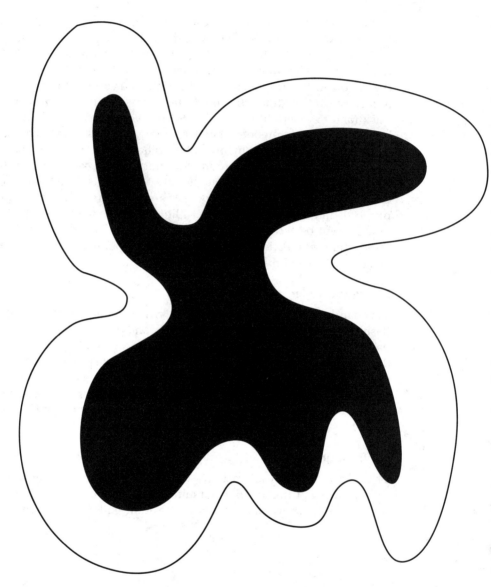

FIGURE 9-2. A complex, convoluted, variable-width track for use in racetrack motility exercises.

because of its similarity to the ocular/motor skills needed in academically oriented tasks (such as reading). You should draw a set of symbols on the left side of a chalkboard (large pieces of paper may also be used) and another set on the right. Place the board at eye level, 3 to 6 feet from the child depending on the size of the presentation. Then draw squiggly lines from the symbols on the left to those on the right. The degree of difficulty will depend on the number of symbols used, the complexity of the path, the number of intersections created, and the angles at the intersections (the smaller the angle, the more difficult the task) (Figs. 9-3 and 9-4).

The symbols may be letters, numbers, geometric forms, or pictures. Consult with the child's teacher to determine the best symbols to use. For example, working on letter recognition, you should use letters that the child consistently knows and place them on the right side of the board. Letters the child needs to learn can be placed on the left side. Tell the child to follow the path from the symbol on the left and to tell you where it leads on the right. The path is to be followed carefully without taking any turns off the road. Initially the patient can use a finger to assist in obtaining more accurate visual fixation skills. The visual tracing paths should not be color coded. If color coding is used, the child can match the beginning and ending symbols using color without any oculomotor/hand-eye activity.

Record player pursuits

The difficulty of this activity can be gradually increased from simple to complex. It requires either a children's record player with variable speeds and a removable cover or a simple motor-driven rheostatically controlled turntable. You should make cardboard "records" about 12 to 14 inches in diameter. A small hole is inserted into the center of each disk. Every "record" can be custom made to meet specific needs of the child. Start the therapy with one colored circle about the size of a quarter (Fig. 9-5, *A*). The following are tracking activities that can be used:

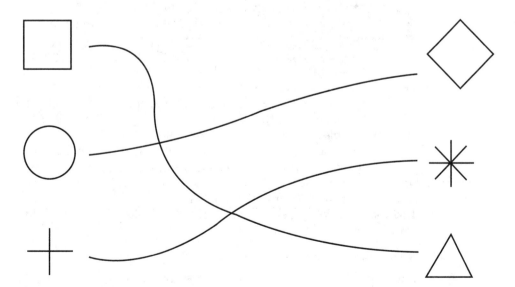

FIGURE 9-3. Groffman tracking trains the accuracy of small saccadic eye movements and fixation skills.

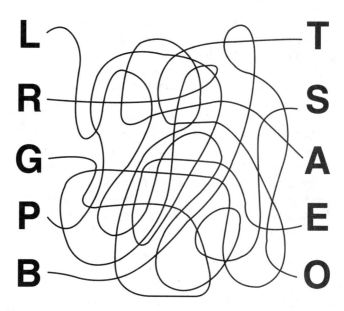

FIGURE 9-4. A Groffman tracking figure with high degree of difficulty.

  Watching the child's eye movements as he/she follows the colored
    circle monocularly
  Holding the flashlight on the circle and having the child indicate
    whenever it moves off the circle
  Instructing the child to hold a pencil or crayon and, at your
    command, move it slowly down to "hit" the circle
  Having the child track the colored circle while he/she keeps a small
    flashlight directed on it

As skills improve with the more simplified "records," you can put
more circles on the disk. Eventually letters, shapes, and/or numbers
may be placed inside the circles (Fig. 9-5 B and C). The child can be
asked to spell words by (1) looking at one letter at a time while you
call out the letter you think he/she is fixating until the word is
correctly completed or (2) using a dowel stick or pen light to point to
a letter as he/she spells the word. Alternatively, the child can use a
pencil or crayon to touch each letter while he/she spells the word.
Numbers can be used to do math problems. The child points to two
numbers that equal 10 or to the number that equals 5×3. This rotating
disk visual-tracking therapy, however, may be limited by the child's
physical and cognitive abilities.

"Lazy Susan" rotations

You may substitute a lazy Susan for the record player activities. It is
best to use three-dimensional figures (such as Sesame Street characters
or a Teenage Mutant Ninja Turtle) to capture and hold fixation.

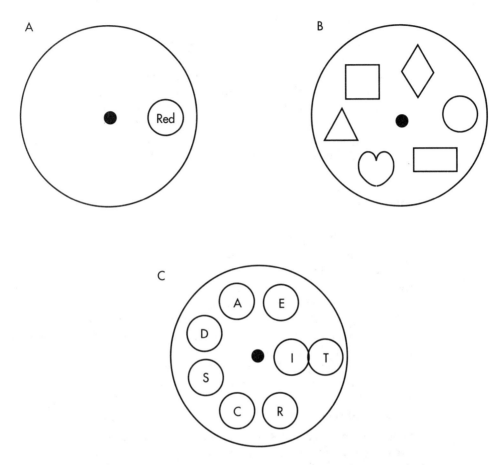

FIGURE 9-5. A number of tracking activities can be used in record player exercises.

The spelling flashlight

In this exercise you and the child face a blank wall in a totally darkened room. You hold a flashlight and slowly move it, writing capital letters. After each letter, the child describes what has been "printed" on the wall. You can help achieve some of his or her teacher's goals by working specifically on letters or numbers that are currently being taught. If the child knows the alphabet, try spelling words the teacher wants him or her to learn. By writing numbers on the wall, you can have the child add or subtract. When he or she becomes proficient in these simple tasks, you may write an entire word. At this stage of therapy you will be not only helping the child develop ocular/motor and cognitive skills but you will also be providing reinforcement of visual memory and visual closure. If the child can handle these, you might attempt to present words in cursive rather than printed format.

Activities to Improve Saccadic Eye Movements

Saccades are important in all academic activities; but for the multiply handicapped child who needs to use a communication device based on eye movements, they are essential for searching the environment for information and for making closure on objects in the peripheral field of view. They are generated on the basis of how far a point being stimulated in the peripheral retina is from the fovea. In adults saccadic movements generally include a major component (between 85% and 90% of the total eye movement) and a small (corrective) minor component (for bringing the fovea onto the target). Several activities are intended to improve the accuracy of a child's saccades.

Object localization

With the child sitting or reclining in a position of relaxation that allows the child to look around, stabilize his or her head and instruct the child to find different objects (a door, a window) in the room. This can be done in the classroom, at home, out of doors, or anywhere the child finds something of interest. Watch the movements of the eyes as he/she searches for the named object. An effective method is to place the child 2 or 3 feet in front of a mirror, facing the mirror, while you stand (or sit or lie) behind the child and watch his or her eyes and the object in space behind you both.

Chalkboard saccadics

Have the child sit 3 to 4 feet from a chalkboard at eye level. In each corner of the board, place a figure or picture of a familiar object. Kneel between the chalkboard and the child but below the child's line of sight and instruct him or her to look at the pictures you have randomly named. If the child has no difficulty with four pictures in the corners, increase the number around the periphery. It is helpful if you have a small diagram of what is on the board so you do not have to keep turning around to see if the child is correct. It is also possible to have the child look at a picture and, on the basis of his eye movements and your diagram, try to guess where he/she is looking.

This activity can also be done with pictures on small cardboard squares attached to the chalkboard with Velcro to allow them to be placed in random order each time the activity is conducted. This eliminates memory components and encourages scanning behaviors. There are many ways to increase the degree of difficulty of the task. You can code each picture on the periphery of the board with a number and write several numbers in the center of the board (Fig. 9-6, A). The child reads a number in the center of the board and looks at the appropriately numbered item on the board. You would stand in front of the child and observe that the task is being done correctly.

A

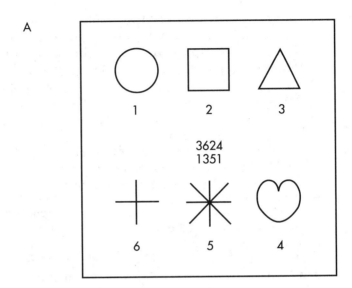

B

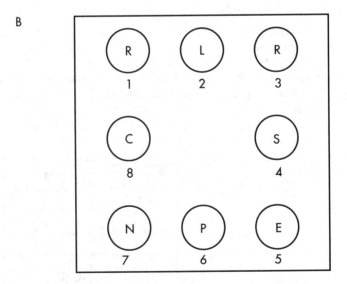

FIGURE 9-6. Educational, speech, or physical therapy goals can be incorporated into chalkboard saccadic exercises.

Visual memory can be incorporated to increase task difficulty by marking two or more numbers on flash cards. As the cards are presented, the child must look at the pictures corresponding to the numbers. To further increase task difficulty, the card can be presented, a short simple activity introduced, and after an interval the child instructed to look at the figures corresponding to the numbers presented on the card. When this visual memory task is being done, no numbers are presented in the center of the board (Fig. 9-6, B) but rather only the symbols. It is easy to incorporate educational, speech, or physical therapy goals into this activity.

Grid activities

Grid activities are an excellent way to build skills necessary for the utilization of electronic language board systems. Although most devices can be customized to the needs of the individual, almost all use some kind of visual scanning behavior to localize a "cell" on the visual display and move a pointer, wand, or light into that cell. Some systems have automated movement of lights from cell to cell until the needed cell is lit. The child must then make a response to stop the light in that cell for expression of needs or wants. The grids can be done at near or far point, with pictures, numbers, letters, symbols, words, or shapes. You can either call out a row and a column and ask the child what is in that cell or call out a stimulus and ask the child where it is. For example (Fig. 9-7), you might ask what is in C-3? (answer: car) or where is "boy"? (answer: D-2).

Tic-tac-toe grids

Another activity that improves saccadic movements and visualization skills utilizes tic-tac-toe boards. The child is taught that the boxes in the grid, from top left to bottom right, are to be described by the numbers 1 to 9 (Fig. 9-8, A). The therapist can then place objects in a single box and ask "What number box is the raisin in?" or "Where is the circle?" (Fig. 9-8, B). An object may be placed in several or all

	1	2	3	4
A	CAT	SAW	CAP	SAD
B	MAN	WHO	ARE	YOU
C	TEN	SIT	CAR	HAT
D	EAR	BOY	WAS	NET

FIGURE 9-7. Grid exercises are an excellent way to build skills necessary for the use of electronic language board systems.

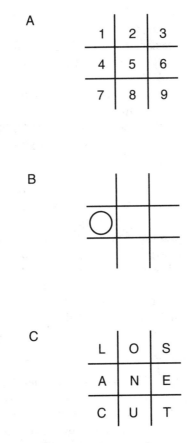

FIGURE 9-8. Tic-tac-toe boards can help saccadic movements and improve visualization skills.

boxes and the child asked to tell you what is in "Box 4?" (Fig. 9-8, C), or where is the "E?" This activity can be made easier or more difficult by decreasing or increasing the number of cells and objects being used. At a much higher cognitive level the child may be given two, three, or four numbers in a visual memory presentation and asked to connect the midpoints of each box "in your mind" and draw what it would look like. For example, connecting 1-7-9 in a nine-cell board would describe the letter L whereas connecting 5-6-9-8 would describe a square.

Cops and robbers

This activity may be used with any child who has sufficient hand control to manipulate a flashlight, or enough head/neck control to manipulate an optical head pointer. It can be completed monocularly or binocularly in a totally darkened room. You pretend to be the "robber" while the child is a "cop" in hot pursuit. You both hold flashlights and face a blank wall. The task is for the cop to catch the robber, who has just "stolen" his favorite possession. As in "follow the leader," it is easier if colored filters are used so there is a clear distinction between the two lights. You place your light at one point on the blank wall. The child then tries to capture it by placing his light directly on top of it so the two lights are superimposed. As soon as this happens, you immediately move your light to some other point on the wall and the child again tries to capture it. When the lights are superimposed, you continue to move your light, etc.

Picture fixations

This activity requires a little more work than most but is rewarding in its effect. The objective is to make up a series of *interesting* 35 mm slides. Animals, family members, school friends and teachers, comic characters, or Sesame Street characters, all of which have saliency for the child, work well. You need to set up two 35 mm slide projectors opposite a blank wall. The child is seated between the two projectors. You alternately present slides on the right and left sides, and the child is asked to look at the picture and, if possible, identify it. He can be instructed to point if it helps maintain visual fixation.

Accommodation

In an earlier work[18] it was observed that "accommodative function is definitely depressed, if present at all, in *severely involved* CP [cerebral palsy] children" but that "monocular amplitude of accommodation and accommodative facility can be improved in this population through standard optometric visual training procedures. It also seems reasonable that if this function can be trained in the severely involved CP child it should be trainable in a more normal population of children with CP."

Accommodative problems are prevalent in the multiply handicapped population; but if training can be administered, results are rewarding. Below are several activities that will be useful for improving the accommodative skills of these children. Keep in mind that the most significant problem in performing accommodative training in this population is that responses are exceptionally difficult to elicit and require a significant amount of time to obtain. Usually the elicitation of a subjective response from the patient takes much longer than the patient's accommodative response to the stimulus. It is often necessary to establish a system which will facilitate subjective responses. For example, something as simple as a smile when the child sees the target can be utilized to indicate when the task has been accomplished. The target can then be removed and the child given as much time as necessary to identify it. Hand or head switches that make a buzzing noise, upward/downward or left and right gazes, vocal noises, etc. may all be used to let the patient communicate to you that the target has been seen. The therapy sequence would be (1) the child makes the accommodative response, (2) the child identifies the target, (3) the child signals that he/she knows what the target is, (4) you remove the target, and (5) the child takes as long as needed to identify it through his/her communication system.

The targets of choice for these exercises are lowercase typewritten letters, numbers, or words on white unlined index cards. The one chosen will depend on the patient's intellectual ability and visual acuity. When none of the targets can be used, line figures of geometric shapes or Bliss symbols reduced on photocopy machines may be utilized. Accommodative training is typically done monocularly until there is equal and adequate function. You should not increase the difficulty of the task unilaterally (in other words, the degree of difficulty should be increased only when *both* eyes can perform well at a given level).

Monocular Accommodative Pushout

Since it is frequently difficult to elicit responses from multiply handicapped individuals, and because the more reliable the responses the more control the therapist has, the "push-out" method is preferred to the "push-up" accommodative method. In the push-up method you go from clarity to blur as the target approaches, which might encourage the child (in an attempt to please you) to report that he/she sees it when in fact it is blurred. In the push-out method you slowly move the target from very close to the eye (assumed blur) to further out (first point at which the child can identify it). The child attempts to accommodate and responds when the target is seen. It is then removed, and the child names it. The distance from the eye is recorded, and the child tries to decrease this. Progress is monitored by comparing the mean distance from the eye at which he/she can identify the target. The smaller the distance, the better will be the response.

Monocular Minus Lens Rock

Using concave lenses and predetermined targets, introduce the appropriate lens power monocularly. Present the target at 16 inches until the patient gives a signal that he/she sees it. Remove both the lens and the target and allow him time to name the target. The starting lens power should be determined by identifying the highest value necessary for the patient to see the target with but a modest degree of difficulty.

Near-Far Monocular Accommodative Rock

Place a distance target about 10 feet from the patient and at eye level. Have the child identify one of the characters on it. Then place a near target card a fixed distance from the eye and have him or her shift gaze to that and signal when it is seen. Remove this and allow the child as much time as necessary to respond. The initial distance for the near target will be the one at which he/she can clearly see the targets with effort. Again, monitor progress by decreasing the distance of the near target and also decreasing the time it takes to make the shifts from near to far to near. Because of the time factor in obtaining responses from the patient, facility training is more difficult (though still possible). The clear response signal is accepted without asking for a subjective response from the patient in terms of target identification. If this method is successful, it is now possible to use plus/minus flippers to train facility. This is first done monocularly. When the patient is ready for binocular flipper training, you need to be careful about suppressions and/or diplopia. These responses are not difficult for patients with verbal skills but become almost impossible when needed from nonverbal patients.

Binocular Fusion Training

As reported in an earlier paper,[6] you usually cannot expect to "cure" strabismus in patients with severe cerebral palsy or other profound disabilities. The exception to this rule is the rare intermittent exotrope with symptomatology. In such cases I attempt duction training, both in and out of instrument, and jump duction vergence facility work. In other patients, however, strabismus is left untreated. Frequently the strabismus is variable and inconsistent over time. I have had patients who during a single evaluation shifted from an esotropia to an exotropia to orthophoria. Pigassou-Albuoy and Flemming[16] have hypothesized that the difficulty in curing strabismus in this population is due to the fact that a significant component of the strabismus is neurological and not "uniquely functional" as in non-affected children.

Perceptual Motor Activities

Visual perception anomalies are commonly found in the handicapped. Normal visual/perceptual development occurs as the child learns body awareness, control, and spatial concepts through active movement. Without the use of normal movement patterns, the child is likely to develop perceptual concepts that are not consistent with the reality of the objective stimulus. Since many patients with disabilities have poor motor abilities, it is not surprising that their interpretation of perceptual space is distorted.

Body Awareness

Being aware of one's body is essential to understanding spatial concepts. Body part identification games with lots of movement and touch to provide feedback are helpful. If the child has enough control of body parts, "touch and go" is an excellent activity for building concepts of body schema (or an awareness that all spatial judgments need to be referenced around an internalized zero point). With the child lying supine, touch a part of his or her body and ask the child to move "only the part touched." For example: "If I touch your arm, I want you to move the arm to shoulder level. If I touch your leg, I want you to slide it out about 2 feet." In order of difficulty (from simplest to most complex) the movements are

1. Homologous: Either both arms *or* both legs
2. Monolateral: One arm *or* one leg
3. Ipsilateral: One arm *and* one leg on the same side
4. Contralateral: One arm *and* one leg on opposite sides

Many multiply handicapped children are unable to make independent body movements. In such cases you can move the child's body parts in an attempt to build awareness and use auditory cues for reinforcement and feedback. For example, "I am going to move both your arms to shoulder level. I am moving your arms higher and higher. Now both arms are at shoulder level."

Movement Through Space

Have the child estimate what needs to be done to get from point A to point B (10 steps or 15 turns of the wheelchair). The child should complete the task and compare his/her estimate with the number of steps it actually took. If he/she can walk, he/she may estimate that it will take seven steps to get from the table to the sink; or if he/she can only creep, the child may estimate that it will take four movements.

Directional Concepts

Concepts of directionality are important in the skills required for reading readiness. Based on the processes of body awareness and bilateralization, they are difficult to establish in non-disabled children but are even more difficult to establish in multiply handicapped children. Confusion in directional concepts reflects an individual's inability to make discriminations around midline and may lead to letter/number reversals and poor academic performance. Activities to help a child establish concepts of directionality include rote memory of right and left, directional arrows, directional maps and movements in space.

Rote memory of right/left

Mark body parts ("L" for left, "R" for right) to assist the child in learning the labels of right and left. These markers should be on the child's body rather than on external objects. If this is done, the child will begin to understand the referencing of directional spatial coordinates against himself/herself. For example, when an educator teaches a child that the right hand is on the side of the classroom where the windows are and the child walks into another room where the windows are on the left, the reference point of "windows" can cause an err. Therefore, the child should learn that these labels of direction are referenced by surroundings.

By playing body part identification games with simple commands ("Show me your right hand," "Show me your left elbow") or, if the child has sufficient motor function, more complex commands ("Touch your left knee with your right hand"), you can build concepts of body awareness as well as auditory motor integration skills. It is also sometimes fun to give an impossible direction and watch what happens ("Touch your right elbow with your right hand"). Children find this amusing.

Directional arrows

Make an arrow on a card. Hold the card up in various orientations and ask the patient which direction the arrow points. This can be done with or without reference marks on the child's hands. As the child starts to develop this skill, the task can be made more difficult. For example, seat the child opposite a chalkboard. In the center of the board and at eye level, make a series of arrows going in the four primary directions (up, down, left, right). You can make one or more rows of arrows depending on the child's ocular/motor skills. Have the child start at the left of a single line or the top left of a multiple-line series and "read" the arrows across in order, naming the direction of each. When the child's skill improves, introduce bidirectional (oblique) arrows.

Directional maps

Make a simple line map using vertical and horizontal lines. The map should show a starting position and lead to some place the child would like to go (Fig. 9-9, A). The child designates with his pencil which way you need to travel. The child must also give you the direction he/she wants you to move and then must watch carefully as you trace over the lines with the pencil. At all corners, he/she must tell you to "Stop" and must then name the new direction. If the child says the wrong direction, you follow that command and continue until he/she says to stop. At that point the child must direct you back to the original "corner" where the error was initiated. The degree of difficulty increases when the four oblique directions are added to the four primary directions (Fig. 9-9 B).

In this activity the child talks about moving the pencil right, left, up, down, etc., which of course in "real" space would be impossible. We move forward/backward and, at junctures, make turns. A much higher cognitive level skill would involve the child's taking a map (such as the one shown in Figure 9-9, A) and, while sitting, "walk" through it saying whether he/she needs to turn right or left at each of the corners. If the child has enough motor function, you can have him or her move through the map in three-dimensional space before

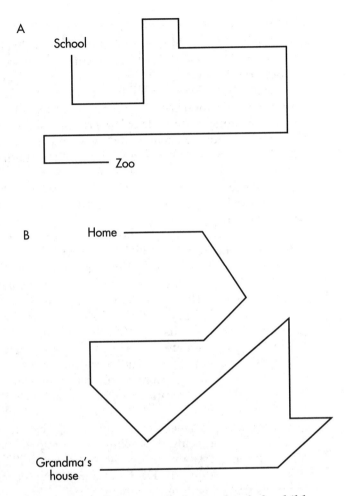

FIGURE 9-9. Directional maps can be used to help children improve their verbal skills.

conducting the higher-level visualization task. Another fun way to do directional maps, which also encourages children to give full verbal directions, is to have them draw their own map and then give verbal instructions to you on what to do (where to start, which direction to go, how large to make your lines). Upon completion of this task, your drawing should look about like the child's original, solely on the basis of his/her verbal instructions. You might peek at the map in case he/she is purposefully giving incomplete or erroneous information.

Moving around in space

You and the child actually move around the room in this activity, following the child's verbal instructions. The movement can be random or goal directed, and you both should do it while naming every direction in which you turn.

Form Perception

At the lowest level, simple three-dimensional shapes can be tactilely manipulated by the child for identification purposes. You ask the child to identify the shapes with and without visual information. In the latter case the shape stimulus is put into a bag and the child, on the basis of tactile information only, identifies it. Boxes with multiple openings through which three-dimensional shapes can be placed are used to foster form-matching and eye-hand coordination skills. Later, geometric shape formers (three-dimensional patterns) may be used to develop the visual/tactual relationships between geometric patterns and movement patterns. The child traces around the former using a finger, crayon, or pencil. As his skill improves, the plastic forms are replaced by thick or textured tape, which allows one to experience the motor patterns necessary to circumscribe the shapes. Eventually the child will be ready for simple form board puzzles.

These puzzles should be done incorporating verbal cues, with the child describing what he/she is doing. Have the child name the shape or tell you where the shape belongs. Use visual scanning and tactile reinforcement. At this point you should start using simple large parquetry block designs. Start with two squares. Then use a square and a triangle, a square and a diamond, a triangle and a diamond. Eventually, introduce more and more pieces for the child to match. Stimulus presentations may be placed physically on the table or incorporated as pictures on index cards. The cards may be left on the table for comparison by the child or flashed (for 3 seconds) to introduce a visual memory component. The child should try to verbalize what is being done while matching the pattern. Parquetry block stimuli may or may not show the contour lines of individual pieces within the design. The latter require high-level visualization of the parts that constitute the whole.

Computers and the Multiply Handicapped Patient

The most compelling device for use in a visual therapy program that deals with persons who have handicaps is the computer. Computers have the capability of drawing out and maintaining a child's attention better than any other device; and they can be adapted to the special needs of numerous patients to train ocular motility, fixation, intersensory matching, hand-eye coordination, perceptual concepts, accommodation, and fusion as well as to achieve educational goals. They also have been used as positive reinforcement for other therapies. They can become an "information prothesis" that is able to amplify or substitute for deficient structures or functions. A computerized environment in the life of a person with physical, mental, sensory disabilities offers not only communication with the outer world but also the opportunity to achieve greater independence in daily or professional activities. (A listing of computer resources appears following the References.)

When modifying a computer for individuals with handicaps, you must take into consideration the extent of the patient's disability. For example, some handicapped persons are able to operate the keyboard with one hand, others with one or two fingers, and still others with a joystick held in one hand or manipulated by the head or the mouth. For these persons there are software and hardware modifications that simplify the data input process. Typing difficulties can be overcome by using membrane-sensitive keyboards whose keys are operated by slight pressure. Extended keyboards with bigger keys or variable keyboard templates are also available. Following are two examples of useful adaptive devices for the multiply handicapped:

1. McIntyre Computer Systems manufactures the "LipStick" (an alternative to the standard Macintosh mouse). It can be used by individuals with little or no hand movement or control and is operated by the lips, chin, cheek, shoulder, arm, hand, or foot. It is simple to use and requires no hardware or software modifications.

2. Unicorn Engineering Inc. manufactures a series of expanded keyboards (Figs. 9-10 to 9-12). The Model II, for example, allows a disabled person to access standard software and also serves as a communication and writing aid. It has 128 touch-sensitive squares that can be grouped together to form larger squares according to the person's needs. Each outputs a character or message (which you have previously defined). When operated with a speech synthesizer, the squares produce a user-definable spoken message or setup that can be saved on disk. Interchangeable overlay sheets may be utilized. Unicorn Keyguards (Fig. 9-13) are helpful in isolating each key on the board so the user can make accurate choices; this prevents unintentional keystrokes. It can also provide greater stability, allowing the user to isolate more closely spaced keys than when it is not used.

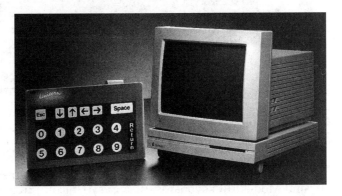

FIGURE 9-10. The Unicorn Engineering Model 510 keyboard. (Courtesy Unicorn Engineering Inc., Richmond, Calif.)

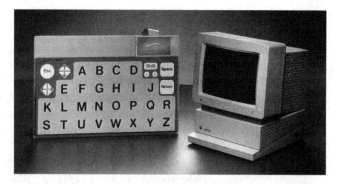

FIGURE 9-11. The Unicorn Engineering Model II expanded keyboard. (Courtesy Unicorn Engineering Inc., Richmond, Calif.)

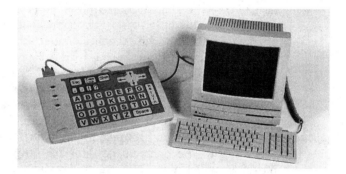

FIGURE 9-12. The Unicorn Engineering IntelliKeys and Smart Keyboard. (Courtesy Unicorn Engineering Inc., Richmond, Calif.)

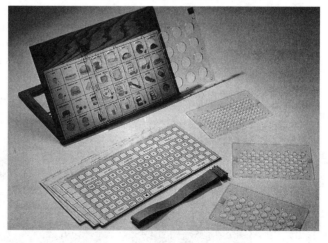

FIGURE 9-13. The Unicorn Engineering keyboards for Model II and Model 510 keyboards. (Courtesy Unicorn Engineering Inc., Richmond, Calif.)

A source of current information in this rapidly expanding and changing field is the bimonthly publication *Closing The Gap* (published in Henderson, Minnesota), which reviews, summarizes, and evaluates new computer software and hardware specifically developed for individuals with special needs.

It provides continuous reports about what is available. In a recent issue, for example, a feature called "DISKoveries" stated that over the past several years there has been an explosion of computer software benefitting children and adults with special needs. Hardware and software programs designed for multiply handicapped persons are constantly undergoing modifications and upgrading so that it is almost impossible to stay abreast of developments. However, keeping in touch with publications such as *Closing The Gap* is very imporant. Remember: The children we serve are very motivated by computer activities and often perform visually on a computer better than they would in any other setting.

Early Emerging Rules

In "Early Emerging Rules" (Laureate Learning Systems*) the rules chosen are negation, prepositions, and plurals. These are usually the earliest learned rules and can be depicted graphically. The graphics, speech, and animation are exceptional and involve the children in the learning process. Each rule offers four levels of training and a game and test option. In the *negation* mode, for example, a picture appears and the auditory output is, "This pig has a hat. Let's make the hat go away." At the press of a switch, the hat is gone and the computer says, "This pig has no hat." Sometimes the negative appears first, "This man has no hair. Make his hair grow." A flick of the switch makes the man grow hair. At a higher level of training two pictures appear (a pig with a hat and one without a hat) (Fig. 9-14). The child must press the switch so a figure sits over the pig with no hat. These games are errorless, well animated, and can be used with very young children. They are powerful tools for a young physically handicapped child because they give control to the child. The child always receives positive verbal and visual rewards for his efforts. A detailed summary of the activity with teacher/therapist comments can be printed at the end of each session for inclusion in the child's record.

Each program, along with others developed by Laureate, encourages fixation skills, saccadic eye movements, visual/motor matching skills, and the development of language.

First

In "First Categories" (Laureate Learning Systems), children are offered 60 nouns in six categories (animals, body parts, clothes, foods,

---

*110 East Spring Street, Winooski, VT 05404, (800) 562-6801.

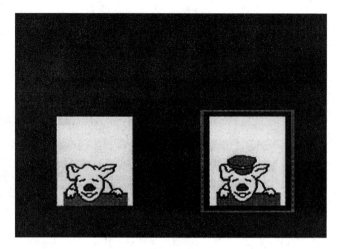

FIGURE 9-14. The "Early Emerging Rules" computer program encourages the development of fixation skills, saccadic eye movements, visual/motor matching skills, and language skills. (Courtesy Laureate Learning Systems, Winooski, Vt. Copyright 1991.)

utensils, and vehicles). Training may be done by inclusion or exclusion, with two or three pictures at a time or with text alone. You decide whether to use speech or animated characters and can customize programs to include a touch window, keyboard, game controller, or single switch. Summary sheets, with your comments, can be printed out. This program improves visual fixation, saccadic skills, category concepts, and retrieval. No reading is required to use it.

Cause and Effect

"Cause and Effect" (MarbleSoft*) has five separate activities. The child can make fish move in water, blow bubbles, change visual effects, move a bee toward a flower, and make letters appear on the screen. You can use this to enhance visual fixation and tracking as well as reinforce the concepts of cause and effect.

My House

"My House" is another Laureate computer program that allows children to understand and express language used in daily activities (Fig. 9-15). Four activities are used to increase understanding of object labels and their functions. Each is carried out using six scenes that represent typical rooms in a house (bedroom, bathroom, dining room,

---

*21805 Zumbrota NE, Cedar, MN 55011, (612) 434-3704.

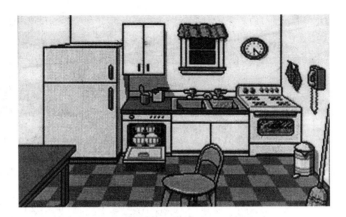

FIGURE 9-15. The "My House" computer program allows children to understand and express language used in daily activities. (Courtesy Laureate Learning Systems, Winooski, Vt. Copyright 1991.)

kitchen, living room, and laundry room). Selections may be made using a touch window, keyboard, or single switch. The activities include (a) discovering labels—select an object in a room, and the computer tells the child what it is; (b) identifying labels—the computer prompts you to find various objects according to their labels (such as "Find the stove"); (c) discovering functions—select an object and the computer will tell you what it does, ("We use a knife to cut food"); and (d) identifying functions—the computer asks the child to find certain objects according to their function ("Where do you put dirty clothes?"). This program is used to enhance visual fixation, scanning eye movements, visual figure/ground, and language skills.

Switches, Pictures, and Music

"Switches, Pictures, and Music" (Technology for Language and Learning, East Rockaway, NY) has high-contrast visual effects and can be programmed to present numerous stimuli. Two pictures flash alternately on the screen as a switch is pressed. It is an excellent way to start training saccadic eye movements and cause-and-effect relationships.

Switch It, See It

"Switch It, See It" (UCLA Intervention Program for Handicapped Children, Los Angeles) presents a moving stimulus that can be used for horizontal, vertical, and diagonal visual tracking. For example, a fire truck and ladder, with a fire fighter on the bottom of the ladder, is pictured; as a switch is depressed, the figure climbs the ladder.

Cause and Effect

Several play options of the "Cause and Effect" (Technology for Language and Learning) program are effective in teaching visual tracking. A few are discussed here.

1. Visual Effects: Designs of various colors appear on the screen against a black background each time the switch is pressed
2. Steps: A stick figure walks up a flight of stairs, one step each time the switch is pressed; when it gets to the top, it parachutes down to the bottom
3. Free Throw: A stick figure at the lower left corner of the screen stands with a basketball in hand, the basket on the right of the screen; at the press of the switch it throws the ball leaving a dotted track to visually follow

Picture Chompers

"Picture Chompers" (MECC),* a keyboard-driven program, teaches the child concepts of color, size, shape, and form matching. It also presents classifications, along with visual differences and similarities. It is a motivating game that develops the ocular motor skills necessary for effective use of electronic communication systems.

Joystick Trainer

"Joystick Trainer" (R.J. Cooper & Associates)** is a program in which the player must be able to move a joystick in the four primary directions. The eight games included are excellent for developing and enhancing hand-eye coordination. The child moves the joystick to drive a bus or a wheelchair through a maze to objects placed at the four corners of the screen.

School Bus Driver, Bowling, and Firehouse Rescue

These three programs, published by Fisher Price,[†] are all joystick computer games that involve moving through simple mazes. They enhance eye-hand coordination.

Body Builder

"Body Builder" (Dunamis)[‡] is a simple program for single switch or keyboard. The child builds a person's body by combining the head, chest, hips, and feet of a weight lifter, grandmother, space man, and ballerina. It can be used for eye-hand coordination and body awareness.

---

*3490 Lexington Avenue North, St Paul, MN 55126, (800) 228-3504.
**24843 Del Prado, Dana Point, CA 92629, (714) 240-1912.
†Aurora, NY.
‡3620 Highway 317, Suwanee, GA 30174, (800) 828-2443.

Build-a-Scene

"Build-a-Scene" (R.J. Cooper & Associates) is a cause-and-effect software program that is switch operated and builds from a blank screen to a colorful scene with every touch of the switch. A voice synthesizer can provide motivating words and sounds with the picture items. Animation occurs frequently to increase the child's interest. The program can be used for development of visual fixation and scanning skills and for perceiving cause-and-effect relationships.

Let's Go Shopping (I and II)

"Let's Go Shopping" (UCLA Intervention Program for Handicapped Children) is switch operated and can be used to train visual attention, scanning, and classification.

Eency Weency Spider Games

"Eeency Weency Spider" (UCLA Intervention Program for Handicapped Children) is also switch operated and uses a competitive game format to build better visual fixation and tracking skills. It is based on a board game that can be played by one to four players.

Sharon's Program Series

"Sharon's Program" (Access Unlimited) uses one of the Unicorn Engineering keyboards or a switch. All 15 musical games are highly motivating and help teach or reinforce important readiness skills using large-print formats. Examples of the programs include Simple Cause and Effect, Fun With Colors, Learning Directions, Big and Small, Same and Different, Scanning Fun, Learning Shapes, Learning Letters, Silly Letters and Numbers, and Learning Sight Words. These are appropriate for the enhancement of visual fixation, tracking, saccadic skills, and visual perceptual skills.

Summary

In view of their significantly high rate of visual/ocular problems, patients with multiple disabilities are seriously underserved by the optometric community. Although they may in many cases be more difficult to treat, numerous opportunities exist for the concerned clinician to improve their visual function and thus the quality of their lives. It is essential that all interested optometric practitioners become involved in the therapeutic aspects of visual anomalies in these patients. The bottom line is: They need and deserve everything that we can provide for them, including vision therapy.

In addition, working with patients who are multiply handicapped can be exceptionally rewarding. Helping a child use a language board to communicate for the first time with the people around him or her and watching the child express the untold story of his/her emotions and feelings are two truly indescribable experiences. The feeling you get when a child can achieve independence by perambulating for the first time in a power wheelchair as a result of something you have provided—greater acuity, a special device, improved rapport with the environment—must be experienced to be appreciated.

REFERENCES

1. Duckman R: The incidence of visual anomalies in a population of cerebral palsied children, *J Am Optom Assoc* 50:1013-1016, 1979.
2. Ronis M: Optometric care for the handicapped, *Optom Vis Sci* 66:12-16, 1989.
3. Correa VI, Poulson CL: Training and generalization of reach-grasp behavior in blind, retarded young children, *J Appl Behav Anal* 17:57-69, 1984.
4. Bader D: Performance changes in a young cerebral palsied child fitted with spectacles, *Can J Optom* 41:25-26, 1979.
5. Bader D, Woodruff ME: The effects of corrective lenses on various behaviors of mentally retarded persons, *Am J Optom Physiol Opt* 57:447-459, 1980.
6. Duckman R: Effectiveness of visual training on a population of cerebral palsied children, *J Am Optom Assoc* 51:607-614, 1980.
7. Harrison W: Assessment and stimulation of vision in multiple-handicapped children, *Br Orthop J* 42:26-31, 1985.
8. Sharav T, Shlomo L: Stimulation of infants with Down syndrome: long-term effects, *Ment Retard* 24(2):81-86, 1986.
9. Holt KS, Reynell JK: *Assessment of cerebral palsy*, Vol 2, London, 1967, Lloyd-Duke.
10. Altman HE, Hiatt R, Deweese MW: Ocular findings in cerebral palsy, *South Med J* 59:1015-1018, 1966.
11. Roberts J: Eye examination findings among children, *Vital Health Stat*, ser 11, no 115, 21, 1971.
12. Lossef S: Ocular findings in cerebral palsy, *Am J Ophthalmol* 54: 1113-1118, 1962.
13. Guibor GP: Some eye defects seen in cerebral palsy, *Am J Phys Med* 32(6)342-347, 1953.
14. Jones MH, Dayton GO: Assessment of visual disorders in cerebral palsy, *Arch Ital Pediatr* 25(3):251-264, 1968.
15. Maino DM, Maino JH, Maino SA: Mental retardation syndrome with associated ocular defects, *J Am Optom Assoc* 61:707-716, 1990.
16. Pigassou-Albuoy R, Flemming A: Amblyopia and strabismus in patients with cerebral palsy, *Ann Ophthalmol* 7:382-387, 1975.
17. Leigh RJ, Zee DS: *Neurology of eye movements*, Philadelphia, 1983, FA Davis.
18. Duckman RH: Accommodation in cerebral palsy: function and remediation, *J Am Optom Assoc* 55:281-283, 1984.

For additonal information on computer applications for therapeutic use please see:

Press L, editor: *Computers and vision therapy programs,* Santa Ana, Ca, 1992, Optometric Extension Program.

Maino D: Computer saccadic and accommodative rock visual therapy program. *Pediatr Optom Vis Therapy* 2(1):3, 1992.

Maino D: Applications in pediatrics, binocular vision, and perception. In Maino J, Maino D, Davidson D, editors: *Computer applications in optometry,* Boston, 1989, Butterworths.

10

Electrodiagnostic Evaluation of the Special-Needs Patient

Don Seibert

Key Terms

electrodiognostic electroretinogram (ERG)	visually evoked potential (VEP)	electro-oculograms (EOG)

Electroretinogram

Background Information

The electroretinogram is a test of the electrical functioning of the retina as it responds to different light stimuli. The neural network that makes up the retina is composed of an electrical hierarchy that, although complex, must obey the laws of conduction, current, and electromagnetic induction. This makes the retina amenable to studying the signals it produces. The rationale for ERG testing is to eventually classify the electrical signature of different disease states to better aid diagnosis and treatment of the patient.

The retina is composed of numerous cell types that work in harmony to create the signal ultimately interpreted by the occipital cortex. Physiologically the retina is called to action when the rod and cone layer is stimulated by a photon of light, causing a hyperpolarization of the photoreceptors. This hyperpolarization sets off a chain of electrical reactions both inhibitory and stimulatory to the bipolar cells of the middle retina (Fig. 10-1). The bipolar cells then stimulate the

Light

Current
flow

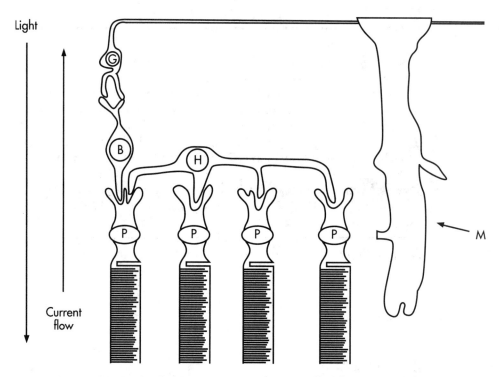

FIGURE 10-1 Ultrastructure of the retina showing the direction of current flow from photoreceptor to ganglion cell after stimulation with a quanta of light. *P,* Photoreceptor; *B,* bipolar cell; *G,* ganglion cell; *M,* Mueller cell.

ganglion cells to respond electrically depending on what type of stimulus it receives. This signal is sent along the nerve fiber layer and eventually makes its way to the occipital cortex for the interpretation of sight.

Whenever a current passes through a cell, a correlating electromagnetic signal is produced that can be received by an antenna. This is the physical basis of the electroretinogram. The retina, with its millions of photoreceptors and electrical matrix, creates an electromagnetic signal both at rest and when stimulated. When at rest, the retina has a natural resting potential created by a constant dark current of sodium ions flowing from the inner to the outer segments of the photoreceptors. When light stimulates the photoreceptor, the Na$^+$ current decreases, causing a relative hyperpolarization of the cell.

The retina has the ability to exist in two separate states, a dark-adapted (scotopic) state and a light-adapted (photopic) state. The scotopic state is a *rod-dominated* response to the surroundings. The retina is extremely sensitive to changes in luminance when in this dark-adapted state. In bright surroundings the retina exists in its light-adapted state. It is much less sensitive to minor fluctuations in light, but it can detect color and visual detail better when in this *cone-dominated* state. These two states work in tandem to allow the eye to see over an extremely wide range of luminance.

There are approximately 130 million rods and 7 million cones in the human retina. As you may know, the rods differ from the cones in many ways. The rods are sensitive to dim light, have poor visual acuity, and do not respond quickly to repeated stimulation (in other words, they have poor temporal summation). They also dark-adapt very slowly, are not sensitive to color, and respond maximally to a wavelength of around 500 nm. By comparison, the cones are more sensitive to bright light, are responsible for the best visual acuity, and have much better temporal summation than rods; they quickly dark-adapt and are responsible for color vision over a wide spectrum of wavelengths. These physiological differentiations are the tools an electrophysiologist uses to electrically dissect the retina and determine its functional status.

A typical ERG response is seen in Figure 10-2. The graph is represented by time along the x axis in milliseconds and voltage along the y axis in microvolts. Initially the resting potential of the eye is around −90 microvolts. This is where the tracing begins. After stimu-

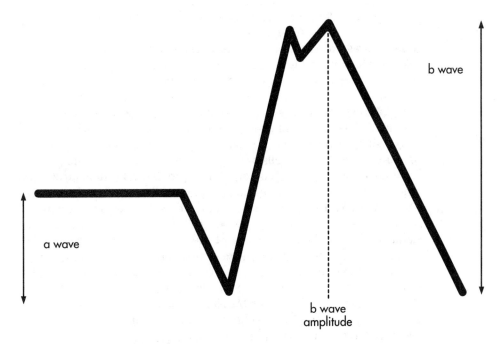

FIGURE 10-2 Typical ERG response showing the a wave and b wave and the latency associated with each.

lation with light, there is a negative deflection that correlates with receptor hyperpolarization. Suddenly there is an upturn in the graph that peaks above the resting potential and returns to approximately the original resting potential. This correlates chronologically with the start of firing of the cells in the middle retina. The large positive deflection is known clinically as the *b* wave. In scientific testing there are many other waveforms present, but they are tested under extremely rigid conditions. In clinical electrophysiology the only waves of significance are the a and b waves.

The heart of electroretinogram testing is in determining the functional status of the rod and cone layer and the middle retinal layers. It was determined early in retinal research that the retina can be easily bisected into an inner and outer portion by occlusion of the central retinal artery. This causes the inner layers (closest to the vitreous) to become anoxic and cease to function and the outer layers (where the photoreceptors are located and fed by the choroid) to remain viable.

If an electroretinogram is attempted on this "bisected" retina, the result is an inherently negatively growing potential. This negative potential measured by an electroretinogram is termed the *receptor potential* because of the cell type causing the response. In clinical electrophysiology the receptor potential correlates with the descending arm of the a wave. The receptor potential extends more negatively than the a wave because there is no b wave to "pull" it in the positive direction. For this reason the latency of the a wave is not usually measured clinically (that is, the b wave gets in the way).

In contrast, a nonbisected retina creates the standard clinical ERG response shown in Figure 10-2. Initially there is a negative growing potential (the a wave) followed by a much stronger and positive growing b wave. Because of the rate and direction that electrical current flows in the retina, it is obvious that the origin of the b wave is the middle layers of the retina, but deciphering the exact cell responsible for the b wave is very difficult. Microelectrode studies[2] reveal that the bipolar cells are both inhibitory *and* stimulatory when stimulated by a photoreceptor. If the bipolar cells depolarize and hyperpolarize in equal numbers, the sum of their electrical discharge should be zero. This is obviously not the case, but the only way to tell it for sure is to measure each bipolar cell discharge after one stimulation and this has not been accomplished at the present time.

It has been determined, however,[3] that the neuroglial Mueller cells located in the middle retina act as a potassium-sensitive electrode that depolarizes in the presence of extracellular K^+, which are released into the extracellular milieu after bipolar cell stimulation. It has become obvious that the b wave results in large part from the large Mueller cell depolarization brought about by the bipolar cells.

When one photoreceptor is stimulated, many bipolar and Mueller cells are stimulated by the horizontal cellular activity of the middle retina. This is the phenomenon thought to be responsible for the large amplitude of the b wave.[4] It should be noted that if a patient has a nonfunctioning ganglion cell layer he can still produce a normal ERG.

The Testing Procedure

The clinical ERG testing procedure appears to be quite complicated at first, but the process is actually relatively simple. First, an antenna is required to measure the signal; and the closer the antenna is to the retina, the stronger the received signal will appear on output.

A number of antenna (from here on called *electrode*) designs have been tried, but most clinics prefer to use one of three types. Some prefer a gold foil electrode that curves over the patient's lid. The patient's cornea should be anesthetized with this kind of foil. A second type, called a Jet electrode, has the wire wrapped around the rim of a polymethyl methacrylate (PMMA) contact lens with a few prongs inserted on the front edge to prevent the patient from blinking and dislodging the lens. I find this lens to be uncomfortable and patients unconsciously blink over the prongs even though the discomfort to them is substantial. Another type of electrode is the monopolar Burian-Allen, which also has the electrode wire wrapped around a PMMA contact lens. The contact lens is mounted on a spring hinge system that prevents it from adversely touching the cornea. The system has a large flange (speculum) mounted on top and bottom that prevents the patient from blinking. This probably is the most comfortable lens to wear and is preferred in our clinic. Any electrical signal must be measured against a reference. Most laboratories generally place a reference electrode covered with conducting gel in the center of the patient's forehead. The ground is usually attached to the patient's earlobe or mastoid bone after being covered with an electrode conducting gel.

CLINICAL PEARL

Another type of electrode is the monopolar Burian-Allen, which also has the electrode wire wrapped around a PMMA contact lens. The contact lens is mounted on a spring hinge system that prevents it from adversely touching the cornea. The system has a large flange (speculum) mounted on top and bottom that prevents the patient from blinking. This probably is the most comfortable lens to wear and is preferred in our clinic.

With the special-population patient the placing of reference electrodes can be difficult. The patient may be uncertain as to what is being done, and this can cause great apprehension. To help alleviate the problem it is advisable to have the parent, guardian, or attendant alongside to calm any fears. Demonstrating the placement of reference electrodes on another person first will show that there is no associated pain. The electrode may be placed on the patient in the dark or light depending on whether the patient seems capable of understanding what the test involves. Sometimes a patient will shy away from the cold conducting gel; so if you feel this is going to be problem, hold the gel and electrode in your hand for a short time to warm them to skin temperature.

CLINICAL PEARL

Demonstrating the placement of reference electrodes on another person first will show that there is no associated pain.

Placement of the measuring electrode is the biggest obstacle in testing the special-population patient. Preferably, it should be done in the dark just before the test begins after 30 minutes of dark adaptation. However, this is not always possible, so the only alternative is to modify or abbreviate the testing protocol and insert the electrode with the room lights on.

After the electrodes have been placed in the proper locations, the patient is ready to be tested. Our usual sequence of testing is as follows:

1. Dark adaptation of both eyes for at least 30 minutes; this has the added effect of calming many special-population patients
2. Placement of the reference electrodes on the cornea, forehead, and earlobe, and then occlusion of the untested eye
3. Movement of the patient (usually a small distance) to the Ganzfeld bowl and situating him comfortably
4. For a flash ERG
   a. Stimulate the scotopic eye with a blue flash and measure its response
   b. Stimulate it with a dim white flash and measure the response
   c. Stimulate it with a bright white flash and measure the response
   d. It should now be essentially light adapted and ready for photopic testing
   e. Stimulate it with a red flash or a flickering red or white light

Because the scotopic response is a rod-dominated response, a blue flash is used first to aid its further isolation. The white flash is utilized to test the evenly illuminated response as well as the largest possible response by the scotopic eye. The scotopic eye is the most sensitive state of retinal adaptation; and when stimulated with a bright flash of white light (all cells responding), the largest a and b wave response seen in ERG testing occurs.

Protocol 2 for testing in a lighted environment is

1. Placement of electrodes on the cornea, forehead, and earlobe and occlusion of the untested eye while the lights are on in the room
2. Movement of the patient (usually a small distance) to the Ganzfeld bowl and situating him comfortably
3. For a flash ERG
   a. Stimulate the photopic eye with a red flash or a flickering red or white light
   b. Turn the room lights and Ganzfeld light off for 1 minute
   c. Stimulate the scotopically moving eye with a blue flash and measure the response
   d. After a few minutes of this procedure, the b wave amplitude should enlarge enough to indicate that the patient has normal scotopic functioning; if after a few minutes there is no growth in amplitude of the responses, it can be concluded that the patient has poor scotopic functioning

Each clinic has its own quirks on ERG testing. For this reason each must establish a set of standard responses, measured from as large a population of age matched normals as possible. To say that any voltage and latency response are standard is not understanding the nature of the test. Each clinic has a testing environment that creates an electrical signature like no other. Therefore to compare numbers between different clinics is not recommended. On the other hand, typical findings can be expected and the numbers seen in Table 10-1 are consistent with the normals seen in many large electrophysiological clinics.

CLINICAL PEARL

Each clinic has its own quirks on ERG testing. For this reason each must establish a set of standardized responses, measured from as large a population of age-matched normals as possible.

TABLE 10-1

Normal b wave latency and amplitude findings consistent with many larger electrodiagnostic clinics*

Test type	b wave latency (msec)	b wave amplitude (μV)
Photopic	23 to 25	100 to 200
Scotopic	45 to 60 white	350 to 600 white
	65 to 70 low blue	150 to 300 low blue
	50 to 60 low white	200 to 350 low white

*Findings will vary from clinic to clinic.

Electroretinographic Stimuli

There are currently two types of commonly performed electroretinograms used as an objective assessment of retinal function—the flash electroretinogram (FERG) and the pattern electroretinogram (PERG).

The FERG merely indicates that the stimulus utilized to evoke the retinal response is generated by a strong flash of light reflected against a surface designed to evenly illuminate the retina (that is, a Ganzfeld bowl). The Ganzfeld bowl closely resembles a standard Goldmann perimeter in appearance.

The PERG utilizes a checkerboard pattern stimulus generated by a special television monitor. The pattern stimulates the macula more than the surrounding retina. The macula will not respond if the check size on the screen is smaller than its threshold visual acuity. Most ERGs performed today use the flash to decipher retinal disease, but the PERG is growing in popularity. If macular function needs to be assessed, the visual evoked potential is still the most popular test.

Standard ERG Responses

When a flash of light stimulates the retina, it creates the typical response seen in Figure 10-2. The clinician looks for proper latency and amplitude in the responses. If the b wave shows repeated abnormalities beyond two standard deviations from the mean responses registered in his clinic, the clinician must call the wave abnormal (Table 10-1). From the above discussion, if there is no a wave present, then based on the electrical path of the retinal tree there will be no b wave present. On the other hand, there may be a normal a wave without a normal b wave. Table 10-2 shows some typical diagnoses characteristic of abnormal electroretinograms. If you suspect one of these diagnoses, a referral for ERG testing is in order. The a wave latencies are not listed because, in a clinical setting, it is impossible to measure them since the b wave starts before the a wave peak amplitude and latency are reached. Clinical measurements are concerned only with b wave amplitude and latency. In years to come the slope of the a wave may show clinical significance, but at present not enough is known about a wave slope for it to be considered clinically significant.

Testing the Special-Needs Patient

Just as the special-population patient requires special adaptations be made for a primary-care eye examination, so he or she needs special considerations when being tested electrophysiologically. Initially the mental and physical status of the patient must be assessed to determine the capacities of the patient.

TABLE 10-2
Typical diagnoses consistent with known ERG anomalous findings

Conditions associated with extinguished ERG	Conditions associated with reduced a and b waves	Conditions associated with normal a wave and reduced b wave
Retinitis pigmentosa (RP) and allied diseases	Some forms of RP and allied diseases	Congenital stationary night blindness with normal fundus
Ophthalmic artery occlusion	Congenital stationary night blindness (CSNB) with normal fundus	Oguchi's disease
Unilateral retinitis pigmentosa		Juvenile retinoschisis
Chorioretinitis	Fundus albipunctatus	Optic atrophy
Metallosis	Drugs (phenothiazines)	Central retinal artery occlusion
Retinal detachment	Retinal detachment	Central retinal vein occlusion
Drugs (chloroquine, phenothiazines)	Vitreous hemorrhage	
Cancer-associated retinopathy (CAR syndrome)	Chorioretinitis	

Based on information from Carr RA, Siegel IM: *Electrodiagnostic testing of the visual system: a clinical guide,* Philadelphia, 1990, FA Davis, 72-78.

For standard electroretinography the patient must sit in a dark room for 30 minutes and be able to remain still, put his or her head on a chin rest, and fixate straight ahead from a few seconds (FERG) up to two minutes (PERG). If it is thought he may not be capable of performing these functions, most clinics can alter their testing procedure to make the testing simpler. But just as it may be difficult to obtain findings during a primary care examination, it may be extremely difficult to test the patient electrophysiologically as well. Generally if the patient has an IQ under 70, ERG testing should not be attempted. If the patient cannot understand simple instructions or communicate properly, or is extremely apprehensive, the ERG should not be attempted unless its results are of an extremely important nature.

CLINICAL PEARL

For standard electroretinography the patient must sit in a dark room for 30 minutes and be able to remain still, put his or her head on a chin rest, and fixate straight ahead from a few seconds (FERG) up to two minutes (PERG).

Some alterations that can be made include inserting the electrode in a lighted room instead of in a darkened room. Protocol 2, above, has worked well in our clinic. Also, if it is thought the patient cannot sit still in a Ganzfeld bowl, most electrodiagnostic clinics still have the handheld Grass photostimulator. The beauty of this instrument is that the tester can hold it by hand so that, even if the patient is not able to keep his head up or fixate very well, a flash electroretinogram can still be obtained.

Visual Evoked Potentials

The VEP (sometimes referred to as the visual evoked response or VER) is the most utilized test in the electrodiagnostic clinic for the special-needs patient. It is the only clinical test available that gives an objective impression of the patient's best visual acuity. It is not the panacea, however. If the patient is moderately cooperative, appropriate responses are obtainable. Its major advantage is that the patient does not have to subjectively respond to be able to tell if he really sees something or not.[7-9,13] Clinically this allows the clinician to detect malingerers and to make an informed assessment of the expected visual acuity for the patient who cannot perform Snellen or other standard visual acuity tests.

The VEP is performed by measuring the occipital cortex voltage response created in Brodmann's areas 17, 18, and 19 with a flash or pattern stimulus. The voltage registered has certain characteristics that define it as a response from the visual system. The whole point of VEP testing is to determine whether the response is present or not.

Patient Preparation

The process of undergoing a VEP can be intimidating, especially for patients with special needs. Many times the patient is anxious about being in a doctor's office and having unfamiliar people around. Every effort should be made to calm the patient and show him/her that the testing will not do damage in any way. Often it is advantageous to show the electrode placement on another person before actually setting the patient up for testing. This shows the younger patient what the test really consists of and can actually speed up the test by increasing patient cooperation. It is highly recommended that the parents stay near their child while the test is being performed.

CLINICAL PEARL

It is highly recommended that the parents stay near their child while the test is being performed.

The electrical setup requires accurate application of reference electrodes at the forehead, a ground electrode usually on one of the ears, and a measuring electrode just above the inion (occipital protuberance) on the scalp. For a three-channel setup two extra electrodes are placed approximately halfway from the occipital vertex to the ear on each side of the inion electrode to better capture optic radiation signals. The electrodes are usually applied after the skin has been rubbed with a mild abrasive and wiped perfectly dry. This aids electrical conduction and improves signal response. Standard electrode gel is placed in the cup of each electrode to add to its signal-recovering ability. It should be stressed that the electrodes are only measuring electrodes and the patient cannot get shocked in any way by the testing equipment.

> ## CLINICAL PEARL
> *It should be stressed that the electrodes are only measuring electrodes and the patient cannot get shocked in any way by the testing equipment.*

Electronic Settings and Signal Averaging

Whenever the visual system is stimulated, it responds by first converting light energy into electrical energy, which is eventually transmitted to the occipital cortex. Once it is received, another electrical signal is produced. The latency from stimulus to cortical reception is in the area of 100 msec for a normal patient. A quality response registered by the occipital cortex is on the order of 5 to 10 µV in size, although this can vary widely between patients. It is an extremely weak signal relative to the natural background noise that occurs from randomly generated ambient electricity. To alleviate this noise from the brain as well as from the surrounding environment, the process of signal averaging must be employed.

Signal averaging involves a number of responses over a specific period. Measuring just one VEP response accurately is almost impossible because of all the ambient electrical noise present. To alleviate this problem, the computer measures a "window" of time on a repetitive scale. Many clinics use a 250 msec (¼ second) window after stimulus presentation to look for the response. After 250 msec the computer window shuts down and will not measure any more electrical activity. If 10 readings or sweeps are taken and are averaged, the random noise during the window will average itself out to zero because theoretically the noise will have a positive voltage half the time and a negative voltage half the time. The tester will be left with only the repeatable, verifiable response he is looking for. Generally, 30 sweeps of the screen is sufficient to get a quality response in a cooperative patient, but more may be required to verify a barely receivable response or the testing of an uncooperative patient. The patient can have a significant effect on the outcome of the reading.

Any movement by the neck muscles creates electrical activity. Any looking away from the stimulus will affect the quality of the response. That is why the patient must be watched for the entirety of the examination to make certain he or she is not wavering his or her eye position. Sometimes to check for malingering, the patient must be given a cycloplegic and then undergo retinoscopy at the time of testing to verify that the stimulus monitor is actually being fixated.

Currently most clinics have taken this procedure one step further.[6] A steady-state VEP is performed by increasing the stimulus rate from 1 to approximately 10 Hz. The result is a repeatable sinusoidal waveform that can easily be distinguished from the ambient noise in all but the most uncooperative patient. Also, a much quicker response measurement is possible and the patient does not have to have as long an attention span. If three consistent readings are obtained, the response is considered valid within a 95% confidence interval.

Types of VEP Stimulation

The retina can be stimulated in many ways to respond. Stimuli can vary in color, luminance, retinal location, and patterns (from lines to checkerboards to shapes)—which all cause different psychological and physiological responses. The VEP is based on foveal stimulation, because the fovea is represented so extensively in the occipital cortex. In other words, the largest occipital response is registered by foveal stimulation and this makes foveal function measurable by electrical means.

There are many types of stimulation currently used for VEPs in the electrophysiology clinic. The most common are flash stimuli, pattern or checkerboard stimuli, red LED (light emitting diode) goggle stimuli, and contrast sensitivity stimuli. The flash stimulus is similar to the ERG in that a large flash of light stimulates the retina to give a massive electrical response. The red LED goggle stimulus is similar to the flash in that it causes a fovea-based response intended to define whether the foveal fibers are functioning all the way to the occipital cortex. Utilizing a red color makes the goggles fovea sensitive, but they will not yield an implied visual acuity. The checkerboard pattern stimulus focuses on the fovea and creates a recognizable pattern. The size of the checks can be changed, and the visual angle they subtend at the nodal point of the eye acts as a minimum angle of resolution stimulus that *implies* the patient's best visual acuity. The same can be said for the contrast sensitivity stimulus. It will change the minimum angle of resolution while maintaining constant illumination on the retina.

Utilization of VEP Stimuli

To investigate the integrity of the visual system, a flash or red-goggle LED is the stimulus of choice for determining whether the signal is reaching the occipital cortex. These stimuli will not tell the clinician what the best predicted visual acuity is, but they will tell if the visual system is intact, even in patients with media opacities. The goggles work even with the patient's lids closed.

If the practitioner wishes to know the best visual acuity that can be attained by a particular patient's visual system, the checkerboard pattern or contrast-sensitivity stimulus must be utilized. The checkerboard pattern is created by a special television monitor with adjustments for contrast and luminosity. It is chosen for its simplistic beauty: half is illuminated and half not at any one moment. As the pattern reverses and the white squares become black and the black white, the average luminosity and contrast of the screen stay exactly the same. What changes is the pattern. The fovea is very sensitive to pattern changes, and the peripheral retina to luminosity changes but not to fine acuity. As the checkerboard changes, the periphery sees the same luminosity and therefore does not respond. The fovea, however, recognizes the pattern change and registers an electrical signal. In this way the pattern VEP is a test of foveal function or implied visual acuity. By constantly reducing the size (visual angle) of the test pattern and correlating the decrease with when the occipital lobe signal is extinguished, an extrapolation of the patient's best visual acuity (minimum angle of resolution) can be attained. An extrapolation is required because no signal is present below 3 μV, the lowest level to which ambient noise can be reduced in most clinics.

Technical factors make presenting a 20/20 stimulus impossible, so large test sizes must be used to determine initially whether a response is present. The testing sequence then calls for reducing the check size to a point where threshold will be reached. Threshold is usually reached when the signal is approximately 3 μV greater than the surrounding noise, because any smaller response cannot be adequately distinguished from the ambient noise. Threshold may also be reached whenever the monitor is incapable of producing any smaller check sizes. The smallest check sizes for a patient seated at 1 m from the monitor is approximately 20/40. Once the threshold is reached, the extrapolation of best visual acuity is compared against a set of age-matched norms to predict the best visual acuity the patient can achieve.

Steady State and Sweep VEP

The problem in the past with trying to get an implied visual acuity on a special-needs patient has been that too often the patient was uncooperative and did not have an attention span of significant duration to undergo transient visual evoked potential studies. Researchers have discovered that if the stimulus rate of the VEP is significantly increased to 8 to 12 Hz a steady-state VEP can be attained. The response is typically a sinusoidal, easily read waveform but it is still subject to electrical complications. A methodology initially introduced[11] to investigate infant VEPs involves employing a steady state VEP of 6 to 12 Hz. Because the signal is oscillating, the stimulus check size (spatial frequency) is constantly changed. This type of testing is termed the *sweep VEP* and has shown promise for instantaneous VEP measurements. It allows immediate extrapolation of the data to an implied visual acuity and has proven much more reliable than the earlier transient (30 to 60 Hz sweep) or steady state (10 Hz) VEP. It should be noted that this is not a commonly performed test and that if you are planning on referring for this type of test you should check with the person to whom you are referring to see whether that individual performs sweep VEPs on a consistent basis and has a set of age-matched norms for the test. The sweep VEP is mainly investigational in nature and requires great skill to be performed correctly.

Optic Nerve Pathology and the VEP

The VEP is most sensitive to pathologic changes in the optic nerve. If the nerve is damaged even slightly, the VEP should be able to detect it. With massive damage the VEP is totally extinguishable; but this is also of little diagnostic value, because simpler tests will elucidate the problem. With much more subtle optic nerve damage the main diagnostic sign is latency of the VEP spike. The spike is significantly lengthened in the presence of a transmission deficit. The lesson to be learned is that if you suspect an optic nerve lesion of subtle character the VEP is the recommended test for this patient. The most common presentation of such a problem is the early manifestation of multiple sclerosis. In fact, as many as 50% of all delayed latency VEPs are eventually diagnosed as multiple sclerosis.

The VEP in Relation to Ocular Disorders

According to Parisi and Bucci,[14] VEP studies may have an investigational role to play in the detection of early primary open-angle glaucoma (POAG). They found an increased latency of the p 100 waveform in patients with POAG but not with ocular hypertension or in nonglaucomatous patients.

In mentally retarded children most of the literature[16-10] indicates that the p 100 wave latency is increased but not by enough to be considered clinically significant and the EEG probably remains a better measure of dysfunction at this time.

PKU and the VEP

An investigational study by Korinthenburg and Fullenkemper[12] has shown that young children with phenylketonuria have increased p 100 latencies when not on a PKU-controlled diet but, after their intake of phenylalanine is curtailed, the VEP returns to its normal value.

Electrooculogram

On a clinical basis the electrooculogram is the least utilized of electrodiagnostic tests, mainly because of its lack of application to a number of common diseases and the small amount of significant information it supplies compared to the ERG and VEP. The EOG functions as an indirect measure of ocular polarity, and that is its main function in clinical and research applications. Clinically the EOG is utilized mostly from detection and monitoring of Best's vitelliform disease; it has not shown promising results in monitoring the changes of age-related macular degeneration.

CLINICAL PEARL

Clinically the EOG is utilized mostly for detection and monitoring of Best's vitelliform disease; it has not shown promising results in monitoring the changes of age-related macular degeneration.

Other disorders in which it shows pathological changes include early chloroquine retinopathy, early siderosis retinae, early diabetic retinopathy, drusen, fundus albipunctatus, and fundus flavimaculatus.

Background Information

The retinal pigment epithelium is an extremely active and important tissue in the maintenance of normal vision. Its apical portion is responsible for phagocytosing the outer segment of the photoreceptors, which allows them to be restimulated by quanta of light. The basal portion is actively involved in the secretion of waste products to the closely appositioned choriocapillaris. In the process of this active physiology the RPE maintains a constant electrical charge that appears to be related to the concentration of extracellular potassium. The important part to remember for electrophysiological testing is that the RPE maintains a relatively negative charge in relation to the cornea. This electrical state makes the electrooculogram possible.

Theory of Testing

As mentioned, the eyeball can be thought of as a dipole battery, with the corneal side being relatively positive and the retinal side relatively negative. In theory, electrodes could be placed on each side of the eye and the potential difference (voltage) between the poles measured. Since this is not practical in a clinical situation, the electrooculogram was invented.

If the eye is extremely abducted, the cornea (positive side) will be closer to the nose and the retinal side closer to the temporal canthus.

If electrodes are placed at the nasal and temporal canthi, they will detect these differences in polarity. Now if the patient extremely adducts the eye, the temporal canthus will detect the more positive charge and the nasal electrode the more negative. As the eye is rotated in the opposite direction, the electrodes will measure the opposite voltages. The amount of voltage registered is directly dependent on the distance from the charge to the electrode. Therefore the registered signal is dependent on the amount of abduction or adduction.

To control eye movements, two light-emitting diodes are placed 30 degrees apart when referenced to the patient inside the Ganzfeld bowl as fixation targets. This constant angle of deviation allows for accurate saccadic movements and eliminates much of the variability in EOG testing. Unfortunately, there is significant variability in ocular polarity *within* the normal population, so much so that a "normal" polarity is very difficult to quantify.

It has been determined that the potential difference across the eyeball is greater when the eye is light adapted than when it is dark adapted. This has been utilized when testing the EOG. If the polarity is measured both in the dark and in the light, a ratio can be established of the greatest polarity in light to the smallest polarity in dark. Arden was the first to set up this ratio, and the term *Arden ratio* is still used today. Some clinicians use the terminology "light peak over dark trough" in place of Arden ratio.

The clinical significance of the Arden ratio is that, although in the normal population the ocular polarity varies greatly, the Arden ratio has been found to be much more consistent, allowing for a table of "norms" to be created. Most clinics deem an Arden ratio of less than 1.65 abnormal and Arden ratios between 1.65 and 1.80 questionable. A ratio above 1.80 is normal, although some clinicians have said they prefer to see the ratio closer to 2.00.

Testing the Special-Needs Patient

If you suspect that a special-needs patient may have one of the previously mentioned diagnoses, a referral for EOG testing is in order. The test consists of attaching electrodes to both inner and outer canthi and a reference electrode to the forehead. After this the patient is seated in the Ganzfeld bowl and the lights are turned out. At 1-minute intervals the LED stimuli turn on and go through a series of back-and-forth movements and the patient views the stimuli, causing him to saccade back and forth. Each minute for 15 minutes this continues, with ocular polarity decreasing as the patient dark-adapts.

The lights are then turned on and the sequence is repeated for another 15 minutes. As the eyes light-adapt, the ocular polarity increases. After light adaptation, the ocular polarity at light adaptation divided by the ocular polarity at dark adaptation is measured, giving the Arden ratio.

In testing the special-needs patient, it is necessary to have only moderate cooperation. The patient should be able to put his head in a Ganzfeld bowl and should not be afraid of the isolation or awkward feelings of electrode placement. The test causes no pain or any discomfort worth mentioning. In fact, the most important factor for ensuring reliable results is merely guaranteeing that the patient is calm and aware of the objectives of the test. Before any referral is made, the clinician should determine that the patient has adequate concentration (of at least a few minutes) and understands that another practitioner will be treating any ocular defects or deficiencies found. The patient can be told that the test will take about 40 minutes and that, to allow for relaxation and the regaining of composure, frequent pauses will be provided during that time.

Conclusion

I hope these pages have made clearer the standard electrophysiological tests and their implications for use with the special-needs patient. There is benefit to be gained from this testing provided the clinician can define exactly

1. What is to be gained by the testing
2. What benefit the patient will realize
3. Whether the patient understands why he or she is being referred
4. Whether the patient is capable of being tested
5. Whether the diagnosis will direct the patient to the proper site for the best treatment

Then you will be in a better position to decide on appropriate referral for electrodiagnostic testing.

REFERENCES

1. Carr RA, Siegel IM: *Electrodiagnostic testing of the visual system: a clinical guide*, Philadelphia, 1990, FA Davis, 13-14.
2. Carr RA, Siegel IM: *op cit*, 13-14.
3. Carr RA, Siegel IM: *op cit*, 13-15.
4. Carr RA, Siegel IM: *op cit*, 15.
5. Carr RA, Siegel IM: *op cit*, 72-78.
6. Carr RA, Siegel IM: *op cit*, 61-62.
7. Creel DJ, Bendel CM, Wiesner GL, et al: Abnormalities of the central visual pathways in Prader-Willi syndrome associated with hypopigmentation, *N Engl J Med* 25:1606-1609, 1986.
8. Ellingson RJ: Development of visual evoked potentials and photic driving responses in normal full term, low risk premature, and trisomy-21 infants during the first year of life, *Electroencephalogr Clin Neurophysiol* 63:309-316, 1986.
9. Gasser T, Pietz J, Schellberg D, Kohler W: Visual evoked potentials of mildly mentally retarded and control children, *Dev Med Child Neurol* 30:638-645, 1988.

10. Giovannini M, Valsasina R, Villani R, et al: Pattern reversal visual evoked potentials in phenylketonuria, *J Inherited Metab Dis* 11:416-421, 1988.

11. Tyler CW. In Heckenlively JR, Arden GB: *Principles and practice of clinical electrophysiology of vision*, St Louis, 1991, Mosby, 408-415.

12. Korinthenberg R, Fullenkemper KU: Evoked potentials and electroencephalography in adolescents with phenylketonuria, *Neuropediatrics* 19:175-178, 1988.

13. Kuroda N, Adachi-Usami E: Evaluation of pattern visual evoked cortical potentials for prescribing spectacles in mentally retarded infants and children, *Doc Ophthalmol* 66:253-259, 1987.

14. Parisi V, Bucci MG: Visual evoked potentials after photostress in patients with primary open-angle glaucoma and ocular hypertension, *Invest Ophthalmol* 33:436-441, 1992.

15. Prager TC, Saad N, Schweitzer FC, et al: Electrode comparison in pattern electroretinography, *Invest Ophthalmol* 33:390-394, 1992.

16. Riise R: Visual function in Laurence-Moon-Bardet-Biedel syndrome: a survey of 26 cases, *Acta Ophthalmol* 65:128-131, 1987.

17. Rizzo JF III, Berson EL, Lesell S: Retinal and neurologic findings in the Laurence-Moon-Bardet-Biedel phenotype, *Ophthalmology* 93:1452-1456, 1986.

18. Rousounis SH, Gaussen TH: Measurement of attention in severely motor impaired infants: a clinical evaluation of a new approach, *Child Care Health Dev* 13:257-268, 1987.

19. Tranebjaerg L, Sjo O, Warburg M: Retinal cone dysfunction and mental retardation associated with a de novo balanced translocation 1;6(q44;q27), *Ophthalmic Paediatr Genet* 7:167-173, 1986.

20. Wenzel D: Evoked potentials in infantile spasms, *Brain Dev* 9:365-368, 1987.

11

The Role of Optometry in Early Intervention

Stanley W. Hatch

Key Terms

Early intervention	Lead poisoning	Public Law 99-457
Drug abuse	Prematurity	Broken Wheel Test
Environmental deprivation	Low birth weight	Random Dot E
	Head Start	

A significant number of preschool children in the United States are at risk for developmental delays and associated problems with health and learning. One response has been to establish early intervention programs that attempt to remedy the effects of these delays. Early intervention centers are becoming increasingly common nationwide. Optometric consultations are frequently sought by parents and the staff of these centers in an attempt to improve the visual development of such children. Thus it is important for optometrists to be familiar with the concept of early intervention and to be able to interact with the team of professionals involved.

This chapter provides an introduction to early intervention programs and the role optometry plays in them. Its objectives are to describe the children and professionals encountered, the prevalence rates of ocular diseases, the nature and effectiveness of on-site screening and examination, the treatment options available, and the influence of early intervention on pediatric populations. It is hoped that after completing the chapter, readers will have attained a functional understanding of early intervention and be able to interact comfortably as members of the team.

What Is Early Intervention?

Early intervention is educational and rehabilitative programs designed for children before they begin elementary school. The programs are usually run as school and day-care activities and are intended for children who, because of medical, environmental, or developmental problems, might not be ready to enter kindergarten. Early intervention attempts to prepare these children for the educational process.

The identification of children at risk for developmental delays and other problems that affect school readiness has increased. Poor prenatal care, the abuse of alcohol, tobacco, or other drugs during pregnancy, environmental deprivation during the preschool years, poor nutrition, and exposure to lead and other toxins have all contributed to an increased number of children with medical and developmental problems (see box on page 285). Prematurity and low birth weight are of added concern because they are associated with learning disability, decreased mental function, and poor health status in school-aged children.[1] Early intervention encompasses a broad range of programs to assist these children—some with small neighborhood staffs that work in church basements, others with a variety of professionals who work in large centers and give educational and rehabilitative care to children with medical problems. The qualifications for acceptance into an early intervention program depend on the program. Perhaps the best known is Head Start, which was developed for children with socioeconomic disadvantages, but others also exist specializing in the diagnosis and treatment of various conditions.

Early Intervention Professionals

A wide variety of professionals participate in early intervention. One prominent member is the preschool teacher. Teachers develop and implement group and individual programs for their students. They design lesson plans for each day and then teach or direct others in the instruction. The teacher may be the most important person in the child's life, since he or she often has more contact with the child than either the parents or other professionals. The teacher becomes part parent, advocate, administrator, coordinator, and friend to the child. For optometric intervention to be successful, communication with the teacher is vital.

Developmental Problems Commonly Encountered in Early Intervention Centers

Learning disability
Perceptual dysfunction
Subnormal IQ (mental retardation)
Gross motor delay
Sensorineural problems
Visual/motor integration dysfunction
Social/environmental deprivation
Congenital syndromes
    Fragile X
    Down
    Cerebral palsy
    Fetal alcohol
    Möbius
    Turner
    Marfan
Prematurity or low birth weight
Complications due to prenatal or perinatal infection
Metabolic disorders
Complications due to trauma or abuse

Preschool teachers are well qualified for this responsibility. Most have obtained a bachelor's degree in elementary education or special education before receiving state certification. The curriculum for elementary education includes courses in child psychology and development, behavior guidance, health and family issues, theories of learning, classroom management, record keeping, and administration, followed by student teaching. Special education requires additional training in the psychology of exceptional children, learning disabilities, and mental retardation as well as in teaching children with physical disabilities and in administration. There is also an internship. The two common routes by which an early intervention teacher enters the field are (first) the traditional one of college after high school, followed by an internship and teaching, and (second) the more expedient one, taken by many older persons, of volunteer teaching followed by vocational education in any of several specialty areas.

Another prominent member of the early intervention team is the teacher's aide. This person acts as a guide, helper, and general assistant for the children in their daily instruction. Although the position does not require formal training, some teacher's aides do attend programs in vocational schools. An advanced position in this area is the child development assistant, who has completed a 9- to 12-month training program and has obtained state certification. Child development assistant programs are available at community colleges and include instruction in basic child behavior, child communication, providing for the physical needs of children, and child health and safety.[2]

Teachers report to the center director or administrator, who is the early intervention program's equivalent of a school principal. This person has obtained a master's degree or its equivalent in education, along with special instruction in developmental psychology or a related field. He or she may be a former teacher who has obtained additional didactical, practical, or research experience, or a practitioner who has designed his or her college curriculum specifically for such a position. In addition to extensive training in special education, he or she has often received courses in statistics and research, school law, school finance, and school administration and has undergone an internship. Center directors carry a great responsibility. They must ensure that teachers develop and implement appropriate programs. They are responsible for the health and safety of each child during school activities. They must arrange for compliance with all government regulations. And they must formulate progress reports and direct projects concerning the center and the children it serves.

Psychologists are present either on the staff full time or available for consultation. They perform psychoeducational testing and make specific recommendations for the children's educational programs. A psychoeducational battery will vary with the examiner depending on philosophy and training, but it usually includes IQ testing, perceptual assessment, achievement tests, and psychological evaluation. A child and/or family may also receive counseling from the psychologist or be recommended for psychiatric evaluation and/or medical treatment. Clinical psychologists must be licensed to practice and usually have obtained a master's or doctorate degree in clinical psychology.

Many health professionals participate in early intervention programs. Physical therapists and occupational therapists play a major role in remedying developmental delays. Physical therapists work to improve or restore motor or orthopedic function and to prevent or minimize physical disability. Physical therapy (like vision therapy) draws on a variety of technological advances and levels of expertise to implement an appropriate program. Another aspect of physical therapy is instruction in the use of prosthetics. A bachelor's degree in physical therapy and a passing score on the national board examination are required for state licensing. The college curriculum is a 5-year program, consisting of 2 years of basic science and liberal arts followed by 3 years of physical therapy training including the study of anatomy, physiology, and treatment methods, followed by an internship.

Occupational therapy concentrates on remediating physical and occupational skills to give disabled persons independence. This could include training in basic skills (such as dressing, toileting, and food preparation). More advanced therapy concentrates on occupational skills, perceptual skills, and rehabilitation for blind children. Occupational therapists do visual perceptual therapy and can be valuable assets in the implementation of certain types of vision therapy. Like physical therapy, occupational therapy requires a 5-year college program consisting of 2 years of liberal arts and 3 years of occupational therapy plus an internship. Occupational therapists must also pass a national board examination and obtain a state license.

The above discussion represents most of the professionals involved in early intervention. Others include nurses, who care for medically fragile children, and each child's pediatrician. For the optometrist, regular communication with the early intervention staff is essential if a child is to receive the best care. It is equally important to place the need for vision care in proper perspective and avoid being overzealous in treating the vision of a child who has other significant health challenges. Being a member of the health profession team means being both active and cooperative to maximize care.

How Should Optometrists Be Involved in Early Intervention?

Public Law 99-457 requires that all early intervention programs include a health assessment for the enrolled child. Vision is an important part of this assessment. Conditions such as decreased visual acuity, significant refractive error, intermittent strabismus, high phorias, and ocular health problems can be detected best by optometric intervention. Routine school screening programs are not appropriate for this age group. It is recommended that screenings or examinations be conducted at the early intervention center. The many advantages of on-site screening/examination include better compliance, improved availability of medical records, decreased no-show rates, and increased levels of parent participation. For screening purposes I use a version of the Modified Clinic Technique shown in the box below.[3,4] The Broken Wheel Test (BWT) for visual acuity,

---

Vision Screening for Early Intervention (modified clinic technique)

Visual acuity (Broken Wheel Test)
Stereopsis (Random Dot E)
Cover test
Extraocular muscle versions
Pupillary evaluation
Retinoscopy
Ophthalmoscopy

CLINICAL PEARL

Photocopies of the Broken Wheel Test and pictures of the Random Dot E can be sent to the center in advance of the screening so the teachers are able to practice with the children.

followed by the Random Dot E (RDE) for stereopsis, works well in that the forced-choice, nonverbal responses are similar. Thus minimum training of patients is required. Photocopies of the BWT and pictures of the RDE can be sent to the center in advance of the screening so teachers are able to practice with the child ahead of time. Even with practice, however, 2- to 3 year-old patients often do not respond well to the tests. For such patients Lighthouse Cards will sometimes yield results (although their validity is not as high as that of the BWT).[4] Comprehensive eye examinations are indicated for those children whose visual acuity cannot be measured.

Comprehensive examination of preschoolers is not difficult at the site (see box on page 289). The BWT, Lighthouse Cards, and Teller Acuity Cards (TAC) are excellent tests and can be easily transported. Handheld instruments, retinoscopy bars, and a trial lens set with handheld tonometer and binocular indirect ophthalmoscope are also easily transported. For certain populations a handheld slit lamp may be required. As any pediatric care provider knows, an assortment of stuffed animals, finger puppets, and (if possible) cartoons on a video cassette recorder provide appropriate fixation devices. I bring Flouress (0.4% benoxinate), 0.5% proparacaine, Cyclomydril (0.2% cyclopentolate, 0.5% phenylephrine), 0.5% and 1.0% cyclopentolate, 0.5% and 1.0% tropicamide, and 2.5% phenylephrine for diagnostic use.

The dilating/cycloplegic regimen will vary depending on associated systemic conditions and the age and weight of the patient.[5] For dilation, 0.5% tropicamide and 2.5% phenylephrine using nasolacrimal occlusion is probably safe in most young children.[6] Cyclopentolate 0.5% with 2.5% phenylephrine has been a standard drug combination for dilation/cylopegia, but tropicamide can be equally effective as a dilating agent and does not lead to rises in blood pressure, heart rate, or emotional status as cyclopentolate sometimes can. For cycloplegia, atropine is the most potent agent; however, I recommend

CLINICAL PEARL

For dilation, 0.5% tropicamide and 2.5% phenylephrine using nasolacrimal occlusion is probably safe for most young children. Cytopentolate 0.5% with phenylephrine 2.5% has been a standard drug combination for dilation, but tropicamide is equally effective and does not lead to increases in blood pressure, heart rate, or emotional status as cyclopentolate sometimes can.

Comprehensive Eye Examination in Early Intervention Centers

Visual acuity (Broken Wheel Test, Lighthouse Cards, Teller Acuity Cards)
Stereopsis (Random Dot E)
Extraocular muscle versions
Pupillary assessment
Confrontation visual fields
Binocular vision
   Hirschberg/Krimsky
   Brückner
   Vertical prism dissociation
   Cover test
   Near-point of convergence
   Prism bar vergence
Refraction
Retinoscopy (dry and cycloplegia)
Ocular health
   Pen light angles
   External examination
   Handheld Goldmann tonometry or Tonopen
   Burton lamp
   Handheld slit lamp examination when indicated
   Direct ophthalmoscopy
   Binocular indirect ophthalmoscopy

---

cyclopentolate because it is faster acting and has less potential for systemic side effects. Atropine results in 0.50 to 1.50 diopters (D) more hyperopia on refraction. In one study,[7] 89% of subjects showed less than 1.50 D difference between atropine and cyclopentolate. By adding 0.50 to 1.25 D of plus to the cyclopentolate refraction, the examiner can determine the full correction for most subjects. Cyclopentolate should be used only in the 0.2% or 0.5% strength with children less than 1 year of age, but two or three instillations 10 minutes apart can be given. This is necessary for babies with dark irides. For toddlers with heart arrhythmias, Down syndrome, abdominal distress, hepatic problems, or other similar conditions, you would use the same regimen as for infants less than 6 months of age. For healthy toddlers, 1% tropicamide with 2.5%

CLINICAL PEARL

Cyclopentolate should be used only in the 0.2% or 0.5% solution with children less than 1 year of age, but two or three instillations 10 minutes apart can be given.

phenylephrine is safe for dilation, and 1% cyclopentolate with 2.5% phenylephrine is safe for cycloplegia and dilation. For children with dark eyes, 0.5% tropicamide, 0.5% cyclopentolate, and 2.5% phenylephrine provides better results when mydriasis and cycloplegia are needed simultaneously.[8] For the child's comfort and to improve ocular absorption, it is important to use anesthetic before multiple instillations.*

CLINICAL PEARL

For toddlers with a heart arrhythmia, Down syndrome, abdominal distress, hepatic problems, or some other unique condition, you would use the same regimen as for infants less than 6 months of age. For healthy toddlers, 1% tropicamide with 2.5% phenylephrine is safe for dilation and 1% cyclopentolate with 2.5% phenylephrine is safe for cycloplegia and dilation. For dark-eyed children, 0.5% tropicamide, 0.5% cyclopentolate, and 2.5% phenylephrine provides a better result when mydriasis and cycloplegia are needed simultaneously. For the child's comfort and to improve ocular absorption, it is important to use anesthetic before multiple instillations.

The ocular conditions most likely to be encountered will vary with the population served. Centers serving children with more severe congenital conditions and medically fragile patients reveal a high prevalence of craniofacial syndromes, strabismus, nasolacrimal conditions, and congenital ocular malformations. In contrast, centers with predominantly healthy children who have mild developmental delays may show few gross ocular problems but many more subtle refractive, binocular, and perceptual dysfunctions. The likelihood of ocular conditions can be inferred from the prevalence of systemic conditions. Communication with the center director before visiting the center is important since the director can provide appropriate information about the children who will be examined.

The role of optometry in early intervention programs was examined by Ciner et al.[12] in a demonstration project between the Pennsylvania College of Optometry and Ken Crest Services of Philadelphia. Ken Crest consists of a group of early intervention centers located throughout metropolitan Philadelphia that serve a large variety of infant and preschool children with developmental delays. Included in

---

*Three reports[9-11] have established that the application of diagnostic agents by spray is effective for purposes of dilation or cycloplegic refraction. I have found spay application to be significantly less traumatic than eyedrops, both for the child and for the examiner, and I highly recommend it for routine use.

this population are medically fragile children who may require full-time nursing care. Children in this program were diagnosed with severe mental retardation, physical disabilities, autism, cerebral palsy, fetal alcohol syndrome, or manifestations of human immunodeficiency virus. Ken Crest centers are geographically distributed so that they are available to many low-income neighborhoods. The demonstration project had three goals: (1) to provide on-site comprehensive eye care for children; (2) to educate staff and parents about vision problems, the services optometrists provide, and the benefits of optometric diagnosis and treatment; and (3) to study the eye/vision dysfunctions of this population and assess new examination/treatment methods.

These goals were accomplished by teams of optometrists, optometric residents, and students traveling to sites one or two times a week. Efforts were made to educate parents about the program. We encouraged parents to be present when their children were examined. Program policies were established to ensure the most accurate eye examinations with minimum disruption of the child's schedule. Examples of these policies included using shorter multiple examinations, allowing the child to become familiar with the lights and instruments, dilating on the second visit, and having the teacher and parents present. These policies provided improved cooperation from the children and led to the collection of more accurate clinic data.

The results of this project demonstrated the need for optometric eye care in the Ken Crest population. Of 135 children examined, 63% (n = 85) had not received any previous eye care. Eighty-one children (60%) had had at least one significant vision problem, and of these only 33 had received examinations. Thus 48 out of 81 children (60%) had substantial vision problems that might have otherwise gone undetected. The prevalence of ocular disease, strabismus, and significant refractive error was found to be higher than in the general population. The box below shows the specific prevalence rates of

---

Prevalence of Ocular Defects in Early Intervention Populations

35% to 40% had significant refractive error
34% had strabismus
29% had ocular disease
19% had nystagmus
Percent of all children seen who had major ocular problems: 60
(n = 135)

See Cinear EB, et al[12] for more information.

these conditions. The results of this study are similar to those documented elsewhere in this text and by those noted by Scheiman[13] and Maino et al.[14]

Optometric Treatment

The management of special populations requires more involvement by the clinician than what is typically found in routine practice. Communication with parents, teachers, nurses, therapists, psychologists, and administrators is important. The optometrist should use this family-oriented approach to assist in the implementation of any therapy. Complete explanations of the vision problems diagnosed and the treatment given will improve compliance. There are distinct advantages to using the early intervention staff in implementing therapy. One reason is that the staff sees the child on a regular basis. Thus, patching or compliance with glasses can at least be accomplished during school hours. Even if little follow-through is completed at home, this can result in significant progress in treating the condition. It is often easy to implement simple vision therapies in the school program. For example, the occupational therapist may have the child in daily visual/motor integration therapy into which active amblyopia treatment can be easily integrated. Furthermore, much of the school and occupational therapy program includes visual perceptual tasks (such as form discrimination, visual memory, and laterality). With some refinement, these programs can be tailored to address specific visual-perceptual problems present.

The disadvantages to working with this population may include poor parental involvement and inadequate funding for services and materials. Referral for conditions that cannot be treated on site is difficult. Long-term treatment or office therapy may be impossible. With these challenges, it is the doctor's responsibility to educate the parent and staff as much as possible and seek alternative treatment procedures to increase compliance.

Is Early Intervention Effective?

Most physicians, psychologists, optometrists, and educators would agree with Levine et al[15] that perinatal events, early health experience, and developmental stimuli are influential in school readiness and subsequent performance. Research over the last 30 years has shown that many factors before elementary school age combine to affect lifetime function. Intellectual competence is largely determined by the age of 4 to 13 years.[16] The formation of social attachments influences future socialization. Children require age-matched language stimulation for language development. Care-giver styles influence personality and temperament. In addition, children with any type of disability are at greater risk for social and emotional problems.[17] Early intervention programs bring these children the necessary contacts. They also provide care-givers who are patient, communicate at the child's level, and give a positive social context for development.

The study of early intervention success has been difficult for several reasons. First, the diagnosis of specific developmental delays is problematical due to the heterogeneity of special populations. Without consensus on the initial problem, evaluating the efficacy of treatment is a matter of controversy. Second, early intervention programs vary greatly, so retrospective research does not provide sufficient consistency to make group comparisons. Third, the utilization of control groups is not always ethically possible because it is unfair to deny children treatment during a critical developmental period. Despite these and other design problems, Guralnick and Bennett[17] have found that programs tailored to specific types of disabilities have the best success. The quality and quantity of programs are also important factors for success. Consistency of implementation and the involvement of parents play important roles. Variations in child achievement tend to be greater in younger age groups with children exhibiting environmental delays responding better than children with biological delays.

Although statistics on success rates vary, it can be concluded that early intervention provides benefits for virtually all individuals with developmental delay. This includes but is not limited to environmental deprivation, mental retardation, prematurity, language and communication disorders, motor handicaps, sensory impairments, and emotional problems. In addition, evidence in support of early intervention continues to build. A randomized controlled study known as the Infant Health and Development Program[18] has revealed higher scores in cognitive function for early intervention participants. Early intervention has shown high rates of placement in kindergarten and success in school, including high graduation rates and entry into the work force.[19]

These findings in the presence of the many biological causes of developmental delay support further development and research. Head Start has continued to receive significant increases in funding even as the U.S. government seeks to reduce spending wherever possible. In 1990, only 47% of the eligible children received early intervention services. In its goals for Healthy People 2000, the U.S. Department of Health and Human Services[20] supports the expansion of early intervention to serve 100% of eligible children. As early intervention expands, it is likely that more studies will become available to appraise its efficacy.

Summary

The preceding has been a brief introduction to optometric involvement in early intervention. As early intervention centers continue to grow, the unique skills of optometrists will be called upon. Since all children enrolled must have health screenings, vision screening and/or examination at early intervention centers should increase in frequency and the role of the optometrist will expand.

REFERENCES

1. McCormick MC, Brooks-Gunn J, Workman-Daniels K, et al: The health and development status of very low–birthweight children at school age, *JAMA* 267:2204-2208, 1992.
2. McCue-Horwitz S, Leaf PJ, Leventhal JM , et al: Identification and management of psychosocial developmental problems in community-based primary care practices, *Pediatrics* 89:480-485, 1992.
3. Schmidt PP: Vision screening. In Rosenbloom AA, Morgan MW (eds): *Principles and practice of pediatric optometry,* Philadelphia, 1990, JB Lippincott, 467-485.
4. Schmidt PP: Allen figure and Broken Wheel visual acuity measurement in preschool children, *J Am Optom Assoc* 63:124-130, 1992.
5. Apt L: Pharmacology. In Isinberg SJ (ed): *The eye in infancy,* Chicago, 1988, Year Book Medical Publishers, 91-99.
6. Bolt B, Benz B, Koerner F, Bossi E: Mydriatic eye-drop combination without systemic effects for premature infants: a prospective double-blind study, *J Pediatr Ophthalmol Strabismus* 29:157-162, 1992.
7. Stolovitch C, Loewenstein A, Nemet P, Lazar M: The use of cyclopentolate versus atropine cycloplegia in esotropic caucasian children, *Binoc Vis Q* 7:93-96, 1992.
8. Nishizawa AR, Orton RB, Cadera W: Comparison of 0.5% cyclopentolate plus 0.5% tropicamide and 1% cyclopentolate alone for mydriasis of dark irides, *Can J Ophthalmol* 23:299-300, 1988.
9. Bartlett JD, Wesson MD, Swiatocha J, Woolley T: Efficacy of pediatric cycloplegic administered as a spray, *J Am Optom Assoc* 64:617-621, 1993.
10. Wesson MD, Bartlett JD, Swiatocha J, Woolley T: Mydriatic efficacy of a cycloplegic spray in a pediatric population, *J Am Optom Assoc* 64:637-640, 1993.
11. Ismail EE, Rouse MW, DeLand PN: A comparison of drop instillation and spray application of 1% cyclopentolate hydrochloride, *Optom Vis Sci* 71:235-241, 1994.
12. Ciner EB, Macks B, Schanel-Klitsch E: A cooperative demonstration project for early intervention vision services, *Occup Ther Pract* 3:42-56, 1991.
13. Scheiman MS: Assessment and management of the exceptional child. In Rosenbloom AA, Morgan MW (eds): *Principles and practice of pediatric optometry,* Philadelphia, 1990, JB Lippincott, 388-419.
14. Maino DM, Maino JH, Maino SA: Mental retardation syndromes with associated ocular defects, *J Am Optom Assoc* 61:707-716, 1990.
15. Levine MD, Brooks R, Shankoff JP: *A pediatric approach to learning disabilities,* New York, 1980, John Wiley & Sons.
16. Bloom BS: *Stability and change in human characteristics,* New York, 1964, John Wiley & Sons.

17. Guralnick MJ, Bennett FC: *The effectiveness of early intervention for at-risk and handicapped children*, Orlando, Fla, 1987, Academic Press.
18. Raney CT, Bryant DM, Wasik BH, et al: Infant health and development program for low birth weight, premature infants: program elements, family participation, and child intervention, *Pediatrics* 89:454-465, 1992.
19. Katcher AL, Haber JS: The pediatrician and early intervention for the developmentally disabled or handicapped child, *Pediatr Rev* 12:305-311, 1991.
20. U.S. Department of Health and Human Services: Healthy people 2000, Boston, 1992, Jones & Bartlett, DHHS Publication no. (PHS) 91-50212.

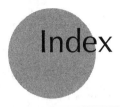

Index

Page numbers in *italic type* refer to figures. Tables are indicated by *t* following page number.